Self-Disclosure in the Therapeutic Relationship

Self-Disclosure in the Therapeutic Relationship

Edited by
George Stricker and Martin Fisher

Derner Institute of Advanced Psychological Studies
Adelphi University
Garden City, New York

Springer Science+Business Media, LLC

Library of Congress Cataloging-in-Publication Data

Self-disclosure in the therapeutic relationship / edited by George Stricker and Martin Fisher.
p. cm.
Includes bibliographical references.
ISBN 978-1-4899-3584-7
1. Psychotherapy. 2. Self-disclosure. I. Stricker, George. II. Fisher, Martin, 1925-
RC480.5.S417 1990
616.89'14--dc20 90-6740
CIP

ISBN 978-1-4899-3584-7 ISBN 978-1-4899-3582-3 (eBook)
DOI 10.1007/978-1-4899-3582-3

Originally published by Plenum Press, New York in 1990
Softcover reprint of the hardcover 1st edition 1990

Contributors

Sabert Basescu, Department of Psychology, New York University, New York, New York 10003, and the Westchester Center for the Study of Psychoanalysis and Psychotherapy, 516 Hommocks Road, Larchmont, New York 10538

Laura S. Brown, 4527 First Avenue NE, Seattle, Washington 98105

Windy Dryden, Department of Psychology, Goldsmiths' College, University of London, New Cross, London SE14 6NW, England

Martin Fisher, Institute of Advanced Psychological Studies, Adelphi University, Garden City, New York 11530

Mary Gail Frawley, Pomona Clinic, Robert L. Yeager Health Complex, Pomona, New York 10970

Arlene Cahn Gordon, 15 Dogwood Drive, West Orange, New Jersey 07052

Lisa R. Greenberg, 428 Franklin Avenue, Nutley, New Jersey 07110

Bede J. Healey, Saint Benedict's Abbey, Atchison, Kansas 66002

James W. Hull, New York Hospital–Cornell Medical Center, Westchester Division, 21 Bloomingdale Road, White Plains, New York 10605

Jonathan M. Jackson, Institute of Advanced Psychological Studies, Adelphi University, Garden City, New York 11530

Adelbert H. Jenkins, Department of Psychology, New York University, New York, New York 10003

Lawrence Josephs, Institute of Advanced Psychological Studies, Adelphi University, Garden City, New York 11530

Robert C. Lane, Institute of Advanced Psychological Studies, Adelphi University, Garden City, New York 11530

Esther Menaker, Postdoctoral Program for Training in Psychoanalysis and Psychotherapy, Department of Psychology, New York University, New York, New York 10003, and Private Practice, 20 West 77 Street, New York, New York 10024

Nicholas Papouchis, Program in Clinical Psychology, Long Island University, Brooklyn Center, Brooklyn, New York 11201

Douglas J. Peddicord, 9402 Sunfall Court, Columbia, Maryland 21046

Judith C. Simon, 329 South San Antonio Road, Los Altos, California 94022

George Stricker, Institute of Advanced Psychological Studies, Adelphi University, Garden City, New York 11530

Sophia Vinogradov, Department of Psychiatry, Pacific Presbyterian Medical Center, San Francisco, California 94115

Lenore E. A. Walker, Walker and Associates, 50 South Steele Street, Suite 850, Denver, Colorado 80209

Irvin D. Yalom, Department of Psychiatry and Behavioral Sciences, Stanford University School of Medicine, Stanford, California 94305

Preface

The editors of the present volume were also privileged to collaborate on an earlier book, *Intimacy,* also published by Plenum Press. In our preface to that volume, we described the importance and essence of intimacy and its centrality in the domain of human relationships.

After reading the contributions to that volume, a number of issues emerged and pressed for elaboration. These questions concerned the nature and parameters of intimacy. The natural extension of these concerns can be found in the current work, *Self-Disclosure in the Therapeutic Relationship.*

The editors, after careful consideration of the theoretical, philosophical, and technical literature, are impressed by the relationship between intimacy and appropriate self-disclosure. Self-disclosure, in this context, refers to those behaviors that allow oneself to be sufficiently revealing so as to become available for an intimate relationship. Levenson has referred to psychotherapy as the demystification of experience wherein intimacy emerges during the time that interpersonal vigilance diminishes through growing feelings of safety. Interpersonal experience can be demystified and detoxified by disclosure, openness, and authentic relatedness.

This is not an easy process. Before one can be open, make contact, or reach out with authenticity, one must be available to oneself. This means making contact with—and accepting—the dark, fearful, and often untouched areas within the person that are often hidden even from oneself. The process of therapy enables those areas to gain consciousness, be tolerated, and be shared with trusted others.

This book is about self-disclosure, with a focus on how it is understood and utilized from a variety of different theoretical orientations and with a variety of different patient groups. We have solicited chapters from a group of well-known and highly regarded authors who, in their chapters, help to display a spectrum of attitudes and ideas about self-disclosure and its role in the therapeutic process.

GEORGE STRICKER
MARTIN FISHER

Contents

PART II. THEORETICAL PERSPECTIVES

PART III. THERAPEUTIC ISSUES

I

Introduction

1

The Shared Experience and Self-Disclosure

Martin Fisher

In a chapter prepared for a book I had previously coedited (1982) I wrote about an approach to psychoanalytic psychotherapy that was referred to as "the shared experience." It was my belief then, as it continues to be now, that when patients present themselves for psychotherapy they are looking for a solution to loneliness or, more specifically, a "cure" for a lack of *intimacy*.

I write this chapter with a particular bias. Regardless of symptom, presenting complaint, or clinical diagnosis, I believe that patients present themselves for psychotherapy because of the inability (with or without awareness) to have and/or to be in intimate relationships. Somewhere, somehow, because of intrapsychic and/or interpersonal deficits, the individual comes to feel his/her aloneness, fear, and vulnerability. The patient, through the transference as well as the real relationship with the therapist, tries to capture (or recapture) this state of grace referred to as intimacy. The openness, closeness, and appropriate dependency that makes up intimate relatedness, will be woven silently or overtly in the patients' attempts at recovery of the lost or disordered self.

How does this alienation from self and others occur? What are the existential manifestations of such a process? One way of conceptualizing this experience of disordered affective and cognitive experiences looks something like the following:

Martin Fisher • Institute of Advanced Psychological Studies, Adelphi University, Garden City, New York 11530.

1. The infant/child is constantly involved in a communication loop with significant others, which produces either positive or negative feedback.
2. Negative feedback results eventually in a psychic withdrawal from the outside and results in the growth of "secrets." (The child is encouraged to keep secret those feelings, ideas, and behaviors that result in some overt or covert form of punishment or rejection.)
3. Early in the development of the ego, an accumulation of "secrets" builds in which the authenticity of the child becomes coarctated and results in an accumulation of negative feelings and ideas that then make up the nucleus of unconscious existence.
4. Since these secrets represent the dreaded aspects of existence (in the eyes of important others), their disclosure would lead to a disaster, that is, a disintegration of the "I" that was created for acceptance and the visibility of the "not I" that the child tried so hard to disguise.
5. The greater the degree of "secrets," the greater the degree of alienation from the self. The greater the alienation of the self, the greater the alienation from others.
6. The greater the alienation from self and others, the greater the loss of real intimacy in interpersonal relatedness. (Fisher, 1982)

At this point, I would like to address myself to the cornerstones of psychoanalytic inquiry, namely, anxiety, transference, and resistance. Specifically, the typical pattern is that under the impetus of anxiety, the individual often utilizes the transference in order to act out the resistance. In like fashion, we now know and understand that this experience of the patient is often met by the counteranxiety, the countertransference, and the counterresistance of the analyst. What then takes place in the arena of psychoanalysis is inextricably woven and interwoven in a combined interaction between patient and analyst. Who is influencing whom, at any given moment, and in what direction, to what end, as a function of that interaction? This is what may be referred to as the psychology of "shared experience" (Woldstein, 1971). I will return to this idea shortly.

Many contributors to the thinking and theorizing of psychoanalysis have referred to this idea of shared experience in a variety of ways. Sullivan (1953) used the term "collaboration" and described it as a mutually rewarding relationship that promotes a reciprocal validation of personal worth. Frank (1977) describes the therapeutic dyad as being

> ...of limited value unless implemented within a relationship characterized by an affectional bond of mutual trust and respect, and where the analyst is willing to fully experience and to be experienced, on an authentically human level. (p. 6)

Searles contends that if the therapist's and patient's mutual therapeutic endeavor is to prove successful, then both patient and therapist must discover "hope" in their collective experience together (in Frank, 1977). Paul Olsen (in Frank, 1977) defines psychotherapy as

> . . . a contact not just between two people engaged in some sort of interpersonal activity on a seesaw of transferential distortions and the "real" relationship but a communion of two souls—a conception for which he expands therapeutic possibilities and, indeed, enriches relationships in general. (p. 141)

Finally, Singer suggests that if the goal of therapy is the growth of the capacity to develop intimate knowledge of one's own personal experience and the comparable knowledge of the experience of others, then the nature of therapeutic intimacy and the resulting exchange must be our starting points for mutual growth (in Frank, 1977, p. 191).

In short, what I and others are calling a shared experience has been referred to in the psychoanalytic literature in a variety of ways; but they essentially describe a similar or identical notion.

First, allow me further to specify the psychodynamic parameters of resistance, which, as a phenomenon, became apparent in the early work of Freud. Attention was paid to resistance as a necessary and intrinsic issue to be confronted in psychoanalysis. In Lecture XIX of the *Introductory Lectures on Psychoanalysis*, Freud (1966) observed:

> Resistances. . . should not be one-sidedly condemned. They include so much of the most important material from the patient's past and bring it back in so convincing a fashion that they become some of the best supports of the analysis if a skillful analyst knows how to give them the right turn. Nevertheless, it remains a remarkable fact that this material is always in the service of the resistance to begin with and brings to the fore a facade that is *hostile to the treatment*. (p. 291) (emphasis mine)

Here then is the cornerstone of much that follows. Resistance, that profound quality of the human psyche to avoid knowing lies at the roots of our endeavors to explore in psychoanalysis. Freud (1966) always felt that one of his great discoveries was the avoidance of knowing which he termed "resistance." He wrote:

> In the first place, then, when we undertake to restore a patient to health, to relieve him of the symptoms of his illness, he meets us with a violent and tenacious resistance which persists throughout the whole length of treatment. This is such a strange fact that we cannot expect it to find much credence. . . . The patient too, produces all the phenomena of this resistance without recognizing it as such, and if we can induce him to take our view of it and to reckon with its existence, that already counts as a great success. Only think of it! The patient, who is suffering so much from his symptoms and is causing those about him to share his sufferings, who is ready to undertake so many sacrifices in time and money, effort and self-discipline in order to be freed from these symptoms—we are to believe that this same

> patient puts up a struggle in the interest of his illness against the person who is helping him. How improbable such an assertion must sound! Yet it is true; and when its improbability is pointed out to us, we need only reply that it is not without analogies. A man who has gone to the dentist because of an unbearable toothache will nevertheless try to hold the dentist back when he approaches the sick tooth with a pair of forceps. (pp. 286–287)

In this description Freud has outlined the profound essence of what sets psychoanalytic inquiry apart from other psychotherapies that are not described as psychodynamic in nature.

In a chapter that I wrote for a previous volume (1982), I point out what seemed to me a critical distinction between the Freudian view of resistance and an existential exploration referred to by Bugental (1965). As significant a place as Freud accords the resistance, existential-analytic theory regards this discovery as even more fundamental. The resistance shown by the patient in the therapeutic session—the ways in which he/she avoids awareness, displaced responsibility, maintains his/her alienation, and so on—is the very pattern through which the patient maintains his/her inauthentic relation to life, is the very source of his nonbeing (p. 88).

> In the above model, Freud implies that the patient's resistance is to the process of psychoanalysis and/or the psychoanalyst and results in the patient's unconscious avoidance of these external forces. Freud emphasizes this idea when he writes: I cannot recommend my colleagues emphatically enough to take as a model in psychoanalytic treatment the surgeon who puts aside his own feelings, including that of human sympathy.... The justification for his coldness in feeling in the analyst is that it is the condition which brings the greatest advantage to both persons involved. (1912/1964)

Freud (1949/1964) makes a clear-cut distinction between analyst and patient, with the analyst invariably being the more "grown-up" of the two. He makes this explicit when he states: "Too many neurotics have remained so infantile that in analysis too they can only be treated as children."

Another view of resistance, more consistent with my own, is expressed by the existential psychoanalyst Bugental (1965). In his book *The Search for Authenticity*, Bugental contends that

> ...the resistance is the shield the patient erects to forestall the feared confrontation with the reality of his being in the world. (Thus, the therapist who thinks of the resistance as a warding off of his own efforts misses the point and confuses the patient.) The therapist's task is to help the patient rediscover the conflict within himself that gave rise to the resistance and other defenses and constrictive maneuvers. (p. 43)

In truth then, the patient resists not the therapist and/or therapy but the dread of discovering himself. As Bugental continues,

> Resistance is the name that we give to the general defensive wall the patient

> puts between himself and the threats that he finds linked to being authentic. Resistance is (simply) anti-authenticity. (p. 43)

We have moved, then, away from the psychoanalyst's couch into the wider and real-life experience of the world.

The existential model of resistance implies threat. Simply stated, it represents the threat of nonbeing. The resistance, then, is humanity's constant effort to avoid the pain of feeling, thinking, or reexperiencing nonbeing. There seems little doubt that the prototype for this potential nonbeing lies in the early traumatic feelings of potential nonbeing that each separation repeatedly arouses in the infant.

In viewing Freud's model, he implies that the patient's resistance is to the process of psychoanalysis and/or the psychoanalyst and results in the patient's unconscious (and sometimes conscious) avoidance of these external forces. In reviewing Bugental's and the existential position the resistance can be seen to be a fear and avoidance of the patient's own self-induced (conscious and unconscious) meeting the real (authentic) self; the fear of discovery, the fear of being seen as, or feeling in some way, damaged. The patient then is avoiding coming to terms with his/her own existence in the belief that he/she is somehow bad and/or damaged and rejectable.

At this time it should be noted that resistance is not confined to the analytic consulting room; neither is the transference phenomenon which is also in the service of the resistance. These two phenomena (transference and resistance) are now readily recognized to be ubiquitous and are present in the individual in therapy as well as in those who never see the inside of a therapy consulting room.

A further extension of the existential view is that humans seek to avoid anxiety—the anxiety of freedom. Freedom represents a world of increased contingencies. An increase in contingencies represents more possibility of failure, rejection, and loss of self-esteem. More pointedly, however, this same acceptance of freedom brings the reality of ultimate nonbeing (death) painfully into awareness.

Think, if you will, what is implied in the existential view of authenticity; authenticity representing the antithesis of resistance. Bugental suggests that the authentic person is, at first, broadly aware of himself, his interpersonal relationships, and all dimensions of his real world. Secondly, the authentic person accepts the fact that life represents choices, that he goes forth to meet those choices, and that decisions are the very stuff of life. And third, the authentic person assumes full responsibility for approaching these contingencies, making decisions, and accepting full responsibility for his acts.

It is agreed that transference is unconscious and distorted (by definition) and arises out of early childhood experiences.

In a recent paper Goldman (1988) refers to the concept of a paradise lost which the child experiences in his/her coming to terms with existence. Goldman suggests that

> ...(for) patients who experience this deep core of sense of essential inner badness or defectiveness, which often borders on a feeling of being personally evil, there is an underlying and almost always unconscious fantasy of having been the wicked destroyer of a preexisting paradise. What I mean by this is that the person unconsciously believes that before his or her conception and birth, there existed a state of *paradisiacal* unity and bliss between the parents and an essential goodness in the family situation that was ruptured by the child's advent and thereby irretrievably lost. This is a specific way in which the child blames him or herself for the pain and difficulty of a family situation structured by narcissistically deprived and damaged parents. (p. 420)

It has been said in the psychoanalytic literature that once a patient is fully capable of "free association" the analysis is over. This idea lies at the heart of the engagement between patient and analyst. Further, it establishes the essence of what brought about the need for the analysis in the first place.

We develop or create "secrets" in childhood in an attempt to avoid *reflection*. Because these secrets move into that sphere, or become part of what we refer to as the unconscious, the secrets are not even known to the patient. Since we have, in effect, gone underground, we have limited our ability to be in or to have intimate relationships. It is my thesis that intimacy is the desired goal in life and that *self-disclosure* is the route to *intimacy*. A clinical example may help illuminate this point.

John, a patient in therapy for three years (three-time-a-week individual psychoanalysis), was having a very difficult time trusting anyone. The evidence was clear in behavioral as well as verbal communications. Early profound experiences were obliterated from his memory. The facts, however, were that, after the death of his father, he had lived in 13 foster homes from age 2 until the age of 12, when he returned to live with his biological mother. His lack of basic trust was so pronounced that he created a world in which he always had to be dominant. This meant controlling people (his wife, four children, the analyst, his professional colleagues, and so forth) lest someone "do him in."

As the characterological layering was peeling off, John reported the following scene. The previous day he had attended the funeral of a friend and neighbor. As the funeral procession formed to leave for the cemetery, his 18-year-old daughter expressed the wish to offer condolences to the daughter of the deceased as she was preparing to enter the funeral car. John immediately explained that this was inappropriate and intrusive. Nevertheless, his daughter proceeded to walk up to the young girl, who in turn expressed great warmth and appreciation at John's daughter's gesture. When his daughter returned to John's side, she commented on the discrepancy between John's advice and the outcome of what she had done. In reply, he admitted that he was ashamed and afraid to do what his daughter had done. Rarely, if ever, had he admitted to anyone so close to him something that might make him seem less than perfect. His daughter's reaction was surprise, delight, and a wish to be closer to her father who acknowledged a possible flaw in his "invincibility."

It is most important to note that the example suggests more than trust in his daughter by John. It demonstrates, even more profoundly, John's basic trust in revealing himself to himself in public. In this example, John decided to "share" his experience with his daughter because of a growing feeling of trust.

I would like to pursue further the notion of the "shared experience." In studying this construct called "shared experience," the idea seemed clearly to be a recreation of a caution that all psychoanalytic therapies attend to; specifically, that the work area or arena of psychoanalytic inquiry lies at the interface of the anxiety, transference, and resistance of the patient and the counteranxiety, countertransference, and counterresistance of the analyst.

This led to my belief that shared experience cannot take place between unequals. Something can only be truly shared by equal co-participants. Yet, if one reviews earlier formulations of psychoanalysis, the opportunity for shared experience disappears. In the id/biological model, the psychoanalyst was expected to be a blank screen intended to encourage regression so as not to distort the patient's transference behavior. In the interpersonal model of psychanalysis, the therapist is expected to be a participant-observer. Although this model includes participation, it would seem more appropriate to have two participant-observers. Just as Sullivan hypothesized that the patient brings into the therapy room many additional people (transferentially from early experience), so does he meet many more people in the therapy room than his psychoanalyst. It is the thesis of this chapter that alienation from self and others is at the root of psychopathology. The modes of inauthentic being come into play as the individual moves further and further away from life and all of the (treacherous) contingencies that we all must face but too often are fearful of. Yalom (1980) describes these life concerns as *freedom, aloneness, meaning,* and *death*. Of course, we as humans have no choice but to engage these issues. But they frighten us into avoiding (or trying to avoid) each of them. As though we could truly avoid death! But we try; and in so doing create an inauthentic life.

When our patients present themselves for psychotherapy, our real task is reclamation. It seems to me that the reclaiming of the self is through the process of coming to terms with and being in an intimate relationship. It seems, then, most obvious that intimacy should occur in therapy, as a prelude for intimacy in life with others, through the process referred to in this chapter as self-disclosure. What is the essence of self-disclosure? Earlier it was suggested that the analysis would end when free-association was fully achieved. Why should this be so difficult to come by? Why are we so afraid of disclosing ourselves? It must be that what we know is too threatening (fear of rejection) or that we no longer consciously are fully aware of those feelings and ideas that we still continue to try and hide. It is as though we must have assurance that who we are, what we say, the ideas we believe in must be guaranteed acceptance, or we face the inevitable fate of rejection (which to the infant is tantamount to death). Bugental (1965) suggested that contingency (choices) is the very stuff of life:

> . . . Once we know all that we need to know in order to make a decision, we no longer make a decision but are determined by what we know. The joy in life comes from making decisions and becoming affirmed. Here then lies the threat in self-disclosure. Will the patient discover that in chance-taking (of opening oneself to another) he or she will be humiliated, rejected, or still worse, destroyed? Or, as I suggested earlier, have these aspects of the self been so thoroughly pushed into the unconscious that without the efforts of psychoanalytic psychotherapy they are not even available for expression?

Clearly, the sense of this essay suggests that alienation, which is a result of withholding thoughts and feelings from others, lies at the root of psychopathology. In order for the individual to reclaim aspects of his/her real self, it is necessary to become self-disclosing to an other, and others in general. I believe that this process can best occur in a relationship that encourages sharing of feelings and ideas. This relationship can best be achieved in an engagement of co-equals in the therapeutic relationship. This last idea is the one that probably raises the most questions. Can therapist and patient truly be in an equal relationship? I believe so.

In a previous paper (1982), I suggested that the paradigm of the dyad in psychoanalysis is the recreation of the relationship between parent and child. I referred, then, to Erickson's (1963) epigenetic diagram of interpersonal ego-psychological formulations. In Erickson's terms, the infant's first psychological task is achieving a sense of "basic trust." The alternate polar solution for the infant is the experience of "basic mistrust." Obviously, for most people the solution of this early period is not absolute, but lies at some point in between. The individual who arrives as a patient some 20 or 30 years later is caught in some dilemma of being unable to trust in human relationships. More importantly, and this issue is critical, in opening himself up to another, the patient is really risking opening up to himself. He must trust the hidden, secretive self to be revealed to the analyst in the context of trust so that his discoveries and revelations will not result in his own rejection (at least) and his psychological death (at worst).

What emerges in the diminished capacity for basic trust appears to be the loss or diminution of intimate relatedness. Distrust encourages "secrets" (banished to the preconscious or unconscious); intimacy (shared experience) encourages openness.

The literature that points to the effect on the infant of mothering (parenting) is rich and voluminous. A. Balint (1965) points out that

> ...maternal love is the almost perfect counterpart to the love for the mother.... Thus, just as the mother is to the child, so is the child to the mother—an object of gratification. And just as the child does not recognize the separate identity of the mother, so the mother looks upon her child as part of herself whose interests are identical with her own. The relation between mother and child is built upon the interdependence of the reciprocal instinctual aims. What Ferenczi said about the relation of man and woman in coitus holds true for his mother-infant relation. He meant that in coitus there can be no question of egoism (love interest of the self) or altruism (love interest of the other); there is only mutuality, i.e., what is good for one is right for the other also. In consequence of the natural interdependence of the reciprocal instinctual aims there is no need to be concerned about the partner's well-being. (p. 101)

M. Balint continues this thinking when he reflects:

> I am rather sad that nobody mentioned the name of Sandor Ferenczi who first called our attention to the fact that the formal elements of transference and the whole analytic situation derive from very early infant-parent relationships.... Perhaps the most important lesson that we can derive from this is that the basis of the infant-parent relationship is in mutual interdependence of the two.... That is, what is libidinal satisfaction for the one, the infant, must be libidinal satisfaction for the mother, and vice versa.... One of the consequences of this idea is that something similar must obtain also in the relationship between the analyst and patient. (p. 145)

More recently, Peterson and Moran (1988) in reviewing "Attachment Theory" as explicated by Bowlby, point out that a number of studies strongly suggest that "...mothers of more securely attached infants appear to be more confident, emotionally stable, and responsive to their infants' attachment behaviors than mothers of insecurely attached infants. Further, mothers suffering from mental illness and those who neglect or abuse their children tend to have insecurely attached infants" (p. 623).

Given the foregoing, it is the thesis of this essay that "shared" experience can only take place between equals. And this equality demands that while the patient can only achieve wholeness (intimacy) through self-disclosure and openness, the therapist too must be engaged in his/her own self-disclosure and openness to his/her patient.

The issue, then, hangs on the notion that no infant child can grow beyond the willingness or capabilities of the parenting figure. In like fashion, no patient can ever move, or grow beyond his or her analyst's (conscious and unconscious) willingness to let him/her move and grow toward greater intimacy.

How, then, does the analyst share or reveal his/her own secrets, feelings, ideas, unconscious, etc.?

Only through an experience of real intimacy can authentic behavior and creation or recreation take place. I have now used the concept of intimacy as synonymous with shared experience. How can anyone truly share an experience, thought, or idea without exposing some of his secret self, unless there exists the potential for intimacy? How can anyone truly expose his authentic, original, changing, and emerging psyche, unless he has experienced himself in a truly intimate relationship? The variable necessary to achieve or approach such a state of grace lies in the concept of basic trust. This climate would then be necessary in the therapy alliance.

With specific regard to trust, the notion of the importance of the mother-child relationship was elaborated by Roy Schafer (1973) in reformulating his position on resistance. He advances the idea that Freud overvalued the concept that resistance has its prototype in the authority of the father in the oedipal situation. Schafer (1973) suggests that

> Freud did not teach us to appreciate the fundamental developmental importance of the infant's prolonged helplessness and of the early danger situations corresponding to this helplessness, especially of the loss of the love object and loss of love.... The prospect of being abandoned by her (mother) physically and emotionally, really or in fantasy, never loses its painful if not terrifying aspect.... Anxiety over losing the mother or her love threatens to undermine the boy's and the girl's very sense of worth or right to exist.... If we think of the analysand as defying the archaic mother's authority too, we will think as well of the growing importance to the child of differentiating himself from his mother.... By dint of these strivings the child establishes and maintains differentiation and wards off its wishing to merge with the mother through incorporation as well as the mother's seductions to merge and her devouring approaches. (p. 270)

A number of possibilities emerge in the repertoire of the psychoanalyst that can be seen as sharing. In our sharing mode, we inevitably reveal ourselves, wittingly or unwittingly. I would suggest that if we *consciously choose* to share, we offer the gift of *intimacy* to our patients. Some of our sharing seems readily apparent. When we engage our patients through *empathy*, we have opened a possibility of sharing. When patients disclose seemingly helpless feelings regarding decisions in their lives we often suggest "alternative solutions." This very behavior is an act of sharing. When we speak to the patient's repressed thoughts or feelings we enter into a mode of sharing and intimacy.

However, the most profound opportunity for sharing, it seems to me, is the essential and significant use of the analyst's countertransference. To understand the implications of the uses of countertransference I refer to the seminal work of H. Racker (1968), in which he contends that

> ...Countertransference reactions of great intensity, even pathological ones, should also serve as tools. Countertransference is the expression of the analyst's identification with the internal objects of the analysand as well as with his id and ego, and may be used as such. Countertransference reactions have specific characteristics (specific contexts, anxieties, and mechanisms from which we may draw conclusions about the specific character of the psychological happenings of the patient. (p. 129)

Racker feels even more strongly that uses of countertransference go beyond revealing of the self of the analyst to the patient. He infers that the reciprocity of transference and countertransference is critical in the unfolding of the analysis. He notes that "...the influence of countertransference upon the analyst's behavior toward the analysand—behavior that affects decisively the position of the analyst as object of the reexperience of childhood, thus (affects) the process of cure" (p. 129).

Most practitioners and students of psychoanalysis are already aware of the strict prohibitions of the early writers and practitioners of psychoanalysis to rid oneself of countertransference so that the analytic enterprise could proceed smoothly and without the interference of the analyst's subjective and objective countertransference issues. There is wider acceptance in more recent writings about theory and practice that countertransference may be the most crucial tool in contacting the patient's repressed and heretofore unavailable feelings and communications in the psychoanalytic arena. Racker clearly represents this later, more recent view.

There are a number of technical issues about how, when, where, and why the analyst in the psychoanalytic dyad would or should reveal countertransference which becomes conscious. This paper will merely suggest that countertransference revealed (timely and appropriately) sets the stage for the psychology of a "shared experience." It is this shared experience that undoes the malignancy of early developmental "secrets" between child and parent. It is this process that makes the products of malignancy benign and therefore safe.

In closing, I refer to a description of psychopathology that was suggested by E. Levinson and elaborated in Group (1977). Levinson proposed three somewhat different major sets within the psychotherapeutic process that need to be addressed if intimacy is to be achieved. He described these as (1) desensitization of experience, in which the achievement of *intimacy* is a direct goal; (2) detoxification of fantasy, which will or should lead to healthy personal experiences from which *intimacy* will ensue; and (3) demystification of experience, wherein *intimacy* emerges as interpersonal vigilance diminishes through feelings of safety (p. 16) (emphasis mine).

Given the expectations of the dynamics of a truly shared experience between patient and therapist, it is my belief that all three descriptions outlined by Levinson are likely (positive) outcomes of a well-conducted psychotherapy encounter. Further, I contend that for a genuine encounter to occur between patient and therapist, and for authentic growth in intimacy to emerge (which is at the heart of the need for therapy to begin with) a truly shared experience must take place. Again, the belief herein suggested is that the encounter between patient and therapist (like that between parent and child) should take place between (psychological) equals: between the co-participants of dyadic psychotherapy. Lastly, that the sharing of experiencing, which leads to *intimacy*, is achieved through the process of (mutual) *self-disclosure*.

An excerpt from a recent volume on *Psychotherapy* (Gilliland *et al.*, 1989) summarizes the point:

> ...the most important element in counseling is the *personhood* of the counselor. The most powerful impact on the client may be that of observing what the counselor *is* and *does*. Counseling is collaborative. It is something two people do together. The counselor must be willing to invite the client to interact with a person (the counselor) who is also struggling, evolving, risking, evaluating self, problem-solving, and experiencing all the normal human emotions from severe grief to ecstasy. It is important for clients to view counselors as people who are competent (*but not perfect*), mature, stable, persevering, and continually learning and growing. It is also important for them to understand that counselors are fallible, and can experience *ambivalence, failure, frustration*, and change.... *Effective counseling cannot be separated from effective living*. (p. 7)

I believe that most patients come to therapy in order to become a "better" human being. Psychotherapy becomes the route to so-called self-improvement. I believe that too many psychotherapists accept this definition of psychotherapy and try to help their patients "improve." I believe that the goal of psychotherapy is *acceptance* of the self as it is. With acceptance of the real self comes a diminution of the need to create a false self and the ability and opportunity to be the authentic self. Once you accept who you really are, you can be or become anyone you want to be.

References

Balint, A. (1965). *Primary love and psychoanalytic technique* (M. Balint ed.) New York: Liveright.

Balint, M. (1965). *Primary love and psychoanalytic technique* (M. Balint ed.) New York: Liveright.

Bugental, J.F.T. (1965). *The search for authenticity*. New York: Holt, Rinehart & Winston.
Eisenbud, R.J. (1977). Personal communication.
Erikson, E. (1963). *Childhood and society*. New York: Norton & Co.
Fisher, M. (1977). The potential for authentic relatedness in group psychoanalysis. *Group Process, 7* (2), 141–150.
Fisher, M. (1983). *Intimacy*. (M. Fisher & G. Stricker Eds.) New York: Plenum.
Frank, K. (1977). The human dimension in psychoanalytic practice. New York: Grune & Stratton.
Freud, S. (1966). *The complete introductory lectures on psychoanalysis*. New York: W.W. Norton. (Originally published, 1917).
Goldman, H.A. (1988). Paradise destroyed: The crime of being born. *Contemporary Psychoanalysis, 24*, (3), 420–450.
Gilland, B.E., James, R.K., & Bowman, J.T. (1989). *Theories and strategies in counseling and psychotherapy* (2nd ed.) Englewood Cliffs: Prentice Hall.
Peterson, R., & Moran, G. (1988). Attachment theory. *Clinical Psychology Review, 8*, (6), 611–636.
Racker, H. (1968). *Transference and countertransference*. New York: International Universities Press.
Schafer, R. (1973). The idea of resistance. *International Journal of Psychoanalysis, 54*, 259.
Wolstein, B. (1971). *Human psyche in psychoanalysis*. Chicago: Ill: C.C. Thomas.
Yalom, I. (1980). *Existential psychotherapy*. New York: Basic Books.

2

Self-Disclosure in Religious Spiritual Direction

ANTECEDENTS AND PARALLELS TO SELF-DISCLOSURE IN PSYCHOTHERAPY

Bede J. Healey

Historical Perspectives of Self-Disclosure

Self-disclosure is a process integral to both psychotherapy and religious experience. Other authors in this book discuss the role of self-disclosure in the therapeutic relationship; I offer an overview of the role of self-disclosure in Judeo-Christian religious experience, with a special emphasis on self-disclosure in the process of Christian spiritual direction.

It is not unusual to consider religion and psychotherapy together. Both are concerned, after all, with healing and the exploration of meaning. From a religious perspective, self-disclosure has a long history. Long before psychology was a discipline, or psychotherapy existed as a profession, the psychological processes that are now associated with psychotherapy were the domain of the priests and healers of society. May (1982) points out that up until the time of the Protestant Reformation, there was little distinction between spiritual and psychological issues. With the discoveries of Freud, May believes psychology and psychiatry became the "new priesthood" (p. 2).

In the Judeo-Christian traditions, religion and religious experience are relationship-based: "Thus the Lord used to speak to Moses face to face, as a man speaks to a friend" (Exodus 33:11, RSV). An integral part

Bede J. Healey • Saint Benedict's Abbey, Atchison, Kansas 66002.

of this relationship is self-disclosure. It is possible to look at the story of the fall of Adam and Eve as a rupture in this relationship, whereby shame and the need to cover up and hide came into being, thus introducing a burden upon humanity that did not previously exist (Gen. 3:1–24). God is self-revelatory, and as a way to heal this rupture, invites humanity to enter a covenant relationship. This covenant is an offer from God of a life-giving relationship. The archetype for this is God's call to Abraham (Gen. 12; 15:18–21). In the Jewish tradition, the priests were the interpreters of the Law, the mediators between God and God's chosen people. Infractions of the Law were disclosed, or confessed (Lev. 5:5; 16:20–24; 26:40–42).

As the people and their religious experience developed, their relationship with God deepened; there evolved a desire to remain on good terms with God. This is reflected in the development of cultic religious practices. Psalm 32 is evidence of this. This psalm is an individual proclamation, probably recited in a ritual setting before a collected community of believers. In part, the psalmist states: "blest is he whose transgression is forgiven...when I declared not my sin, my body wasted away...I acknowledged my sin to thee and I did not hide my iniquity...then thou didst forgive the guilt of my sin." In the psalm God replies, "I will instruct you and teach you the way you should go. I will counsel you with my eye upon you." A more recent, and poetic translation (Sullivan, 1983) of the psalm ends with the line: "We tell You, all of us You set free" (p. 32). The sense of freedom that results from self-disclosure is clear.

In this psalm we see self-disclosure ritualized. While here it is directly between God and the individual, the very practice of ritual celebration brings others in as mediators (Lev. 16:20–24). It is only a small step then to utilize other people as mediators of this "counsel." Hence, it is possible to see these practices as precursors to the practice of spiritual direction.

Rabbi Arthur Green, a prominent writer on Jewish spirituality, notes both the rich history of the master–disciple relationship in Jewish mystical spirituality, and the in-depth knowledge of religious psychology of these masters. Unfortunately, there was a historical tendency to refrain from speaking of one's personal experience with God. It was not considered appropriate to do so publicly, and was only passed on in a one-to-one basis, to a "pupil both wise and already intuitively open to such matters" (1988, p. 8). Thus, there is a lack of "confessions," the telling of one's personal spiritual experiences, in Jewish spiritual literature. Yet this is a heritage of the Jewish faith, and Green argues for renewed interest and development of a richer faith experience by tapping into the Jewish mystical and master–disciple traditions, which involve disclosing and sharing of one's experiences with others.

In the Christian tradition, these themes have been further developed, and the focus is on God's actual manifestation in Jesus Christ. Jesus revealed himself as both God and a human being, inviting others to a relationship with him (Matthew 11:28). There is a clear expression in the Gospels of the master–disciple relationship between Jesus and his followers (Luke 5:5; 9:49; Matthew 8:23). Indeed, in the Western tradition, the evolution of religious experience can be seen as an ever-increasing disclosure of God to humankind, with a concomitant reciprocal disclosure of humanity to God. More often than not this disclosure is mediated by another human being. Indeed, Jesus, as God and human being, is the primary source of this disclosure and mediation.

This is not primarily the case in the Eastern tradition, where there is an emphasis on impersonality. Buddhist traditions are centered on meditative practices to help an individual become one with the void. The master–disciple relationship is central to the process, but according to Acharya (1982), this relationship is not comparable to the place spiritual sonship has in the Christian tradition. The end result is not toward union with God, but toward emptiness (see McDargh's (1984) discussion for a comparison and contrast of Christian and Eastern religious experience).

Conditions for Self-Disclosure

For the present discussion, self-disclosure should be seen as a process, i.e., a means toward an end. Self-disclosure is a means toward the development of some type of intimacy. There are two important elements, two necessary preconditions, before self-disclosure can take place. The first condition is a relationship. The second is trust.

Self-disclosure cannot happen without a relationship. It may seem unnecessary to state the obvious, but I do this for two reasons. One is to call to mind the essential relatedness of humanity, one to another, and that the quality of these relationships will determine whether authentic self-disclosure will take place. The other reason is that it is important to remember that in religious experience, particularly in Western traditions, relationships are essential. Even in the case of hermits, there is usually an extended period of community living. For example, the Rule of St. Benedict, a rule for living the monastic life, holds that only after living with others in the monastery for a long time may the monk seek the solitary way of life. The monk is prepared for this by the "help and guidance of many" (RB 1:3–5; Fry, 1981). During this period, the future hermit is generally under the tutelage of an experienced spiritual guide. It is after such a relational experience that one takes up the life of a hermit as a means to develop a more intense relationship with God.

Further, relationships can provide multiple levels of meaning. Often, relationships with others are the vehicle for experiencing and understanding one's relationship with God. In the Jewish tradition, prophets and priests were the mediators of God's will and way to His people. In the later Hassidic tradition the spiritual master is also defined in terms of a relationship. In discussing this point, Rabbi Arthur Green states, "It's not that he [the master] knows the esoteric Torah that nobody else knows, but he knows *this* disciple's Torah, because he knows this discipline so well and stands in relationship to him" (Ware, 1974, p. 314).

In the Christian tradition, the relationship of Son and Father is given central prominence (Matthew 5:45; 5:48; 10:21; 10:31), and this is taken up in full force by the desert fathers and mothers of the fourth and fifth centuries. Regarding relationships, it is important to note that especially in the Christian tradition, spiritual direction is not a dyadic relationship. It is triadic; God is always present as the third person, "for where two or three come together in my name, there am I with them" (Matthew 18:20). This has special implications for self-disclosure in the Christian tradition. Again and again in the literature on spiritual direction, the presence of God is emphasized, and the role of the director is described as one of facilitating the directee's relationship with God. Indeed, the notion of a dyadic versus a triadic relationship is a primary distinction between therapy and spiritual direction.

In addition, it is important to note the collective, communal nature of religion and religious experience. The relationship with God is both individual and communal, and one self-discloses both as an individual, and as a member of a community. There are ritual self-disclosing practices of both an individual and a communal nature in almost all Judeo-Christian religions. These include the Yom Kippur services and attendant practices in the Jewish faith, and the confession and penance celebrations, as well as the practice of spiritual direction, in the Christian traditions. Communal rituals help promote identity and solidarity. They also help promote the acceptance of the basic human condition, described by various authors as being weak, wounded, in need of help, and incomplete.

The second necessary condition for self-disclosure flows from the first, the need for trust. Without a sense of acceptance by another person and trust in that person's ability and desire to be with oneself, authentic self-disclosure will not take place. While trust is basic to the development of a relationship, other elements are also necessary. Witness what some people say are the necessary prerequisites of someone who aspires to be a spiritual director:

"Have a loving patience."
"Be a fellow searcher."

"...hospitality; openness; an ability to welcome all of life."

"Have an applied knowledge of both psychological and spiritual areas."

"Be in full communion with the whole of your humanity."

"...provide an environment out of which a person can pay attention and allow this intuitive noticing to become an important part of his/her life" (Edwards, 1980, p. 127).

Self-Disclosure in Religion and Psychotherapy

Broadly speaking, psychotherapy is concerned with the growth and development of the individual to enable him or her to live more freely, unencumbered by the myriad maladaptive patterns that tend to restrict, confine, and limit one's potential. In the psychotherapeutic process, self-disclosure promotes intimacy, which allows therapy to proceed.

As a religious practice, self-disclosure ultimately promotes intimacy with (or a clearer vision of) God. This intimacy is mediated in most cases by others, although there are strong mystical traditions in all religions that attest that God's presence can be directly experienced. An additional point is that this process of developing a closer relationship with God is often concomitant with (some might say preceded by) a deeper understanding of oneself. It is at this level that parallels between religious experience and psychotherapy become clearer.

Lonsdale (1985) has listed some of the different ways Christians have conceived of the director in spiritual direction: "guide, companion, soul friend, spiritual father or mother, fellow pilgrim, 'God's usher,' 'artist of ongoing faith' " (p. 94). The master–disciple and guru–disciple models appear to be less popular outside of monastic and Eastern traditions (although, in the monastic tradition, there is also a strong influence of motherhood/fatherhood, and this will be elaborated below), yet, as Lonsdale points out, early dependence can lead to a mature freedom if this is carefully handled. In all of these models, being with, and disclosing to, another are essential to the process of spiritual direction.

Schneiders (1984), and Connolly (1975) highlight an interesting trend in present-day spiritual direction, that of an experiential approach to both understanding and transmitting the essentials of this field. Schneiders makes the point that by speaking about and focusing on the present experience in the process of spiritual direction, this anchors the practice in the present cultural milieu. I would add that it also accentuates the relationship, and ultimately, the self-disclosing aspect of spiritual direction. A weakness of this approach is a lack of interest in, or knowledge of the long history of the many traditions of spiritual direction.

How Spiritual Direction Differs from Psychotherapy

What is spiritual direction, and how does it differ from psychotherapy? Indeed, there is considerable overlap, and a number of authors have written on this subject (Walsh, 1976; Doran, 1979). Many writers believe it is important to separate one from the other. McCarty (1976) believes that it is important to differentiate spiritual direction from psychotherapy so as not to trivialize either. Geromel (1977) compares and contrasts therapy and spiritual direction, using Yalom's (1975) conceptualizations as a starting point. In his article, Geromel states that the difference is in intent and focus, and that this difference transcends methodology. Leech (1977) devotes an entire chapter to exploring the relationship among spiritual direction, counseling, and psychotherapy. His extended discussion precludes a simple statement outlining the differences of each; for Leech, there is no easy dividing point between what is spiritual and what is psychological. There is significant overlap between these areas. Leech points out the many parallels between the various practices of spiritual direction throughout the ages, and the different psychotherapeutic techniques. The parallels are noteworthy in that, at least in some respects, the two areas are more alike than different.

Barry and Connolly (1982) state that spiritual direction "is concerned with helping a person directly with his or her relationship with God" (p. 5). Dyckman and Carroll (1981) define spiritual direction as "an interpersonal relationship in which one person assists others to reflect on their own experience in light of who they are called to become in fidelity to the Gospel" (p. 20). The process involves objectification and articulation of experience, as well as discernment, seeking to know God's will for a person by interpretation of his/her experience in the light of faith. Objectification and articulation are processes that may be used in psychotherapy and counseling, while discernment is principally restricted to spiritual direction. Self-disclosure is the ground from which objectification and articulation can take place.

Connolly (1975) points out the function of attitude change that is operative in both spiritual direction and therapy. This attitude change leads to problem solving. Spiritual direction and therapy both deal with development and require a trusting relationship. The difference between the two, Connolly believes, lies in who or what is responsible for the positive changes that take place. "In counseling, insight, healing, and new directions result basically from the relationship between counselor and client. In direction they result basically from the directee's relationship with the Lord" (p. 119). Integrity and freedom are important to both relationships. In spiritual direction these are to be developed between the director and the directee, but the director is primarily a facilitator of the primary relationship, that of God and the directee.

May (1982) points out that there have been periods when "psychological phenomena were seen in only spiritual terms," and then another, more recent period where "spirituality was often seen in psychological terms" (p. 4). He differentiates the two in terms of content and intent. Regarding content, psychotherapy focuses on the emotional and mental processes. Spiritual direction focuses on prayer, the relationship with God, and religious experiences. The intent of psychotherapy, according to May, is to encourage more efficient living, and to achieve a sense of self-mastery both over oneself and one's life circumstances. Spiritual direction's intent is to foster a sense of freedom from attachments and a surrender to God and God's will. An attachment can be anything in a person's life that clouds his or her vision and sense of God's will. As a person becomes less concerned with nonessentials, that person will be able to attend to what is essential, a deeper understanding of what that person believes to be God's will for him or her.

None of the other attempts at differentiation seem as useful and as clear as May's distinction of content and intent. The benefit of this approach toward distinguishing psychotherapy from spiritual direction is that one can consider the tools as not belonging to either, but being common to both. This is consonant with Leech's notion of the similarities between the two approaches mentioned previously.

Self-Disclosure in Spiritual Direction

What is the nature of spiritual direction, and in particular, what is the role of self-disclosure in the process? McCarty (1976) provides a framework for understanding the purpose of self-disclosure in spiritual direction. It is to help the individual keep honest in his or her search, to work continually at the process of unmasking, striving for inner freedom and openhandedness in one's relationship with God. Again, the process is similar to therapy, but the intent and final purpose are different. The honesty is greatly facilitated by authentic self-disclosure.

Thomas Merton (1960), a Cistercian monk of our day, has this to say regarding the experience of spiritual direction:

> What we need to do is bring the director into contact with our real self, as best we can, and not fear to let him see what is false in our false self. Now this right way implies a relaxed, humble attitude in which we let go of ourselves, and renounce our unconscious efforts to maintain a facade. (p. 24)

Certainly Merton, even though he does not use the word, places great emphasis on the importance of self-disclosure. This is nothing new or unique to Merton. Nemeck and Coombs (1985), in their discussion of the topic, provide quotations of similar sayings, including that of St. John Climacus, a seventh century ascetical writer: "Lay bare your wound to your spiritual physician. Without being ashamed say: 'Here is my fault, Father. Here is my illness' " (p. 67), and of St. Basil, a fourth century monk, who admonishes one of his followers to "reveal the secrets of his heart... By practicing such openness, we shall gradually be made perfect" (p. 68). Self-disclosure, then, can be seen to be the cornerstone and foundation of the practice of spiritual direction. These writers, some of whom lived hundreds of years before our time, were well aware of the difficulty in self-disclosing and the reluctance to speak freely, thus the exhortations to lay bare the heart. The sayings of the Desert Fathers, a collection of stories from desert monks who lived in the first few centuries of the Common Era, reveal this as well.

The Desert Fathers

As mentioned previously, the original relationship between God and humanity and the Judeo-Christian tradition was filial. The monks of the desert, in the fourth and fifth centuries, developed the theme of spiritual fatherhood and motherhood to the fullest. This tradition is still strong in many current monastic communities, although present-day spiritual direction in other areas generally is less focused on the father/son, mother/daughter relationship. Yet, some understanding of this period will shed light on the development of spiritual direction, and on the essential nature of self-disclosure in this process.

Ward (1975) states that the relationship between a spiritual father, or 'abba,' and his son was 'vital,' that is, life-giving. The son would approach the father and ask for a 'word.' This word "was not a theological explanation, nor was it 'counseling,'... it was a word that was part of a relationship, a word which would give life to the disciple if it were received" (p. xxii).

Essential to the relationship was authentic self-disclosure. There is the story of a brother who had difficulties in revealing his troubling thoughts to his abba. His abba, guessing this, continued to encourage the brother and give him advice. The brother was able to talk of his problems and receive help (Louf, 1982). This practice was not primarily the confession of sins, but the exploration of those deeply lurking thoughts usually told to no one. Abba Poemen sees this as important, and puts it succinctly (Louf, 1982):

> Does he who knows he is losing his soul need to inquire? Hidden thoughts are to be questioned, and it is the elder's task to test them; as for visible flaws, there is no need to inquire, but to remove them right away. (p. 46)

One can see the similarity here between this statement and the belief in psychoanalytic theory that it is often the offhand comments or seemingly innocuous thoughts that can have the most meaning.

Merton (1968), in summarizing the value of understanding the Desert tradition for present-day spiritual direction, states:

> The Master does not merely lecture or instruct. He has to know and analyze the inmost thoughts of the disciple. The most important part of direction is the openness with which the disciple manifests to the spiritual Father not only all his acts, but all his thoughts. (p. 17)

To make his point Merton then quotes St. Anthony: "The monk must make known to the elders every step he takes and every drop of water he drinks in his cell, to see if he is not doing wrong" (p. 17).

The totality of self-disclosure is thus emphasized.

Self-Disclosure in Practice

What is this experience of self-disclosing and receiving spiritual direction like? Wilson (1982) describes his experience as a spiritual son. He emphasizes the necessity for trust in one's spiritual father. Wilson makes the case that the self in the fledgling initiate to religious life is undeveloped, and that at first, the son turns himself over to the father, whose self is more fully developed. He states, "Left to his many desires, often conflicting and sometimes totally destructive, the confused self of the young disciple would often follow wrong and hurtful impulses. So he chooses to follow the directives of the more achieved self of the spiritual father" (p. 229). Implicit in this is the necessity of disclosing to the spiritual father these "many desires." Thus, self-disclosure leads to reflective understanding, and further growth in the development of the true self of which Merton speaks. It is important to keep in mind that the use of the word 'self' does not necessarily have a specific meaning, such as is found in the writings of Kohut. Wilson, in particular, provides no particular theoretical base for his understanding of the experience of spiritual sonship, but, in my reading, he takes a developmental approach, and there is a literalness to his use of the terms father and son. Still, there is to be no imposition of the father's ideas upon the son, but rather the father nurtures the growth of his son as if he were his (the father's) true self. Wilson's wording is slightly ambiguous. He seems to be making the point that, through the son's disclosing to the father, and through their shared working to understand the meaning of these disclosed thoughts and desires, a deeper understanding of God and God's will for the son will result.

Conclusion

Self-disclosure is integral to the religious practice of spiritual direction, and is a common element in both direction and therapy. While religion can claim historical precedence, psychotherapy has done much recently to increase our understanding of the role and uses of self-disclosure. My reading of the literature shows a willingness on the part of religion to use (too willingly? see Kemp, 1985) psychotherapy's advances and apply them to the practice of spiritual direction. May (1982) feels that a too-ready application of psychological principles closes one off from the rich spiritual heritage of the Western spiritual tradition. Psychotherapy, on the other hand, has not been as willing to carefully consider the role of self-disclosure in spiritual direction as developed in religious circles. Again, for hundreds of years, the religious tradition provided for both an individual's psychological and spiritual needs. A careful look at the accumulated wisdom of the centuries could prove helpful to the practice of psychotherapy.

McNamara, for example, believes the Christian tradition is fundamentally oriented toward individuation, and provides an outline for the process, which eventually leads to wholeness of both the individual and society. Perhaps overstating the point, McNamara (1975) writes:

> The early Christian diagnosis of man makes Freud's comparable attempt seem like a very weak cup of tea indeed. The discoveries of analytical psychology do little else than repeat, in modern phraseology, and with detailed empirical evidence, the principle injunctions of the Christian way. (pp. 404–405)

Geromel (1977) offers a similar view:

> . . . I felt that the insights of psychotherapy would provide "new" material for spiritual direction. This is obviously not the case. Much of our "new" insights have been known for centuries. . . . It is, I believe, one of the "heresies" of our time to believe that we are the discoverers of new information, and that what went before does not relate to the present. (p. 763)

It has only been recently that there has been a revival of interest in the rich traditions of the religious and spiritual past. Perhaps, as the ideas and sources become more readily available, further exploration of the psychological principles developed over the centuries by the various spiritual traditions will take place.

References

Acharya, F. (1982). The guru: The spiritual father in the Hindu tradition. In J.R. Sommerfeldt (Ed.), *Abba: Guides to wholeness and holiness East and West*. Kalamazoo, Mich: Cistercian Publications.

Barry, W.A., & Connolly, W.J. (1982). *The practice of spiritual direction*. New York: Seabury Press.

Callahan, A. (1988). Traditions of spiritual guidance: Thomas Merton as spiritual guide. *The Way, 28*, 164–175.

Connolly, W.J. (1975). Contemporary spiritual direction: Scope and principles, an introductory essay. *Studies in the Spirituality of Jesuits, 7*, 95–124.

Doran, R.M. (1979). Jungian psychology and Christian spirituality: 1. *Review for Religious, 38*, 497–510.

Dyckman, K.M., & Carroll, L.P. (1981). *Inviting the mystic, supporting the prophet*. New York: Paulist Press.

Edwards, T. (1980). *Spiritual friend*. New York: Paulist Press.

Fry, T. (Ed) (1981). *RB 1980: The Rule of Saint Benedict*. Collegeville, Minn: Liturgical Press.

Geromel, E. (1977). Depth psychotherapy and spiritual direction. *Review for Religious, 36*, 753–763.

Green, A. (1988). Rethinking theology: Language, experience, and reality. *Reconstructionist, 54*, (Sept.), 8–13,30.

Kemp, H.V. (1985). Psychotherapy as a religious process: A historical heritage. In E.M. Stern (Ed.), *Psychotherapy and the religiously committed patient*. New York: Haworth Press.

Leech, K. (1977). *Soul friend: The practice of Christian spirituality*. San Francisco: Harper & Row.

Lonsdale, D. (1985). Bookshelf. *The Way Supplement, 54*, 94–103.

Louf, A. (1982). Spiritual fatherhood in the literature of the desert. In J.R. Sommerfeldt (Ed.), *Abba: Guides to wholeness and holiness East and West*. Kalamazoo, Mich: Cistercian Publications.

May, G. (1982). *Care of mind, care of spirit*. San Francisco: Harper & Row.

McCarty, S. (1976). On entering spiritual direction. *Review for Religious, 35*, 854–857.

McDargh, J. (1984). The life of the self in Christian spirituality and contemporary psychoanalysis. *Horizons, 11*, 344–60.

McNamara, W. (1975). Psychology and the Christian mystical tradition. In C. Tart, (Ed.), *Transpersonal psychologies*. New York: Harper & Row.

Merton, T. (1968). The spiritual father in desert tradition. *Cistercian Studies, 3*, 3–23.

Merton, T. (1960). *Spiritual direction and meditation*. Collegeville, Minn: Liturgical Press.

Nemeck, F.K., & Coombs, M.T. (1985). *The way of spiritual direction*. Wilmington, Del: Michael Glazier.

Schneiders, S.M. (1984). Horizons on spiritual direction. *Horizons, 11*, 100–112.

Sullivan, F.P. (1983). *Lyric psalms: Half a psalter*. Washington DC: Pastoral Press.

Walsh, W.J. (1976). Reality therapy and spiritual direction. *Review for Religious, 35*, 372–385.

Ward, B. (1975). *The sayings of the desert fathers*. Kalamazoo, Mich: Cistercian Publications.

Ward, B. (1984). Spiritual direction in the desert fathers. *The Way, 24*, 61–69.

Ware, K. (1974). The spiritual father in Orthodox Christianity. *Cross Currents, 24*, 296–320.

Wilson, W. (1982). Spiritual sonship: A report on experience. In J.R. Sommerfeldt (Ed.), *Abba: Guides to wholeness and holiness East and West*. Kalamazoo, Mich: Cistercian Publications.

Yalom, I. (1975). *The theory and practice of group psychotherapy*. New York: Basic Books.

II

Theoretical Perspectives

3

Self-Disclosure and Classical Psychoanalysis

Robert C. Lane and James W. Hull

The Problem of Self-Revelation

Fenichel (1945) pointed out the paradoxical nature of the patient's experience around self-disclosure, describing the wish to conceal as the essence of resistance: the patient who has entered therapy to reveal himself to the doctor in order to learn more about himself continually acts out the wish to conceal. The issue of self-disclosure has been hardly less problematic for the psychoanalytically oriented practitioner, leading to a number of intense debates in the history of psychoanalysis.

These debates have revolved around questions such as the following: Should the patient be the only member of the dyad to self-disclose, or should the therapist also engage in self-revelation? Does personal self-revelation make the therapist seem more humane, leading to greater self-revelation on the patient's part (referred to by Jourard (1971) as the "dyadic effect"), thereby enhancing therapeutic progress? How much and what types of personal information should the therapist share? Are there situations or types of patients for whom self-revelation might have an opposite effect, setting back the therapy or even harming the patient? Does therapist candor, authenticity, and openness mean the same thing to all practitioners and all patients? How should the decision around self-disclosure be influenced by variables such as the age and

Robert C. Lane • Institute of Advanced Psychological Studies, Adelphi University, Garden City, New York 11530. **James W. Hull** • New York Hospital–Cornell Medical Center, Westchester Division, 21 Bloomingdale Road, White Plains, New York 10605.

sex of the patient, and the stage of therapy? Other more technical questions, such as those regarding the nature, intensity, and timing of self-revelation, also have been raised.

Currently there exits a strong polarization among therapists of different schools regarding these issues. Dissatisfaction with classical psychoanalysis has included the criticism that its practitioners, most of whom eschew self-revelation, can be aloof, nonresponsive, and seemingly unavailable. The various therapies of the human potential movement (Murphy, 1958) have been one outgrowth of such criticism. Many of these approaches advocate "therapist's transparency," a willingness to share immediate impressions as well as past experience with the patient. This is said to make the therapist more humane, to bind therapist and patient together in an exchange of intimacies. The therapist provides a model for personal growth, facilitating spontaneous, genuine, and even "creative" being (Culbert, 1961; Trilling, 1975). Examples of such approaches include humanistic/existential therapy, client-centered therapy, sensitivity training and the encounter movement, experiential therapy, gestalt therapy, bioenergetics, and some varieties of cognitive-affective therapy.

Family therapists also have argued for the usefulness of self-disclosure. Whitaker related success in family therapy mainly to the therapist's self-involvement in the process, including the sharing of unique personal reactions, confusion, and uncertainties (Whitaker & Malone, 1953; Napier & Whitaker, 1978; Whitaker & Keith, 1981). He argued that self-disclosure might be the only strategy that could rescue a family treatment from impasse, but cautioned that it could produce harmful effects for therapist and family alike. Others who have made similar points include Garfield (1987) and Watzlawick (1978).

While these voices have echoed across the current professional scene, many psychoanalysts have continued to advocate the neutrality and anonymity of the "blank screen," feeling that self-revelation may contaminate the transference and interfere with its resolution. Expressions of the analyst's personal opinions, attitudes, and feelings still are seen by many as a sign of countertransference difficulties. Texts on psychoanalytic technique commonly espouse this position (e.g., Fenichel, 1945; Fine, 1982; Glover, 1955; Greenson, 1967; Langs, 1982; Menninger, 1958; Strean, 1982). The psychoanalytic community has not been unanimous in its rejection of self-revelation, however, and in recent years some analysts have begun to explore how judicious self-disclosure may further the work of analysis. This has led to a rediscovery of the early writings of Ferenczi.

In the present chapter we discuss the problem of therapist self-disclosure from the perspective of classical psychoanalysis, tracing the historical debate and current controversy around the benefits and costs of such intervention. We will not take up the question of patient self-disclosure, and also will limit ourselves to comments about individual psychotherapy. Many new approaches advocating therapist self-revelation have evolved from the group therapy field and in this sense our comments may not be directly applicable to those modalities where therapist self-disclosure is most common. Nevertheless, we feel that psychoanalytic thinking about self-disclosure in the analytic relationship highlights central issues and problems that can be applied usefully to other therapeutic modalities.

Self-Disclosure and the Early Analysts

Freud (1915) felt that the patient needs a safe environment for personal self-disclosure, including reassurances that his or her communications will be confidential and no punishment will result from saying whatever comes to mind. Thoughts, feelings, impulses, dreams, fantasies, and traumatic memories are to be revealed to an objective, understanding, and empathic listener. In this way the power of the patient's critical superego is reduced, fostering the emergence of unconscious material. With the development of healthier ego controls the patient is slowly freed from the debilitating anxiety that keeps him or her from living more fully.

In his writings on technique Freud (1912) advocated a policy of strict nondisclosure on the part of the analyst. The analyst should remain "opaque to his patients, like a mirror and show them nothing but what is shown to him" (p. 118). In this paper, he also warned against too much intimacy on the part of the doctor. Later (1919) he stated that, "the patient must be left with unfulfilled wishes in abundance, deny(ing) him precisely those satisfactions which he desires most intensely and (has) expressed most importunately" (p. 164). Privation and frustration, fostered in part by a non-revealing stance, are used to maintain the patient's motivation for carrying on the work of analysis. "The patient's need and longing should be allowed to persist. . . in order that they may serve as a force impelling the patient to work and make changes" (Freud, 1919, pp. 164–165).

Although his writings are clear in their recommendation for abstinence and neutrality on the analyst's part, records of how Freud actually worked indicate his "sovereign readiness to disregard his own rules" (Gay, 1988, p. 292). There was a personal and compassionate element to his demeanor in the consulting room, which he felt to be unobjectionable, an aspect of the human relationship between patient and doctor that is separate from the work of analysis. Gay (1988) provides many examples of Freud's self-revelations and "non-neutral" behavior with patients. For example, his analysis of Eitington, which was one of the first training analyses, was conducted during leisurely strolls around Vienna. At times Freud gave gifts to patients, and he was known to remit fees when a patient fell on hard times. His decision to analyze his daughter Anna directly contradicted earlier technical recommendations regarding neutrality and the need to function as a blank screen. He assisted Max Graf in the analysis of his own young son (Little Hans), and later when Jung began to analyze his wife Freud encouraged him, thinking that he might meet with some success. The Rat Man was provided with a meal when he arrived for a session hungry, and other solicitous behavior was directed toward Wortis (1954), Doolittle (1956), Blanton (1971), and Kardiner (1977).

Freud's self-disclosure with patients finds its complement in his writings for other professionals. In *The Interpretation of Dreams* (1900) he reported and analyzed some of his own most revealing dreams, often reporting highly embarrassing childhood memories which were uncovered by his associates. For example, the discussion of the dream of Count Thun includes memories of an incident when he was seven or eight and urinated on the floor of his parents' bedroom, prompting his father to predict he never would amount to anything. Gay (1988) also describes how self-revelation and "wild analysis" were a regular part of the culture and collegial interaction of the early analytic community. While on the ship to America, Freud and Jones passed the time by analyzing each other's dreams. Offhand interpretations of colleagues' personalities, dreams, and slips of the tongue were common, with diagnosis of paranoia and homosexuality freely given. "They all practiced in their circle the kind of wild analysis they decried in outsiders as tactless, unscientific and counterproductive. . . . Freud played this game with the rest" (Gay, 1988, p. 235).

Freud's abandonment of the seduction theory led him to emphasize intrapsychic conflicts and minimize the role of the actual environment in the causation of neurosis. By contrast, Ferenczi placed increasing emphasis on the role of real trauma in pathogenesis (Lum, 1988a,b). In his clinical diary he maintained that psychoanalysis placed too great an emphasis on the role of fantasy, and whenever analysis went deeply enough a traumatic-hysterical basis of neurosis could be uncovered. He drew a parallel between the child traumatized by the hypocrisy of adults, the mental patient traumatized by the hypocrisy of society, and the analysand whose trauma is revived by the technical rigidity of the analyst. The analyst's hypocrisy consists of the denial of countertransference feelings, and it is this that reactivates the earliest traumas of the patient.

In order to deal with the reactivation of early traumas in analysis, Ferenczi proposed a number of technical innovations that departed significantly from the method outlined by Freud. He first experimented with an "active technique," in which privation and absence of gratification were carried to an extreme. He imposed restrictions on patients in the areas of sex, food, drinking, and smoking in the hope of gaining insight into the damming up of libido and releasing "inaccessible unconscious material" (Lum, 1988a,b), but discovered this usually led to increased anxiety, rage, and defiance (Thompson, 1964).

Ferenczi's later experiments focused on the development of a "relaxation technique." Abandoning the authoritarian and "cold" stance of the classical analyst, as well as his earlier "active technique" of privation and abstinence, Ferenczi transformed the analytic setting into one of indulgence. Instead of functioning as a mirror, passively and at times aloofly reflecting the patient's reactions, the analyst should adopt a stance of warmth and participation. He must become a "good" loving mother, empathic, involved, highly sensitive, and responsive to the patient's needs. The goal was removal of anxiety and a reliving and discharge of feelings related to the original trauma experienced at the hands of the parents. Of paramount importance were the analyst's sincerity, authenticity, and truthfulness, so that the original insincerity of the parents would not be repeated. The analyst's real personality, his ability and willingness to be a new and healthy parent, would help undo the original childhood traumas.

In this search for truth the analyst must be willing to face himself, giving free rein to self-criticism and accepting the possibility that the patient's accusations have a reality basis. Ferenczi believed that the analysand could accurately perceive the analyst's errors, resistances, and blind spots. Responsibility for failure to make progress should not be placed solely on the patient, but rather on the therapist–patient interaction and the transference–countertransference exchange. The therapist should admit his mistakes and say, "I'm sorry," but Ferenczi went even further, advocating that the therapist "unmask his professional hypocrisy" by revealing his own secrets, resistances, annoyances, and shortcomings to the patient, making his disturbance fully conscious and discussing it with the patient (Ludmer, 1988; Zaslow, 1988).

Reciprocity was carried to the point of having his patients analyze him, termed "mutual analysis" (Dupont, 1988). In his diary Ferenczi states that when an analyst is unable to help the patient because of his own blind spots, he at least has the obligation to provide guideposts by acquainting the patient with his own weaknesses and feelings. This technique of mutual analysis was originally the idea of one of his patients, a woman who had been in analysis for two years and whose treatment was stalemated. Ferenczi first found this patient disagreeable and in overcompensation had yielded to all her wishes. She came to believe that he was in love with her and that she had found the ideal lover. Frightened by this, he retreated, interpreting the negative emotions she should be feeling toward him. She responded with the same interpretations directed toward him, which he felt were not unjustified. He decided to express his feelings freely to her, and noted that she began to make progress again in her sessions. Carrying the experiment further, he scheduled double sessions or alternating sessions, one for her and one for him.

Gradually Ferenczi became aware of the problems of mutual analysis, including the patient's wish to deflect attention from herself, the impossibility of letting oneself be analyzed by every patient, the need to respect patients' sensibilities, and the problem posed by the discretion owed to other patients. He specified the limitations of mutual analysis: it should be practiced strictly according to the needs of the patient, and no further than necessary for the patient. Eventually he considered letting himself be analyzed only after the patient's analysis was completed. When his patient began to develop delusional ideas about their collaboration, suggesting they prolong it indefinitely and that without it Ferenczi would lose his therapeutic skill, he terminated the experiment. In reflecting on this experience he concluded that mutual analysis was only a technique "of last resort," when the training analysis had been incomplete.

Lum (1988a,b) documents Freud's strong disapproval of Ferenczi's technical innovations. Freud felt that Ferenczi was obsessed, first with the need to cure by extreme deprivation (active technique) and later with the need to cure by love (relaxation technique). He chastised Ferenczi particularly about rumors that he permitted kissing. The analytic community at the time reacted with amazement and extreme criticism. More recent evaluations have been less condemning. Rachman (1988) points out that in addition to challenging the classical position that the analyst should be a "mirror," Ferenczi was the first dissident analyst to offer an alternative to the Oedipus complex. Ferenczi was one of the first psychoanalysts to call attention to the crucial importance of the earliest mother-child relationship. In identifying early affect deprivation as one cause of infant death, he predated Spitz' (1946) work on marasmus. Finally, in his emphasis on the analyst as a human partner in the therapeutic exchange, with a focus on transference–countertransference dilemmas, he paved the way for later interpersonal and self psychological pioneers such as Sullivan, Fromm, and Kohut.

Contemporary Views on Self-Disclosure

Ehrenberg (1984) has taken up the question of self-disclosure from the perspective of the interpersonal analyst in her discussion of "direct effective engagement." Arguing that expressing affective reactions to the patient may "add a new dimension to analytic interaction," she shows how the analyst's shared countertransference responses may help patients become aware of their own repetition compulsions and actual impact on others. "The transference-countertransference drama, as it develops in the immediate relationship, (is a)...window to the past, as well as a prism or lens, not a barrier." Judicious use of countertransference also may help the patient see that the analyst has real feelings, supporting the experience of empathy and understanding. It encourages the patient to assume responsibility for his or her participation, or lack of it, in events both inside and outside the sessions. Ehrenberg cautions that too much or too little affective participation on the part of the analyst can destroy the relationship. Not responding affectively can lead to a feeling of abandonment, transference/countertransference collusion, increased resistance, and detachment. For her the important questions are: (1) When to react? (2) How much to share of one's reaction? and (3) When would it be helpful to the patient, encouraging further exploration, and when would it be burdensome to have such material shared?

In his discussion of Ehrenberg's paper, Spence (1984) agrees that the important question is when is it useful and when is it a mistake to share such responses, and to "what extent does a focus on the here and now violate the assumption of the basic rule and put the patient unnecessarily at risk?" He stresses the need to clarify the concept of neutrality, pointing out that its meaning might be very different for different patients. Breger (1984) also agrees it is crucial to clarify concepts such as "neutrality," "abstinence," and "gratification," since each analytic contact is different and must be understood on its own terms. He feels that interventions in which the therapist communicates emotional reactions of acceptance, empathy, and encouragement are especially potent. Utilizing self-disclosure to help resolve a transference–countertransference impasse is seen as an intervention "fraught with danger," and demanding considerable experience; "such moments are not for the beginner." Breger feels that communicating negative feelings directly to the patient almost always is a mistake; "it is most often felt as criticism...and a betrayal of the very openness that one has encouraged..."

Khan (1986) presents what is perhaps the most vivid example of current analytic work in which self-disclosure is used to an extreme. With his patient Khan violated many of the usual ground rules, so that classical analysts would not consider this psychoanalysis at all. The patient's outrageousness had first manifested itself when he farted during his fifth birthday party. His mother was disgusted with him, both for the farting and for the behavior that followed, including his refusal to go out or go to school for weeks at a time. After her three-month hospitalization during which he was cared for by his grandparents, she returned home to find him "filthy" and stated, "it took four months to straighten him out." He withdrew, didn't participate in games, just stayed in his room reading and gluing together pebbles that he had collected. In later life this man perfected the art of quietly provoking others. For example, he was spiteful with his employees, leaving out crucial details in his instructions to them, so that they never knew what had to be done.

Khan carried out two analyses with this patient, with a three-year period intervening during which Khan fought a life-threatening battle with cancer that required the removal of half his larynx and many operations. When the patient began his second analysis, Khan shared the details of this illness. He stated, "I no longer have the strength or motivation of three years ago to devote energy and talent to someone who wants to play games...Thank you for coming...I can refer you." And later, "I have been fighting death for two years and more and have made it back to the living and working...but I was damaged in my physique. Now I make the demands." In this way Khan conveyed that he felt under no obligation to save the patient or be blackmailed by suicidal threats.

Khan acted capriciously in an attempt to change the tempo and "unsettle" this patient. He kept the patient waiting for some appointments, permitted him to leave one appointment after only 30 minutes and kept him for over two hours during another. He demanded three hours' notice if the patient was going to cancel his second session, a number made up on the spot with no explanation given to the patient. He said he was determined to conduct the analysis as if the patient were five years old, and not be cowed by the patient's provocativeness. When the patient brought up the subject of money, Khan let him know that he was not intimidated by financial considerations, stating, "My father has taken care that I should never need to earn money...I don't need this, I can go to my estates." When the patient challenged him by saying it was little wonder that he was having trouble in the British Psychoanalytic Society, Khan said he didn't give a damn, he was in demand all over the world and even if he were not he could return to his family's ancestral estates in Pakistan. He discussed his butler, chauffeur, and the staff of his Pakistan estate with his patient.

In commenting on this case Khan describes the effective ego state of outrage and outrageousness as a distinct syndrome, related to the cumulative trauma that can result from supposed "good-enough mothering" (Khan, 1963). When the child is raised as a "cot baby," to be clean, tidy, and good, but with an excess of inhibition and a restriction of spontaneity, outrage, and outrageousness may result. The aggression of such patients, often first manifested in adolescence, is not overt but is turned into provocativeness and devious spitefulness. Such "pretend care" also leads to a considerable amount of unrelatedness, particularly in later life. Kahn feels that clinical handling is difficult "because interpretation is an alibi the analyst uses to cover his incapacity to deal with the patient's conduct. The patient knows how to exploit the analyst's technique to his advantage, with compliance, without reaching that authenticity which is his personal self." In dealing with such patients Khan is himself ready to act out in an "interpretative" manner. "When the patient needs me to hold him by acting (managing his private life) I act."

The major current spokesman for a traditional stance of restraint with regard to self-disclosure is Langs (1982). He spells out necessary conditions for an ideal therapeutic framework, the "definitive rules of relatedness" through which a healthy therapeutic symbiosis may be constituted and maintained. Practitioners are divided into those who "adhere to all fundamental tenets," or move as close as possible to the ideal therapeutic situation, and those who "modify one or another of the basic ground rules...(thus creating)...a deviant treatment setting." Breaks in the frame and a lack of adherence to these ground rules lead to pathological forms of relatedness. Langs feels that such deviations "virtually always" serve as "inappropriately seductive element(s)" that may evoke powerful unconscious sexual and aggressive dynamics. They function as "powerful adaptation-evoking" therapeutic contexts to which patients respond through "derivative communications" that the therapist may easily misunderstand.

The basic ground rules include the therapist's neutrality and anonymity, and the need for total privacy and confidentiality of the treatment process. Neutrality, which insures the patient's safety, means confining one's interventions to silences, interpretations, reconstructions, and the establishment and management of the ground rules or framework. Interventions such as questions, clarifications, and confrontations, proposed as a means of fostering patient openness, are lacking in neutrality and interfere with the patient's free association. Personal opinions, self-revelations, directives, and unnecessary reassurances are to be especially avoided. While these may provide momentary relief, they always have a pathological effect and provide the basis for "therapeutic misalliances."

According to Langs, anonymity provides full opportunity for projection by the patient and lends a sense of safety to the therapeutic relationship. It signals the therapist's willingness to forgo and renounce pathological needs and repel any tendencies to misuse the relationship for pathological satisfaction. Total anonymity is impossible and absurd, but the therapist should not be deterred from striving for relative anonymity, with self-revelations confined to those implicit in the setting. Patients should be accepted for treatment only when there has been no prior contact, so that relative anonymity has not been compromised. Magazines, artwork, books, and furnishings in the therapist's office, as well as the therapist's own personal appearance, should be minimally self-revealing. Seeing the patient in a home office, revealing aspects of one's personal life such as vacation plans, political preferences, or hobbies and interests, or disclosure of information about the therapist's state of health or the reason for sudden cancellations are to be avoided. Langs feels that self-revelations exist on a continuum, anchored at one end by those "that are inevitable, humanly necessary, and do not interfere with the therapeutic relationship" and at the other end by "a multiplicity of deliberate self-revelations that clearly disturb the ideal therapeutic environment and the relationship between the patient and therapist." Most self-revelations, both deliberate and inadvertent, fall between these two extremes.

Other contemporary analytic writers have taken a conservative, although somewhat less rigid, position on the issue of self-revelation. Anna Freud (1954) stated, "I feel still that we should leave room somewhere for the realization that the analyst and patient are also two real people, of equal adult status, in a real personal relationship to each other..." (p. 618). Gitelson (1952) emphasized that an impasse may develop if the analyst does not understand or avoids the patient's discovery of him as a real person. Greenson (1967) saw the nontransference or real relationship as an essential part of the working alliance "which makes it possible for the patient to work purposefully in the analytic situation" (p. 46), despite transference impulses. He recommends self-disclosure around errors in technique, but stresses the need to analyze the patient's reactions to mistakes and the analyst's discussion of them. Weiner (1972) outlined situations where self-disclosure is contraindicated, including a poor therapeutic alliance and a state of negative transference. He stated, "If a patient has some need to see me as a real person with whom a real relationship can be established, such as an adolescent or an adult with a borderline personality, I will often accede to his wish for historical information" (p. 48). Even then, however, Weiner (1969) felt the therapist should eschew total exposure, having an obligation both to himself and his patients to offer professional competence rather than personal idiosyncrasies.

Special Events

Some events during psychotherapy by their very nature lead to therapist self-disclosure. Examples are serious illness in the analyst, pregnancy and birth, and marriage. Most of the literature to date has dealt with illnesses in the analyst. Rosner (1986) identifies this as one situation where self-disclosure may be necessary for the patient's emotional health. To regard serious illness as no different than separations due to vacation or minor illness represents denial on the part of the analyst. Not revealing information gives the patient's fantasies free rein, there is no opportunity to deal with distortions, and the failure to reveal information, especially when it can provide relief, and runs the risk of introducing real issues of exclusion, abandonment, and rejection. On the other hand, divulging information prevents the emergence of transference distortions and may greatly complicate the patient's working through of hostility toward the analyst. Crucial technical questions include: Who should inform the patient that sessions are to be cancelled? How much factual information should be provided? Should different patients be provided with different amounts of information, based on their personality and the stage of their analysis?

With regard to the patient's reactions to the analyst's illness, Dewald (1982) identified the problem as "the need adequately to explore the full gamut of the patient's responses, affects and associations to the illness, and to do this in the face of countertransference temptations either defensively to promote premature closure and evasion of more threatening affects, or to use the experience for exhibitionistic, masochistic, narcissistic or other neurotic satisfaction" (p. 361). He argued that too much information may inhibit the patient's fantasies and reactions, thereby interfering with the analysis, while too little information may overburden the patient's adaptive capacity. He attempted to vary his approach to the needs of each patient and the phase of therapy: some factual material was offered to those in the beginning phase so that they would not drop out, while the least factual information was provided to those in the middle phase. He felt that patients in the terminal phase "didn't need information."

Abend (1982) maintained that how much factual information is offered should depend on how well the patient can maintain analytic productivity "in the absence of factual information." He feels that most analysts who have written on this topic have arrived at a solution close to Dewald's, but cautions analysts to be aware of their own unconscious needs that may be served by the transmission of factual information about illness, even when it seems technically correct to provide such information and the subsequent analytic work appears unimpeded or even enhanced by the disclosure.

Another event that leads inevitably to self-disclosure is pregnancy. Lax (1969) described pregnancy as "...a personal event in the life of the analyst that cannot be hidden from the patient and intrudes into the analytic situation. The so-called anonymity and neutrality of the analyst is interfered with" (p. 363). She related experiences with several patients during her own pregnancy to illustrate that each responded with a reactivation of those infantile conflicts most relevant to his or her pathology. Fear of sibling rivalry and concerns about femininity are especially likely to be aroused in the analyst. Lax concluded that pregnancy did "not necessarily interfere with the unfolding of a pattern of infantile conflicts characteristic for a given patient" (p. 372). Paluszny and Poznanski (1971) point out the wide variation in patients' reactions to the analyst's pregnancy. Benedek (1973) discussed the reactions of staff in a residential treatment center to the analyst's pregnancy.

Several writers have addressed the topic of "extra-analytic contacts" when patients suddenly meet the analyst outside the session and learn something about his or her private life. Tarnower (1966) delineated conflicting motives and wishes that such events can mobilize. Weiss (1975) stressed the importance of analyzing these contacts in order to avoid disruptive transference effects. He feels that when understood and interpreted properly, especially with good timing, these occurrences can be helpful in mobilizing, highlighting, and clarifying transference phenomena. Katz (1978), writing of his experiences with patients after they had seen him in a community play, also felt that transference and resistance could be managed in such contacts. Strean (1981) delineated three types of extra-analytic contact: those actively brought about by the patient, accidental contacts, and contacts anticipated by the analyst but not by the patient. He argues that extra-analytic contact can interfere with or heighten latent transference, countertransference, and resistance, as well as "serve(ing) as an index of therapeutic progress." Such meetings are interpersonal events "not to be encouraged or discouraged but thoroughly analyzed." In discussing this paper Green (1982) feels it is erroneous to believe such events may be disregarded as long as they are analyzed. His position is close to that of Langs (1976), who stated that extra-analytic contact always modifies the transference, offers neurotic gratifications, reinforces resistances, and undermines basic therapeutic work.

Discussion

Psychoanalysts have concerned themselves with the problem of self-revelation since the earliest days of Freud. Self-disclosure was a regular part of Freud's demeanor in the consulting room, and in their early congresses and informal social gatherings. Analysts revealed much about themselves, sometimes too much, making self-disclosure a regular feature of their informal professional culture. In addition, many early writers followed Freud's example of using partially disguised self-revelation to illustrate theoretical points, and from the beginning there were bold experiments in technique such as those of Ferenczi.

Our own position on this issue might be described as one of "tempered" restraint. We agree that the best environment for therapy is provided when the analyst assumes a neutral stance, when physical and social contact are avoided, and the analyst's own conflicts do not intrude into the patient's hour. The revelation of personal feelings, the telling of anecdotes, and other forms of self-disclosure, usually hinder the therapeutic process. We feel that a willingness to share one's past or present experience with the patient does not make the analyst more genuine or humane, neither "unshackling" the patient nor providing a model for spontaneous relating. It is naive to believe that self-disclosure will bind analyst and patient together in "an exchange of intimacies."

On the other hand, we describe our position as one of "tempered" restraint because some self-revelation always is present in analysis, and that in certain special circumstances judicious self-revelation may further the work of analysis. To try to eliminate self-disclosure completely strikes us as unrealistic and probably undesirable. Langs has pointed out that complete anonymity is impossible, suggesting instead that the therapist strive for "relative anonymity." We do not go as far as Langs in giving prescriptions regarding pictures on the desk, paintings on the wall, or clothing that the therapist wears. Close approximations to complete anonymity run the risk of moving the analytic encounter away from its origins in, and ultimate impact on, everyday human experience. As Anna Freud and others have pointed out, the patient's discovery of the analyst as a real person may be a crucial phase of every analysis that is carried toward completion.

Regarding "affective engagement," it seems to us that it should be used very sparingly, and not until the analyst is quite clear about what is going on in the transference. As Breger (1986) stated, such moments are "not for beginners," and the use of countertransference to resolve therapeutic impasses can be very dangerous. Interventions of this type should be intentional and planned with a clear rationale. For example, in certain situations of crisis innocuous self-disclosure of related experience by the analyst may convey an element of relatedness, empathy, and hope to the patient. Freud provides examples of this type of intervention, such as sharing the details of his granddaughter's death in response to Hilda Doolittle's attempt to work through the death of a loved one (Gay, 1988). We recognize, however, that many classical analysts would object to such technique.

In summary, we accept that much of the analyst's personality inevitably is revealed despite his or her best intentions, and feel that sometimes limited and judicious self-disclosure may further the work of analysis. Self-disclosure by the analyst should be regarded as one aspect, perhaps even a central dimension of the ongoing analytic encounter, to be monitored and studied in the same way that the analyst studies the ebb and flow of transference, countertransference, and resistance.

References

Abend, S.M. (1982). Serious illness in the analyst: Countertransference considerations. *Journal of the American Psychoanalytic Association, 30*, 365–379.

Benedek, E. (1973). Fourth world of the pregnant therapist. *Journal American Medical Women's Association, 28*, 365.

Blanton, S. (1971). *Diary of my analysis with Sigmund Freud*. New York: Hawthorne Books.

Breger, L. (1984). Discussion of D. Ehrenberg, Psychoanalytic engagement II: Affective considerations. *Contemporary Psychoanalysis, 20*, 583–589.

Culbert, S.A. (1961). The therapeutic process of self-disclosure. In J.T. Hunt & T.M. Tomlinson (Eds.), *New directions in client-centered therapy*. Boston: Houghton Mifflin.

Dewald, P.A. (1982). Serious illness in the analyst: Transference, countertransference, and reality responses. *Journal of the American Psychoanalytic Association, 30*, 347–363.

Doolittle, H. (1956). *Tribute to Freud with unpublished letters to the author*. New York: Pantheon Press.

Dupont, J. (Ed.). (1988). *The clinical diary of Sandor Ferenczi*. M. Balint & N. Jackson, trans. Cambridge: Harvard University Press.

Ehrenberg, D. (1984). Psychoanalytic engagement II: Affective considerations. *Contemporary Psychoanalysis, 20*, 560–583.

Fenichel, O. (1945). *The psychoanalytic theory of neurosis*. New York: W.W. Norton.

Ferenczi, S. (1933). Confusion of tongues between adults and the child. *International Journal of Psychoanalysis, 30*, 225–230.

Fine, R. (1982). *The healing of the mind*. New York: The Free Press.

Freud, A. (1954). The widening scope of indications for psychoanalysis: Discussion. *Journal of the American Psychoanalytic Association, 2*, 607–620.

Freud, S. (1900). The interpretation of dreams. *Standard edition*, Vol. 4. London: Hawthorne Press.

Freud, S. (1912). Recommendations to physicians practicing psychoanalysis. *Standard edition*, Vol. 12. London: Hogarth Press.

Freud, S. (1919). Lines of advance in psychoanalytic therapy. *Standard edition*, Vol. 17. London: Hogarth Press.

Garfield, R. (1987). On self-disclosure: The vulnerable therapist. *Contemporary Family Therapy, 9*, 58–78.

Gay, P. (1988). *Freud: A life for our time*. New York: W.W. Norton.

Gitelson, M. (1952). The emotional positions of the analyst in the psychoanalytic situation. *International Journal of Psychoanalysis, 33*, 1.

Glover, E. (1955). *The technique of psychoanalysis*. New York: International Universities Press.

Greene, M. (1982). Discussion of H.S. Strean, Extra-analytic contacts: Theoretical and clinical considerations. In H.S. Strean (Ed.), *Controversy in psychotherapy*. Metuchen, NJ: Scarecrow Press.

Greenson, R. (1967). *The technique and practice of psychoanalysis*. New York: International Universities Press.
Jourard, S. (1971). *Self-disclosure: An experimental analysis of the transparent self*. New York: Wiley-Interscience.
Kardiner, A. (1977). *My analysis with Freud*. New York: Simon & Schuster.
Katz, J.B. (1978). A psychoanalyst's anonymity: Fiddler behind the couch. *Bulletin of the Menninger Clinic, 42*, 520–524.
Khan, M. (1963). The concept of cumulative trauma. In *The privacy of the self*. London: Hogarth Press, 1974.
Khan, M. (1986). Outrageousness, compliance and authenticity. *Contemporary Psychoanalysis, 22*, 629–652.
Langs, R. (1976). The therapeutic relationship and deviations in technique. *International Journal of Psychoanalytic Psychotherapy, 4*, 106–141.
Langs, R. (1982). *Psychotherapy: A Basic Text*. New York: Jason Aronson.
Lax, R.F. (1969). Some considerations about transference and counter-transference manifestations evoked by the analyst's pregnancy. *International Journal of Psychoanalysis, 50*, 363.
Ludmer, R.I. (1988). Creativity and the self. (Discussion of S. Ferenczi, *Confusion of tongues between adults and the child*.) *Contemporary Psychoanalysis, 24*, 234–239.
Lum, W.B. (1988a). Sandor Ferenczi (1873–1933)—The father of the empathic-interpersonal approach. Part I: Introduction and early analytic years. *Journal of the American Academy of Psychoanalysis, 16*, 131–153.
Lum, W.B. (1988b). Sandor Ferenczi (1873–1933)—The father of the empathic-interpersonal approach. Part II: Evolving technique, final contributions and legacy. *Journal American Academy of Psychoanalysis, 16*, 317–347.
Menninger, K. (1958). *Theory of psychoanalytic technique*. New York: Basic Books.
Murphy, G. (1958). *Human potentialities*. New York: Basic Books.
Napier, A.Y., & Whitaker, C. (1978). *The family crucible*. New York: Harper & Row.
Paluszny, M., & Poznanski, E. (1971). Reactions of patients during pregnancy of the psychotherapist. *Child Psychiatry Human Development, 1*, 266.
Rachman, A.W. (1988). The rule of empathy: Sandor Ferenczi's pioneering contributions to the empathic method in psychoanalysis. *Journal of the American Academy of Psychoanalysis, 16*, 1–27.
Rosner, S. (1986). The seriously ill or dying analyst and the limits of neutrality. *Psychoanalytic Psychology, 3*, 357–371.
Spence, D. (1984). Discussion of D.B. Ehrenberg, Psychoanalytic engagement, II: Affective considerations. *Contemporary Psychoanalysis, 20*, 589–595.
Spitz, R.A., & Wolf, K.M. (1946). Anaclitic depression: An inquiry into the genesis of psychiatric conditions in early childhood. *Psychoanalytic Study of the Child, 2*, 313–342.
Strean, H.S. (1981). Extra-analytic contacts: Theoretical and clinical considerations. *Psychoanalytic Quarterly, 50*, 238–259.
Strean, H.S. (1982). *Controversy in psychotherapy*. Metuchen, NJ: Scarecrow Press.
Tarnower, W. (1966). Extra-analytic contacts between the psychoanalyst and the patient. *Psychoanalytic Quarterly, 35*, 399–413.
Thompson, C. (1964). Sandor Ferenczi, 1873–1933. In M. Green (Ed.), *The collected papers of Clara Thompson*. New York: Basic Books.
Trilling, L. (1975). *Sincerity and authenticity*. Cambridge: Harvard University Press.
Watzlawick, P. (1978). *The language of change*. New York: Basic Books.
Weiner, M.F. (1969). In defense of the therapist. *Psychosomatics, 10*, 156.
Weiner, M.F. (1972). Self-exposure by the therapist as a therapeutic technique. *American Journal of Psychotherapy, 26*, 42.
Weiss, S.S. (1975). The effect on the transference of "special events" occurring during psychoanalysis. *International Journal of Psychoanalysis, 56*, 69–75.

Whitaker, C., & Keith, D. (1981). Symbolic-experiential family therapy. In A. Gurman & D. Kniskern (Eds.), *Handbook of family therapy*. New York: Brunner/Mazel.
Whitaker, C., & Malone, T. (1953). *The roots of psychotherapy*. New York: Blakiston.
Wortis, J. (1954). *Fragments of an analysis with Freud*. New York: Simon & Schuster.
Zaslow, S. (1988). Comments on "Confusion of Tongues." [Review of S. Ferenczi, *Confusion of tongues between adults and the child*.) *Contemporary Psychoanalysis, 24*, 211–225.

4

Show and Tell

REFLECTIONS ON THE ANALYST'S SELF-DISCLOSURE

Sabert Basescu

The classical analytic stance has been that of the blank screen, with the analyst maintaining anonymity. This article discusses the conceptual bases for this position and how these conceptual issues are undergoing modification. These changes impact upon the role of analytic anonymity and consequently upon the nature of the analyst's self-disclosure. The article focuses on the writer's personal experience with self-disclosure in the context of therapeutic work.

The public's image of the typical psychoanalyst has been given expression in many jokes and satirical comments such as "He always answers a question with a question," or "I knew he was alive because I could hear him breathing." That image has been consistent with the classical analytic role of the blank screen who discloses no personal facts, reveals no emotions, but simply mirrors the projections of the patient. My intention in this presentation is briefly to discuss the conceptual issues that have sustained this analytic stance and how our understanding of those issues is changing, the impact of these changes on the concept of analytic anonymity and, finally, the nature of the analyst's self-disclosure—especially my own.

Although Freud, the clinician, grossly violated most of the thera-

Sabert Basescu • Department of Psychology, New York University, New York, New York 10003, and the Westchester Center for the Study of Psychoanalysis and Psychotherapy, 516 Hommocks Road, Larchmont, New York 10538. Versions of this paper were presented at The Manhattan Institute for Psychoanalysis on November 20, 1987, and at the NYU Postdoctoral Program for Psychoanalysis on February 5, 1988.

peutic dictates of Freud, the metapsychologist, it is Freud, the theorist, unfortunately, who has been the source of most of the structure of clinical psychoanalysis. Freud, the theorist, made fantasy the primary focus of psychoanalytic inquiry. Fantasy in this sense is not simply the imagined elaboration of experience, but rather the symbolic reflection of intrapsychic processes, wishes, and defenses, and their distorting impact on experience.

If fantasy is all-important and reality more or less irrelevant, it follows that the less reality offered by the therapist, the freer play afforded to the patient's fantasy. Increasingly, however, the question has been raised whether the primary data of psychoanalysis are facts or fantasies. Do intrapsychic symbolizations have a life of their own or are fantasies a function of the person's reality experiences? As Levenson (1981) puts it, "Who dreams the dream? Does the dream perhaps dream the dreamer?" (p. 486). Interpersonalists answer the question one way and Freudians the other. Although theoretical allegiance has been the main basis for choosing one's answer, recent infant research may provide some independent evidence. Daniel Stern (1985) writes: "...infants from the beginning mainly experience reality...It is the actual shape of interpersonal reality, specified by the interpersonal variants that really exist, that help determine the developmental course. Coping operations occur as reality-based adaptations" (p. 255).

Perhaps a more clinically cogent way of discussing the same issue is in terms of the concept of transference. Is transference a one-person or two-person affair? (Gill, 1984). Those who hold to the one-person model see the patient's distorting perceptions of the analyst as coming whole cloth from the patient's past experience as structured by his or her intrapsychic dynamisms. The intruding realities of the analyst's person and personality can serve only to obfuscate the portrait of the life to be explained. Therefore, it behooves the analyst to do all in his or her power to minimize them.

Those who hold to the two-person model see transference as interactional. That is, transference is regarded as the patient's attempt to arrive at a plausible understanding of the analytic relationship and is more or less influenced by the analyst's behavior. The concern is less with the patient's distortions and more with constriction in modes of understanding. For example, a patient said, "I was trying to read the meaning of changes in your tone of voice last time when we were talking about makeup appointments. It felt like you thought I was a pest." I said, "You read correctly that something was going on with me, but it had to do with my realizing I was uncertain as to when I wanted to make the appointment." He said, "I'm glad you told me. It's so easy to feel crazy—like adults aren't supposed to react to changes in the tone of voice."

According to Levenson (1981), "The interpersonal therapist must grapple with the *real* matrix of events and personalities in which every therapy is embedded. It is not a question of what the patient has projected 'onto' the therapist, but of really *who* the therapist is and *what* he brings to the therapy encounter" (p. 492). I would modify that to read that it is at least as much one as the other.

Psychoanalysis, as a nondirective discipline, has traditionally maintained the importance of the therapist's neutrality. The issue of neutrality is relevant here in that the means by which it has usually been operationalized is therapist anonymity. By avoiding disclosure of values, feelings, judgments, and personal experiences, the therapist is presumed to convey neutrality. This has always reminded me of the issue of stimulus constancy in experimental psychology. Does stimulus constancy refer to properties of the stimulus or perceptions of the observer?

Assuming the value of neutrality, how is it best conveyed? Here is an excerpt from a session. The patient, a well-trained and experienced analyst, was speaking of her work and describing how she is plagued by self-doubts—thoughts of not doing enough for her patients or not doing something right. I said that I thought the problem was not so much the self-doubting questions—we all have those—but the consequences. "For you it's life and death, for me there'll be other chances."

In the following session she said she had a dream that night. "A nice dream. I was dressing in a different style—a checked blouse, blue and aqua, more comfortable and stylish. It made me very happy. It was such a happy dream. I was dressing more like women I admire—effortlessly. I just found things in my closet and realized they could go together. It was a color I like but never wear. I tend to wear somber tones. I don't like to—I'm ambivalent about calling attention to myself." She spontaneously went on to say, "I feel the dream is related to the last session. It was relieving when you said last time that for you the consequences aren't dire. You said something about yourself. That's meaningful to me. I feel you care about me. For me, anonymity of my therapist duplicates my background with my parents. I never knew anything about my parents' experience of themselves. I remember being thrilled once that my mother colored in my coloring book. I have only one or two memories of my father revealing something about himself. Your anonymity is not background but a constant stimulus. It's not freeing. It's provocative."

Whatever the other messages conveyed in this, one seems to be that if I show my true colors, she feels freer to show hers. This is consistent with Jourard's (1971) research findings that the best way to foster self-disclosure is to model it: "... Intimate self-disclosure begets intimate self-disclosure" (p. 17). Greenberg (1986) makes the point that personal revelations may enhance or detract from neutrality. There is no fixed relationship between the two. He goes on "...the analyst who maintains a posture of aloofness—that is, the analyst who has confused the behavior of anonymity with the goal of neutrality—offers the patient no context within which to appreciate the nature of his transference" (p. 85).

But there is even a further question as to the desirability of the neutral stance itself—especially when it doesn't reflect the true state of the analyst's feelings—and how often is it that we analysts feel truly neutral? Wachtel (1987) suggests, "For some patients, the stance of neutrality can contribute to their tendency to invalidate their own perceptions and even to doubt their own sanity" (p. 66). The increasing recognition and acknowledgment that the analytic relationship is a fully human encounter between two, more alike than different, fallible human beings, imply that neutrality may be primarily a technical fiction, more honored in the breach, rather than an analytic attribute.

However, what indisputably is an analytic attribute is the striving to analyze and understand deviations from neutrality, which may or may not be countertransferential, and to deal with them openly in the context of the therapeutic relationship. Ehrenberg (1982) observes, "What defines an analytic relationship is that our impact, whether the result of deliberate interventions or the result of inadvertent aspects of our participation, must be explicitly clarified...The hallmark of an analytic relationship is that it is essential that there be no covert manipulation and that the patient be cognizant of whatever critical transactions have occurred, as well as their impact" (p. 540). It is by virtue of this openness that the essential attribute of psychoanalytic neutrality is maintained, namely, that control of the patient's life remains in the patient's hands, not in the analyst's.

Anonymity of the analyst is considered essential to another central dynamic of traditional psychoanalysis, the formation of the transference neurosis. The analyst scrupulously refrains from any self-disclosure in order to avoid providing substitute gratifications that the patient may get from the transference. This condition of abstinence fosters the process of regression that lies at the core of the transference neurosis. It can certainly result in an intensification of affect, but a question has been raised about the nature of the regression. The theory holds that the regression is temporal—to an earlier time in the person's history; but critics claim that the regression is structural—to a lower level of personality integration. Structural regression may be quite dangerous—particularly to people whose personality integration is shaky to start with. Aside from the danger, however, there is much uncertainty about the relationship between transference neurosis and change. It may well be that people get better in spite of a transference neurosis, rather than because of one.

To attribute change to a corrective emotional experience has, until recently, constituted a denigration of the therapy involved. Furthermore, it has generally presumed a degree of self-revealing participation on the part of the therapist, which has contributed to the feeling of denigration. True change comes about through interpretation and insight. However, with the advent of the deficit theory of psychotherapy, alongside that of conflict theory, the corrective emotional experience has attained an area of legitimacy. According to Kohut (1984), the patient "...contrary to his experience in childhood, [requires the] sustaining echo of empathic resonance [from the therapist, and if this constitutes a] corrective emotional experience,...so be it" (p. 78). That is a somewhat defiant claim, as if anticipating criticism. But, increasingly, therapeutic impact is attributed to the relationship, not primarily by making up for missed parenting, but by providing a protected arena in which the patterns of interpersonal experience can be confronted and illuminated.

To summarize thus far, as our understanding of conceptual issues in psychoanalysis has expanded and modified, so too has our conception of the role of the therapist. The issues that seem most germaine to the quality of the therapist's participation in the analytic process are the nature of the data of psychoanalysis, the conception of transference, the place of neutrality, the role of the transference neurosis, and the impact of a corrective emotional experience. The changes in our understanding of these issues have resulted in an evolving conception of the analyst's role from mirror, to participant observer, to human being, or, as Michels (1986) put it, "from authority to collaborator" (p. 488). Each succeeding role does not displace the former, as in the Kuhnian sense of a succeeding paradigm overthrowing a former one (1962), but rather exists alongside the others. That is, most analysts seem to function in each role at some time with the same patient and to varying degrees with different patients. Of course, the analyst's theoretical allegiance might be expected to govern the predominance of one role over others. However, on the basis of my experience working with people who have told me about previous analyses with analysts whose theoretical positions are known, I advise you not to presume too much. In any case, each succeeding role does involve a greater degree of self-disclosure on the part of the analyst than the former one. I now turn to the nature of that self-disclosure.

It is obvious that anonymity as such is always a matter of degree. Analysts show themselves all the time in their dress, in their office surroundings, in their manner of speaking, in the way they establish time and money ground rules, and in the myriad ways of being that are publicly observable. One person knew when my eyeglass prescription changed. Another took me to task for the horrible painting I had on my office wall. (Since I was a part-time tenant in someone else's office at the time, I was sorely tempted to disclaim any responsibility for the painting that I didn't like either.) Somebody was pleased that I didn't wear a tie. Somebody else assumed I was going to a bar mitzvah when I did wear one. (It was actually a funeral.) My books have been criticized. My plants have been taken to mean that I'm good at making people grow. My cough meant I was getting a cold. My eyes showed I was tired. My car proved I didn't know much about cars, and the loud voice on the other end of the phone indicated I was a henpecked husband. Not all of such conclusions are accurate, but some are, and some are more accurate than I initially gave them credit for being.

There are further, perhaps more profound, ways in which analysts reveal themselves inadvertently. The questions asked and not asked, the content focused upon, the connections made, the fleeting and not-so-fleeting emotions invariably displayed, the facts remembered and the facts forgotten—all convey information about the analyst's interests, values, theories, anxieties, and emotions. Singer (1968) claims that analysts are, at times, reluctant to make correct interpretations. "The more to the point and the more penetrating the interpretation, the more obvious it will be that the therapist is talking and understanding from the depth of his own psychological life.... It takes one to know one, and in his correct interpretation the therapist reveals that he is one" (p. 369).

Patients come to know their analysts through the shared experience of the therapeutic relationship. The quality of that subjective knowing is not simply dependent upon knowing about objective facts of the analyst's personal life. Singer maintains that patients' readiness to know their analysts—that is, to make use of the experience that is always available to them—is a measure of their psychological health (1977).

So much for showing, which takes place whether we wish it or not. Now about telling, which is deliberate, intentional, and chosen, although it may also be experienced as driven, compelled, or manipulated. What analysts tell their patients about themselves runs the full range of personal facts, opinions, feelings, reactions, associations, memories, experiences, fantasies, and dreams. Very few analysts tell all, but some "wild" analysts do. It's a safe bet, however, that all analysts tell something. The motivations, circumstances, and rationales vary tremendously, as do the therapeutic consequences.

For example, Masud Kahn (1986) informed his patients of his brother's death. He writes, "...Analysts rarely speak about events in their personal life that affect their work mutatively. The death of my brother had changed my whole outlook on life, and I knew my patients would sense it; so I told them as much. It is not a question of transference or countertransference, but actually real, lived life that makes our fatedness or destiny, and about which we are often somewhat devious, both with ourselves and others" (p. 644). Similarly, Singer (1971) reports that when his wife became seriously ill, requiring him frequently to cancel appointments, he told his patients the reason.

One analytic candidate I was supervising learned suddenly that she had a cancerous growth and had to have a mastectomy. In discussing how best to inform her patients, she decided she would tell them in general terms that she would be out for some weeks for surgery but she did not feel comfortable being more specific than that. However, when she returned to work after the surgery and was confronted by her patients' fantasies—especially the fantasies that were correct or near correct—she was unable to contain her own distress and burst into tears. At that point she told them the fuller story.

Some years ago I had a back condition that left me unable to sit, although I could stand or lie down comfortably enough. I chose to continue working and informed the people I was seeing that I would have to use the couch myself for about a month. I could discern no disruptive impact on the work and have since talked with a number of other analysts who have had similar experiences with similar results.

In none of these situations or a host of others like them have I heard of destructive consequences for the analysis. One might anticipate that the analyst's misfortune or infirmity would mobilize sadistic, vengeful, or hostile impulses or, conversely, inhibit them. People do react in highly individual ways; but a common theme seems to be the desire to be helpful. The asymmetrical structure of the analytic relationship, with the patient expected to be needy and the analyst helpful, can induce a humiliating sense of uselessness in the patient, without the opportunity for reality-oriented and constructive relatedness (see Singer, 1971). A woman dreamed that when she came for her session, she found me on the couch with a fever and she put a cool, damp washcloth on my forehead. We both understood the dream to mean that she wanted to be helpful to me as I was to her.

One moral to be drawn from these experiences is that when the analyst's life impacts upon his or her work, it is in the service of clarifying the patient's attempts to make sense out of the relationship to acknowledge the facts of life. However, there are dangers in such disclosures, having less to do with the patient's ability to handle the facts and more to do with the analyst's motives in disclosing them. If the analyst is exploiting the patient by eliciting sympathy, warding off criticism or anger, or manipulating a feeling of intimacy, then the disclosures are likely to be destructively double-binding.

Other occasions on which I have found it useful to tell of events in my life have to do with my feeling that some messages are better conveyed through recounting experiences than by saying what you mean.

That is, in order to convey that I understand something that has been told me, I might briefly tell of a similar experience that I've had. Or when working with someone who feels so separate and different from the rest of the human race, I might say something about myself that bridges their feeling of distance.

One woman said, "I had a bad weekend. Other people are stable. I'm so up and down. I hide my rockiness." I said, "Don't we all." She: "You too?" I: "Does that surprise you?" She: "Well, I guess not. You're human too." I understood that to mean she also felt human, at least for the moment. On another occasion she expressed her anguish that something was so wrong with her because her therapy took so long. I said I was in analysis for eight years, and that was only the first time. She said she felt better knowing that I didn't feel she was taking too long and wasn't fed up with her. I am aware that she may have meant something was wrong with me because her therapy took so long, and that's an issue we have also dealt with.

There are those inevitable times when the analyst's personal issues intrude upon the work and disrupt the patient's understanding of what's happening. The most likely outcome is for the patient to assume the blame and experience self-contempt. At such times it is essential that the analyst acknowledge the intrusion. Ehrenberg (1984) puts it: "No matter how entangled analysts find themselves they must be able to re-establish the analytic integrity of the relationship. The process of so doing actually becomes the medium of the analytic work, and may involve making the analyst's reactions explicit to engage the patient in a collaborative way" (p. 563).

Prior to my taking a brief out-of-town trip, a man who knew where I was going wished me a good time and began to tell me of interesting things to do there. I somewhat brusquely replied that I'd been there before. In the session following my return he said he was angry and had been upset for hours after the previous session, feeling rejected by me, as if something were wrong with him. Although these were characteristic reactions of his, I suggested that there might be other possible explanations. I went on to say that I did cut him off because I was not going to have that kind of vacation and felt somewhat deprived about it. He said it helped to know that and I said that he was always ready to see something wrong with himself. Sometimes there were things wrong with others.

Michels (1983) asserts, "The primary data of psychoanalysis are neither what happens in childhood nor what happens in adult life, and not even the cause–effect relationship between them; the primary data are what the patient says in the analyst's presence, how the analyst responds, and how the patient can make constructive use of the experiential and dialectical process" (p. 61). This points to what I think is the predominant arena of analysts' self-disclosure, namely, what the analyst says about his or her reactions to what transpires in the relationship between the two people. It is predominant in importance, in relevance to the therapeutic work, and in frequency of occurrence. It is also probably the least controversial area of analysts' self-disclosure.

The patient–therapist relationship is the most immediate and experientially cogent arena in which to explore the patterns of interpersonal relatedness and the role that each person plays in actively creating and maintaining these patterns. What is unique about psychoanalysis, as opposed to other therapies, is the focus on this relationship, the nature and structure of which colors the way in which all other experiences are dealt with in the analysis. That is, it acts like a filter system through which other experiences are seen and processed. The exploration of this filter system itself is the primary work of psychoanalysis.

The direct person-to-person encounter between patient and analyst "creates a history together, experienced as relevant engagement, and characterized by wholeness and complexity" (Held-Weiss, 1986, p. 3). The truthfulness with which the participants can explore and acknowledge what it is that's going on between them empowers the relationship to be an agent for change. Lichtenberg (1986) describes it as "...the combination of the unique interaction of a relationship with tensions at its junction and the joint search for meaning that constitute an analysis, or rather that constitute the curative experience that a successful analysis is" (p. 73).

The mutuality of relevant self-revelation works against the mystification of experience in the relationship and allows for the development of intimacy and trust. In that context unattended-to or anxiety-laden aspects of relatedness can be acknowledged and clarified, and resistance overcome. Wolf (1983) suggests that, "Since in essence, resistance is nothing but fear of being traumatically injured again, the decisive event of its analysis is the moment when the analysand has gained courage from these self-revelations of the analyst to know that the analyst does not need to feed on the patient to achieve cohesion and harmony" (p. 500).

As I have written elsewhere (Basescu, 1987), I at times feel prompted to express something I'm thinking or feeling in a session; but I almost always respond to a patient's questioning me about it. If I am asked, I generally answer. For example, a man, himself a therapist, previously told me that he looks to see if I am glad to see him. This time, as he scrutinizes me when I come to the waiting room, something strikes me funny, and I can't stop myself from broadly smiling as he enters the office. He asks me why I'm smiling and I tell him it's because he's scrutinizing me. He says, "That's no answer. I realize you don't have to answer me." I say, "Your looking at me had a whimsical quality that struck me funny." He says, "That's an answer. Thanks. That helps me know something about myself." When I asked him what it helped him know he told me that often people don't take him seriously and that perhaps he doesn't present himself as serious.

A woman, who is familiar with psychotherapeutic literature but not in the profession herself asked me if I would give her a reprint or reference for anything I've written. I told her I didn't care what she read but I didn't want to give her what she asked for. She asked why not, saying that she could get it on her own and this would simply save her some trouble. That made sense to me but I still didn't feel right about doing it, although I wasn't clear why. She pressed for a reason and I said, "Well, let's see if I can be clear about it. It's because I don't want to participate in or reinforce something that I don't know the meaning of. My job is to analyze the meaning, not to collude with it." She said, "I understand that," and then told me she wanted something of mine to have while I was away on vacation. That then was what we dealt with.

I generally find that the process of answering questions about what is going on with me at the moment helps clarify for both of us what's happening. It often has the additional consequence of enabling further exploration of the patient's experience. It conveys a respectful attitude toward the other and enhances the spirit of collaboration.

Another class of personal reactions that I tend readily to express are those that are discrepant with what seems to be going on. I've said things like, "You're smiling while you tell me this, but I feel sad. I wonder why," or, "I feel like I'm listening to a lecture," or "I have the feeling of being buttered up." I think it is fairly common for analysts to rely on their own reactive emotional sensibilities for clues to understanding the less obvious aspects of what is being enacted. Disclosing these feeling reactions invites an experiential exploration of more than meets the eye. It also conveys to the other person the kind of impact he or she is having.

Vulnerable people tend to defend themselves against humiliation in ways that often bring about the very hurts they are trying to avoid. The therapeutic relationship affords a unique opportunity to experience these defensive patterns and their consequences in a context that allows for learning, not simply blind repetition. I saw a woman who was in therapy with me, a therapist herself, at a professional meeting. From her look and manner I gathered she would be more comfortable if I kept my distance, which I did. In the session following she told me how hurt she was that I was so unfriendly, as if I were letting her know that she should make no mistake about the boundaries of our relationship. I told her how

I had felt warned away by her appearance and thought I was complying with her wishes. This led to our discussing other aspects of the same pattern. I observed that she never expressed interest in any aspect of my life, such as where I went on vacation or if I enjoyed it. She explained that she was fearful of my seeing her as intrusive and slapping her down for it. Her stance was that of rigid avoidance to forestall rejection. Her impact was that of indifference.

In thinking about the way I say things to people in therapy sessions, I realize that sometimes I know in advance what I'm going to say and sometimes I don't. I may formulate something or mull it over momentarily before I say it, or it may just come out. A woman said to me critically that she never knew what to expect from me. I said, "That makes two of us," and that just came out. Two weeks later she said my remark stuck with her and she realized that unless you're rigid you don't always know what you're going to say.

This bears upon the issue of the therapist's spontaneity. I think that when I'm working effectively I am functioning spontaneously—and that does not refer to whether or not I mull things over before I say them. It refers to functioning freely in the mode appropriate to being the analyst in a psychoanalytic relationship. One's way of being is influenced by the nature of the relationship, as in a marriage or friendship, or in a classroom or social gathering. The different structures elicit different modes of being and different behaviors. The differences are a function of varying meanings, purposes, and intentions. The manifestations of spontaneity vary as well.

While there clearly may be detrimental consequences to the analyst's self-disclosures under the best of circumstances, I think most problems are not caused by the analyst's true spontaneity but by the lack of it. That is, inappropriate self-disclosures are those compulsively driven by the analyst's personal needs or they are responses to the patient's intimidating manipulations. If the analyst is operating out of countertransferential reactions, such as needing to impress the patient, or being defensive, seductive, hostile, controlling, fearful, or placating, then personal revelations are likely to be intrusive, diverting, burdensome, inhibiting, or otherwise countertherapeutic. Saying whatever comes to mind may be the mark of thoughtless impulsivity. Being fully present, available, and freely responsive to the ongoing interpersonal interactions are, to my mind, the hallmarks of spontaneity.

The fact that the distinctions are often difficult to make has led many analysts to warn against self-disclosures. Gill (1983), for example, is concerned that the analyst's subjective experience may be defensive and that revealing it may result in shutting off further inquiry into the patient's experience. He is wary about changing the patient's analysis into mutual analysis. He emphasizes the importance of the analyst being especially alert to the patient's experience of any of the analyst's revelations—a point with which I would strongly concur.

On the other hand, there are those like Coltart (1986), who writes, "If we are too protective of our self-presentation and of what we consider grimly to be the sacred rules of True Psychoanalysis, then we may suffocate something in the patient, in ourselves, and in the process" (p. 197). Or, as Symington (1986) refers to owning and expressing his feeling reactions to the patient: "Again when I acted from personal freedom rather than follow some specific technical regulation. . . then therapeutic shifts occurred. . . My contention is that the inner act of freedom in the analyst causes a therapeutic shift in the patient and new insight, new learning and development in the analyst" (p. 260).

Clearly, the analyst's self-disclosure is an intervention that can cut both ways. However, we can no longer use what was always a mythologically conceived position of anonymity as a way out. We are who we are. It will show and we will tell, each of us in our own individual way. Wolstein (1987) puts it: "Every psychoanalyst must seek a perspective and create a technique that allow the deeply private gift of talent to show itself; the inner voice gives a psychoanalyst the uniqueness of self and the wholeness of personality" (p. 348). It behooves each of us, in keeping with our professional responsibility to our patients, to do what we can to insure that our showing and telling are primarily in the service of the therapeutic enterprise, and not simply acts of self-indulgence.

One final word. In recent years I have written a number of self-centered papers on my work as an analyst—on the anxieties of the analyst (1977), the inner experience of the analyst (1987), and now this one. Therefore, it was heartening for me to read that in research on therapy outcomes, eight times as much outcome variance was accounted for by therapist differences as by treatment differences. Luborsky (1987) concluded: "The study of forms of treatment may be drastically less enlightening than the study of therapists, yet there are phenomenally more studies of the former" (p. 58). I took that as justification for my focus in these papers.

References

Basescu, S. (1977). Anxieties of the analyst: An autobiographical account. In K.A. Frank (Ed.), *The human dimension in psychoanalytic practice*. New York: Grune & Stratton.

Basescu, S. (1987). Behind the "seens": The inner experience of at least one psychoanalyst. *Psychoanalytic Psychology, 4*, 3.

Coltart, N. (1986). 'Slouching toward Bethlehem. . .' or thinking the unthinkable in psychoanalysis. In G. Kohon, (Ed.), *The British school of psychoanalysis, the independent tradition*. New Haven & London: Yale University Press.

Ehrenberg, D. (1982). Psychoanalytic engagement: The transaction as primary data. *Contemporary Psychoanalysis, 18*, 4.

Ehrenberg, D. (1984). Psychoanalytic engagement II: Affective considerations. *Contemporary Psychoanalysis, 20*, 4.

Gill, M. (1983). The interpersonal paradigm and the degree of the therapist's involvement. *Contemporary Psychoanalysis, 19*, 2.

Gill, M. (1984). Psychoanalysis and psychotherapy: A revision. *International Review of Psychoanalysis, 11*, 161–179.

Greenberg, J. (1986). The problem of analytic neutrality. *Contemporary Psychoanalysis, 22*, 1.

Held-Weiss, R. (1986). A note of spontaneity in the analyst. *Contemporary Psychoanalysis, 22*, 1.

Jourard, S. (1971). *Self-disclosure: An experimental analysis of the transparent self*. New York: Wiley.

Kahn, M.R. (1986). Outrageousness, complaining and authenticity. *Contemporary Psychoanalysis, 22*, 4.

Kohut, H. (1984). *How does analysis cure*. (A. Goldberg & P.E. Stepansky, Eds.). Chicago: University of Chicago Press.

Kuhn, T. (1962). *The structure of scientific revolutions*. Chicago: University of Chicago Press.

Levenson, E. (1981). Facts or fantasies: On the nature of psychoanalytic data. *Contemporary Psychoanalysis, 17*, 4.

Lichtenberg, J. (1986). The tension between unrestricted personal revelation and circumscribed personal revelation. *Contemporary Psychoanalysis, 22*, 1.

Luborsky, L. (1987). Research can affect clinical practise—A happy turnaround. *The Clinical Psychologist, 40*, 3.

Michels, R. (1983). Contemporary views of interpretation in psychoanalysis. *Psychiatry update, VII*. (L. Grinspoon, Ed.). Washington, D.C.: American Psychiatric Press.

Michels, R. (1986). How psychoanalysis changes. *Journal of the American Academy of Psychoanalysis, 14*, 3.

Singer, E. (1968). The reluctance to interpret. *Uses of interpretation in treatment*. (E. Hammer, Ed.). New York: Grune & Stratton.

Singer, E. (1971). The patient aids the analyst. *In the name of life*. (B. Landis & E. Tauber, Eds.). New York: Holt, Rinehart & Winston.

Singer, E. (1977). The fiction of analytic anonymity. *The human dimension in psychoanalytic practice*. (K.A. Frank, Ed.). New York: Grune & Stratton.

Stern, D. (1985). *The interpersonal world of the infant*. New York: Basic Books.

Symington, N. (1986). The analyst's act of freedom as agent of therapeutic change. *The British school of psychoanalysis. The independent tradition*. (G. Kohon, Ed.). New Haven & London: Yale University Press.

Wachtel, P.(1986). On the limits of therapeutic neutrality. *Contemporary Psychoanalysis, 22*, 1.

Wolf, E.S. (1983). Concluding statement. *The future of psychoanalysis. Essays in honor of Kohut*. (A. Goldberg, Ed.). New York: International Universities Press.

Wolstein, B. (1987). Experience, interpretation, self-knowledge. *Contemporary Psychoanalysis, 23*, 2.

5

Self-Disclosure in Rational-Emotive Therapy

Windy Dryden

In this chapter I will first outline briefly the basic principles of rational-emotive therapy; then consider how rational-emotive therapists view client and therapist self-disclosure; and, finally, deal with common obstacles to such self-disclosure and how these may be overcome.

The Basic Principles of Rational-Emotive Therapy

Rational-emotive therapy holds that people are disturbed not by events but by their view of events. More specifically the theory postulates that when people are psychologically healthy, they adhere to nondogmatic preferences even though events may go against their preferences (e.g., "I want to be approved by Susan but I don't have to be. It is unfortunate that Susan doesn't like me"). However, when people become psychologically disturbed they tend to make absolute demands out of their preferences (e.g., "Susan must like me. It's terrible that she doesn't"). When people think in such rigid ways they tend to draw irrational conclusions from their dogmatic premises (i.e., their *musts*). Thus they tend to conclude that whenever they do not get what they think they *must* that (1) it is *awful* (meaning more than 100% bad); (2) they *cannot stand* it (meaning that they can never be happy again as long as the "awful" events in their life are present); and (3) they, other people,

Windy Dryden • Department of Psychology, Goldsmiths' College, University of London, New Cross, London SE14 6NW, England.

and/or life conditions are *damnable.* A basic goal of rational-emotive therapists is to help their clients to identify (1) their disturbed emotions and self-defeating behaviors; (2) the events that trigger the irrational beliefs that lead to these disturbed emotions and behaviors; and (3) the irrational beliefs, to which they devoutly cling. After helping clients to identify such irrational beliefs, rational-emotive therapists then encourage them to dispute their irrational beliefs vigorously by using various cognitive, emotive, and behavioral means (Ellis & Dryden, 1987).

The role of rational-emotive therapists in the therapeutic process is usually a direct and educative one. RET therapists strive to teach their clients the ABC theory of emotional disturbance and educate them in their active role in disputing their own irrational beliefs cognitively, emotively, and behaviorally.

The RET Approach to Client Self-Disclosure

RET is a structured approach to psychotherapy and, as such, RET therapists generally encourage their clients to disclose themselves, using the ABC framework of psychological disturbance (where A = the *A*ctivating event, B = *B*elief, and C = Emotional and Behavioral Consequences of those beliefs). However, it is recognized that some clients do benefit from disclosing their problems and their feelings about them in a fairly unstructured way in the early stage of therapy.

A typical sequence of structuring client self-disclosure in RET is as follows. First the therapist asks the client to focus on one psychological problem at a time. This may be a problem that the client finds most distressing in his life or one that he wishes to address first in psychotherapy. When both therapist and client agree on the nature of the client's problem in broad terms, the therapist then attempts to assess the client's problem according to the ABC framework. Typically, the therapist starts with C, the client's major disturbed emotional response. Here the RET therapist will encourage her client to be as specific as he can about this emotional response. In general, when clients disclose their emotional problems in vague terms such as "I feel upset," "I feel bad," and "I felt miserable," RET therapists attempt to help them to clarify these problems and, in particular, whether the negative emotion was appropriate or inappropriate to the activating event at A.

According to RET theory, appropriate negative emotions stem from clients' rational, undogmatic beliefs which are normally expressed in the form of wishes, wants, and preferences. Major negative emotions that stem from these rational beliefs are sadness, concern, annoyance, and regret—emotions that are constructive responses to negative life events and that help people adjust to those events and then to move on with their lives. Such emotions are distinguished from inappropriate negative emotions which, according to RET theory, stem from dogmatic irrational beliefs. Such emotions are anxiety, depression, anger, and guilt—emotions that are seen as being unconstructive responses to negative life events and that inhibit people from adjusting to those events and from getting on with their lives.

While helping the client to distinguish his inappropriate from his appropriate negative emotions at *C*, the therapist will often help the client to distinguish between irrational or rational beliefs at *B*. Assuming that the client has a disturbed inappropriate negative emotion at *C*, the RET therapist will proceed to encourage the client to disclose what was the triggering activating event at *A* in the ABC framework. Here the RET therapist will encourage her client to disclose a *specific* example of the activating event; this is because the client, in real life, reacted to a *specific* activating event and his irrational belief was in fact triggered by such a specific event. The therapist will discourage her client from describing activating events in vague or overly discursive terms, since such disclosures will not aid the identification of specific irrational beliefs at *B*, later in the assessment process.

At this phase of assessment a particularly powerful intervention tool is the use of "inference chaining" (Moore, 1983). In RET theory, *A* stands not only for the event but also for the client's interpretations or inferences about the event, and it often occurs that clients make themselves disturbed not so much about the actual event but about the inferences that they make about the event. In inference chaining the therapist seeks to help the client to identify and disclose the most relevant inference in the chain (i.e., the one that served as a trigger for the irrational belief).

A brief example of inference chaining follows:

Therapist: So at point C you felt anxious. Now what were you anxious about? (Here the therapist encourages the client to disclose what it was about A that he was disturbed about.)

Client: I was anxious because I thought that the woman might reject me.

Therapist: And what would be anxiety-provoking in your mind if she did reject you?

Client: All my friends would see this and they would laugh at me.

Therapist: And what would be anxiety-provoking about that in your mind?

Client: Well, if my friends would laugh at me, I would gain the reputation of being a wimp.

Therapist: And if people generally thought of you as a wimp...?

Client: Oh my God, I couldn't stand it, that would really be horrible.

In this clinical exchange it can be seen that while the initial reported *A* was rejection, the client was really anxious about the psychological implications of this rejection. Thus, using inference chaining, the therapist structured the client's self-disclosure in a way that helped the client to identify the core aspect of *A* that served as a trigger for his irrational belief: "I must not be thought of as a wimp."

After assessing both *C* and *A*, RET therapists then encourage their clients to identify and disclose the irrational beliefs that account for their psychological disturbance at *C*. There are two major strategies that can be used to identify such irrational beliefs. First is through the use of such open-ended questions as "What were you telling yourself about that experience to make yourself feel anxious?" The problem about this strategy is that clients then disclose aspects of their thought processes that are not irrational beliefs. Thus, they may often disclose automatic thoughts (not in the form of irrational beliefs) and inferences or interpretations that again do not lie at the core of their emotional problem. If this occurs, the rational-emotive therapist will explain to the client why that particular thought would not be sufficient to account for his emotional problem. Through the subsequent use of guided questions and short didactic explanations, the therapist is generally successful in helping the client to identify the major *must* in his thinking which did account for *C*.

A second strategy at this point is to ask questions that are guided by RET theory. Instead of asking: "What were you telling yourself about that experience at *A* to cause your anxiety to point C?" the therapist asks such questions as: "What *must* were you telling yourself about *A* that caused C?" The danger of using such a strategy is that the therapist may put words into the client's mouth. However, the advantage of this type of theory-guided question is that it encourages the client to identify efficiently the *musts* in his thinking.

At this point the RET therapist has two major tasks. First, while encouraging disclosure of the client's irrational beliefs the therapist will educate the latter concerning the important distinctions between rational and irrational beliefs. Second, it is helpful if the therapist encourages her client to disclose his irrational beliefs both in the form of a premise, i.e., the musts and demands, and the conclusions derived from such premises (i.e., awfulizing, I can't stand it-itis, and damnation).

When the client can see the relationship between his irrational beliefs and his emotional problems at point *C*, the therapist is then in a position to help him to dispute his irrational beliefs and to encourage him to practice doing this outside therapy sessions. To facilitate this the therapist often encourages the client to undertake certain homework assignments, the goal of which is to encourage the client to begin to internalize his new rational philosophy. As therapy proceeds the client's self-disclosure tends to center on (1) reporting back on his experiences of doing homework assignments, and (2) bringing up new problems that are approached in a similar way to that outlined.

It can be seen, then, that rational-emotive therapists do not give their clients free rein to disclose themselves in whatever way they choose. If given such free rein, clients will often bring up irrelevancies, sidetrack themselves, and generally discourage themselves from adopting a problem-solving approach towards their psychological problems. Having said this, the use of clinical flexibility is advised in varying the structure of RET according to the therapeutic requirements of given clients at given points in the therapeutic process. Thus, some clients will require and benefit from a less structured approach on the part of their therapists if they are to disclose their concerns in a meaningful way. This is particularly the case if they are ashamed about disclosing certain experiences.

In addition, the more a client is successful at using RET methods during the middle and end phases of therapy, the less the therapist's role is a direct one and the more she will encourage the client to structure his disclosures for himself during this period. Here the therapist may do little more than to make interventions such as, "OK, that was your *A*, now what was your irrational belief?... Fine, how did you challenge that?... Good, what was the result of doing that?... Fine, what homework assignment did you give yourself?... that sounded good." The purpose of this gradual shift in therapeutic style from "active-directive" to "prompting-encouraging" is twofold. First, it helps the client to gain increasing control over the therapeutic process. Second, it encourages the client to be his own therapist so that he can disclose his problems to himself and use the RET method of problem assessment and solution to help himself.

Therapist Self-Disclosure in RET

One of the basic aspects of the therapist's role in RET is to educate the client in the ABCs of his emotions (Dryden, 1987). As such however, the therapist will freely disclose her own experiences in the service of making that educational experience a memorable one for her client.

In order to understand fully the RET position on therapist self-disclosure, it is first necessary to outline the RET view of human fallibility (Ellis, 1972) since this is central to such understanding. The RET theory of human fallibility states that all humans are equal in humanity, that there are neither good humans nor bad humans and that no human being is more valuable or more worthy than any other. All people are equal in humanity although they may be unequal in terms of their different traits, behaviors, thoughts, feelings, etc. Thus the RET therapist does not see herself as being more valuable than her client, although she will tend to consider that she is more knowledgeable about understanding emotional problems.

Given that the effective RET therapist would accept herself for her errors and flaws and for past and present emotional disturbances, she will, as often as is therapeutically advisable, show her client how she upset herself about experiences similar to those with which her client is concerned and how she used RET to overcome such emotional disturbances. Note that in choosing this mode of self-disclosure, the RET therapist is providing her client with a coping model of overcoming emotional disturbance and not with a mastery model. The therapist who employs a mastery model approach to self-disclosure will stress that she has never experienced a problem similar to the client's because she thinks rationally about similar events with which the client is struggling. This approach is unproductive because it unduly emphasizes the inequality between therapist and client and deemphasizes their shared humanity.

A coping model of self-disclosure, on the other hand, where the therapist outlines that she too has experienced or is currently experiencing similar emotional disturbances but is able to get over these by using RET methods and techniques, indicates to the client that both therapist and client share the same experiences, although one is more adept at present in overcoming them than the other. Such a coping model emphasizes the shared humanity of the therapist and client while not belaboring the inequality that exists between therapist and client in the therapeutic enterprise. The therapist who utilizes the coping model of self-disclosure can furthermore outline the *process* of solving emotional problems for the client, and as such self-disclosure can often be a powerful therapeutic tool.

Let me use a personal example to illustrate this. I used to have a very bad stammer and was not only ashamed about this but also anxious about speaking in public because I was scared that if I revealed my stammering in public, other people would laugh at me and I would severely condemn myself if this occurred. I often disclose this fact to clients who not only experience similar problems concerning stammering but who also have problems that are exacerbated by their anxiety that these problems may be revealed publicly. My self-disclosure is often along these lines:

"You know, as we find out more about your problem I am myself reminded of a problem that I used to have which in certain ways is quite similar to yours. I don't know if you've noticed but I have a stammer—here the client usually says, 'Well yes, I have noticed it but it's really not that noticeable' (indeed, I rarely stammer these days although I still have a slight speech hesitancy). I used to have a very bad stammer and hid myself away because I used to tell myself, "I must not stammer in public. It would be terrible if I did and I couldn't stand it if other people were to see me stammer and to think badly of me." Well, I struggled with this problem for many years and received much inadequate help from various speech therapists. However, it wasn't until I heard a radio program on which a noted entertainer outlined his own approach to overcoming his stammering problem that I started to overcome mine. This man told how he decided to force himself to speak up in public while reminding himself that if he stammered, he stammered, too bad. This was the first good piece of advice I'd heard on overcoming anxiety about stammering and I resolved to apply this myself. Indeed, although I did not realize it, I used the principles of RET which I'm now going to teach you. What I did was to force myself to enter situations and speak up, but before I did so I prepared myself by telling myself that there is no reason why I must not stammer, and if I did, too bad. On occasion I would speak more vehemently to myself and say things like; "If I stammer, I stammer, fuck it!" The more I internalized these beliefs, the more I was able to go into situations and speak up. It certainly wasn't easy and I did have setbacks, but I persisted and now I can speak without anxiety in a variety of public situations, including radio and television. I still make myself anxious at times, but when I do, I look for and dispute my irrational beliefs in a very powerful and vigorous way and push myself forward on the basis of my rational beliefs. Even on the odd occasions when I cop out, I refuse to condemn myself and fully accept myself as a person who has opted out at a given moment. So you see, I too have experienced similar problems but have managed to help myself enormously. So I have a lot of faith that if you apply similar techniques you could also gain a lot of benefit from these methods."

While I have presented this personal self-disclosure in uninterrupted form, in practice, parts of it are interspersed with dialogue with the client concerning what he or she can learn from my experience.

It should be noted that this self-disclosure illustrates for the client the rational-emotive approach to therapeutic change. In this personal example I show the client (1) how to identify a personal problem; (2) how to identify the rational belief that underpins the problem; (3) the importance of repetitive and forceful disputing of this belief in situations in which the problem occurs; (4) that setbacks will occur and that under certain circumstances, people will choose to avoid rather than confront their problems; and (5) the importance of accepting themselves when this happens. When the therapist discloses personal information for educative purposes it is important that she ask her client what he can learn from her experience. It should not be forgotten that the purpose of therapist self-disclosure is to aid the learning process of the client. It is not an opportunity for the therapist to boast about her achievements in overcoming personal problems. Rather, the philosophy that should preferably underpin therapist self-disclosure is: "You and I are equal in humanity. At the moment I have more experience and skills in overcoming emotional problems but you can learn this too. It is difficult, but if you persist with it you can experience as much benefit as I did."

Cautions

While therapist self-disclosure does have great therapeutic merits, therapists should not disclose themselves indiscriminately to their clients; and I will now outline circumstances in which it may be preferable for therapists not to disclose themselves to their clients.

First, therapist self-disclosure, like any form of therapist communication, needs to be considered within the wider framework of the therapeutic alliance (Bordin, 1979). For example, in my experience, it is probably not wise for therapists to disclose their own problems and how they overcame them at a very early stage in the therapeutic process. This is so mainly because clients may not view such early self-disclosure as appropriate therapist behavior, and this may threaten the therapeutic alliance (Dies, 1973). This being so, some clients will, however, experience benefit from early therapist self-disclosure and therapists need to use their therapeutic judgment and their knowledge of their client as guides concerning the wisdom of making such disclosures.

Second, RET therapists are cautioned against disclosing themselves to clients who seek a formal relationship with their therapist. I made this mistake once when I disclosed a piece of personal information to a client who responded in this way: "Well, young man, that's all very interesting but I'm not paying you good money to hear about your problems, will you please address yourself to mine." This client wanted her therapist to act in a formal manner and did not value the use of therapist self-disclosure which, parenthetically, does seem to be associated with therapist informality. This is perhaps one reason why RET therapists in general favor therapist self-disclosure in that they favor adopting, whenever possible, an informal therapeutic role with their clients.

Third, RET therapists should be wary about disclosing themselves to clients who might use such information to harm themselves, or their therapists. For example, there are clients who idealize their therapists and for whom disclosure of therapist fallibility may come as a very painful blow, with the result that such clients may make themselves (albeit needlessly) depressed and anxious about this. Other clients may distort the content and the purpose of therapist self-disclosure to discredit the therapist in his or her community. It is difficult for RET therapists to predict which clients will have such negative responses to therapist self-disclosure; but it is possible to gain such information, and certain signs in the clients' psychopathology may provide clues for therapists in this respect.

For example, if a client has a history of extreme anger and vengefulness when their view of a person is threatened, this is perhaps a clue that the therapist may not wish to disclose personal information to the client that may threaten the client's view of the therapist. However, it should be noted that unless there are signs to the contrary, RET therapists do tend to use self-disclosure whenever therapeutically advisable and will often take risks (although not foolhardy risks) in this regard. Of course RET therapists can never guarantee that their self-disclosures will have positive effects. Therapists who demand certainty that their clients will react favorably to their disclosures will probably never self-disclose. Given the fact that RET therapists are not afraid to take calculated risks in therapy, they will take the chance of gaining therapeutic leverage by disclosing their problems and how they overcame them after disputing any demands they may have about this being acceptable to the client.

Now that I have outlined the value and risks of therapist self-disclosure in RET, I would like to emphasize how important it is for therapists to elicit feedback from their clients concerning the impact of their self-disclosures (Beck, Rush, Shaw, & Emery, 1979). Thus at the end of a session during which I have disclosed to a client some of my problems and how I have overcome them, I generally ask the client what impact this had on him, how he felt about my disclosure, what he learned from my disclosure, and whether or not he preferred me to disclose this information. If the therapist establishes her own system of feedback with the client, then it is possible to gauge the likely future benefit of therapist self-disclosure with that client. When a client indicates that therapist self-disclosure is not helpful, then that is perhaps a good guide for the therapist not to disclose her problems and the way she overcame them in future to that client.

Disclosing Personal Reactions to the Client

While I have so far focused on one major feature of therapist self-disclosure, namely disclosure of problems and how these have been overcome, there is another aspect of self-disclosure that I would like to address in this chapter—the issue of providing clients with feedback concerning one's personal reactions to them. When clients talk about such issues as not getting on with people, I look for possible ways in which they may antagonize people by monitoring my own reactions to them in the therapy session. It sometimes occurs that I get a clear indication that a client's mode of interaction with me may, if reproduced with other people, lead these other people to shun the client.

For example, one of my clients developed the habit of putting his feet up on my furniture. His presenting problem was that he felt quite lonely and didn't get on with people. I not only shared with him my reaction of displeasure whenever he did this, but was also keen to show him that while I disapproved of his behavior, I did accept him as a person. I told him that while I did not demand that he must not under any circumstances continue to put his feet on my furniture, I would, if he continued to do so, exercise my right to terminate the therapeutic relationship. Later on in the therapeutic process he told me that he really valued my feedback on his interpersonal behavior (although he did not appreciate it at the time!) because he could see in a very clear way the negative impact that he was having on other people.

In this example I have stressed an important aspect of the RET approach to disclosing personal reactions to clients—namely, that it is important to make a distinction between the person's behavior from the person as a whole and to teach this principle to the client. While the client is encouraged to take responsibility for his behavior, he is shown that he does not equal his behavior. Thus when the therapist brings to the client's attention some problematic aspect of his behavior she demonstrates unconditional acceptance of the client as a person but takes a no-nonsense approach to drawing attention to the negative aspects of the client's behavior.

RET therapists are again advised to use clinical judgment before disclosing their personal reactions to their clients. For example, clients who very easily upset themselves about even minor criticisms need to be quite adept at using RET methods to overcome such strong reactions before therapists disclose their negative reactions to problematic aspects of their clients' interpersonal behavior. This is true whether or not such clients ask for such feedback.

In general, whenever clients ask me for my opinion of them, I use this as an opportunity to teach them RET, particularly if I do have a negative reaction to them, and I sometimes disclose this reaction without being asked, as in the example just provided. Such disclosure needs to be made tactfully, and it is important for the therapist to pay attention to the language she uses to disclose her negative reactions to aspects of her clients' behavior. In addition to showing the client that he does not equal his behavior, it is also important that the client be shown that, although he is acting in a way that the therapist finds negative, he does not have to continue to act that way, and that the therapist has faith and confidence that he can improve his behavior. I have personally found the combination of *both* disclosing negative reactions about certain aspects of my clients' behavior in the context of teaching the RET position on (1) the difference between the person and his acts, and (2) the possibility of change *and* providing encouragement, to be especially therapeutic.

Overcoming Obstacles to Disclosure in Clients and Therapists

There are many reasons that both clients and therapists do not disclose their experiences, feelings, and problems during the therapeutic process and, in this concluding section, I outline some of the main explanations for disclosure avoidance and what RET therapists can do about this phenomenon.

Clients

In my experience there are three main reasons clients do not disclose their experiences and problems to their therapists in RET: (1) shame, (2) need for the therapist's approval, and (3) reluctance to participate in the therapeutic process.

When clients are ashamed about disclosing their experiences to their therapists they tend to believe that they *must* not have these problems in the first place and that they are in some way unworthy individuals for having them. Thus, rather than disclose both the nature of their original problem to themselves and their therapist, they unwittingly give themselves a second problem (i.e., shame about the original problem) that accounts for their disclosure avoidance. If this is the case, it is important for the RET therapist to deal with the client's shame about the problem before encouraging him to disclose the nature of this problem. If the client does admit to feeling shame, one way of doing this is to label the client's problem "X" and help the client to see that "X" is really the activating event (*A* in the ABC framework) and the feeling at *C* is shame. The client can then be helped to identify the irrational beliefs at *B* that underpin his experience of shame. If this assessment proves to be correct and the client acknowledges that this is the case, then the RET therapist can deal with the irrational beliefs about the undisclosed problem without having to know what the problem is. Then, having been helped to overcome his shame about the problem, the client may find it easier to disclose the problem to his therapist.

The second reason a client avoids disclosure of his problems is that he fears that if he discloses the problem to the therapist she would somehow disapprove of him and he would condemn himself because he thinks he needs the therapist's approval. First, it is important to ascertain that this is the reason the client does not disclose the true nature of his problems and, if so, this is again dealt with using the ABC framework, with A = the prospect of losing the therapist's approval, B = "I need the therapist's approval and I am less worthy if I don't have it," and C = anxiety. Then the therapist can help the client to dispute and change the irrational beliefs that underpin the anxiety that stops him from disclosing the true nature of his problems. Once again, if this proves successful, the client is likely to disclose his problems after he has overcome his need for the therapist's approval.

The final reason for the client's unwillingness to disclose his problems to his therapist is a general reluctance to being a client in the first place. This often occurs when the client is told that if he does not participate in the therapeutic process, he will incur a penalty, for example, from the courts, or from his partner who may leave the relationship. My approach to this situation is to show the client that there is no reason he has to disclose his problems to me or to participate fully in the therapeutic process and that he has every right not to do so. However, I also point out to the client that since he is choosing to attend, even under duress, he might as well work on a problem as defined by him rather than work on a problem that has been defined for him by a third party. Once the client sees that I am on his side and not on the side of the referring agent, he is more likely to see me as an ally and begin to use the therapeutic process for his own benefit rather than for the benefit of others.

Therapists

RET therapists are usually quite willing to disclose not only their problems and how they have overcome them but also their personal reactions to their clients; although, as I have suggested, such disclosure needs to be made in the context of sound clinical decision making. However, some RET therapists are reluctant to employ self-disclosure in this way and, in my experience in supervising such therapists, there are three main reasons that this occurs: (1) a need to be seen as thoroughly competent by the client; (2) a need for the client's approval; and (3) the belief that therapists should not have psychological problems.

When RET therapists believe that they have to be competent under all conditions, they tend to avoid the appropriate use of therapist self-disclosure because they predict that if they disclose that they have had emotional problems, even though they have overcome them, their clients will judge them as being incompetent; and if this was the case, they would condemn themselves for this. While supervising therapists who have this belief, I have used a double-barreled approach to this problem. First, I encourage the therapist concerned to assume that her worst fear is realized, i.e., that if she discloses herself to her clients they will indeed see her as being incompetent as a therapist. Having encouraged her to imagine that her worst fear has come true, I then help her to see that it is her beliefs (*B*) about this situation (*A*) that leads to her reluctance to self-disclosure at C. I then help her to identify and to challenge the irrational belief that underpins this experience, namely: "I must be seen as a competent therapist, otherwise I'm unworthy." When this has been done, the therapist is in a better position to reassess logically the likelihood that her clients will actually see her as incompetent. Here I use both my own example of past self-disclosure to clients (as outlined earlier in this chapter) and the fact that Albert Ellis (the founder of RET) also employs self-disclosure to show that competent RET therapists do self-disclose and that there seems to be little evidence that our clients generally see us as less competent (although some may have done so in the past).

The second reason RET therapists are reluctant to self-disclose is their need for their clients' approval. This is related to the need to be seen as competent; but here the therapist is more concerned with the approval of her clients than with their judgments of her competence. Again I suggest a double-barreled approach to this issue—helping the therapist first to identify and challenge her irrational beliefs before helping her to reevaluate the likelihood that her clients will disapprove of her if she does disclose to them some of her personal experiences.

Finally—and this is perhaps more true of novice therapists than more experienced ones—I find that some RET therapists have a dire need to see themselves as thoroughly mentally healthy. This is, in fact, a paradox, since if they demand that they *must* have perfect mental health, they are in fact disturbed because of the very existence of such a demand. This need to be problem-free stems partly from a misunderstanding of what it means to be a therapist. Being a therapist does not mean that one must be free of all psychological problems; rather that one has such problems, but can use RET techniques to overcome them. The approach to helping a therapist overcome this rigidity is quite similar to what has already been outlined in this chapter. I first encourage her to assume that her unrealistic expectation is true, namely that good therapists do not have any emotional problems. Then I help her to see that there is no reason why she *must* be a good therapist by this criterion and, if she is not, she can still accept herself and continue to overcome her problems. I then help her to reevaluate her unrealistic expectation and encourage her to see that being a good therapist does not mean being problem-free but means, in part, that one can apply what one is teaching others to oneself and one's own life situation. In using RET to help RET therapists in these ways, it is my experience that they become less anxious about disclosing themselves to their clients and do so appropriately and therapeutically during the process of RET.

References

Beck, A.T., Rush, A.J., Shaw, B.F., & Emery, G. (1979). *Cognitive therapy of depression*. New York: Guilford.

Bordin, E.S. (1979). The generalizability of the psychoanalytic concept of the working alliance. *Psychotherapy: Theory, Research and Practice, 16*, 252–260.

Dies, R.R. (1973). Group therapist self-disclosure: An evaluation by clients. *Journal of Counseling Psychology, 20*, 344–348.

Dryden, W. (1987). *Counselling individuals: The rational-emotive approach*. London: Taylor & Francis.

Ellis, A. (1972). Psychotherapy and the value of a human being. In W. Davis (Ed.), *Value and valuation: Aetiological studies in honor of Robert A. Hartman*. Knoxville: University of Tennessee Press.

Ellis, A., & Dryden, W. (1987). *The practice of rational-emotive therapy*. New York: Springer.

Moore, R.H. (1983). Inference as "A" in RET. *British Journal of Cognitive Psychotherapy, 1* (2), 17–23.

6

Self-Disclosure in Psychotherapy and the Psychology of the Self

Lawrence Josephs

A chapter on the psychology of the self is particularly apropos in a book on the role of self-disclosure in psychotherapy, for how better to grasp the nature of the self that is disclosed in the act of self-disclosure than through the insights of a school of thought devoted to the systematic study of the self? Self-disclosure in psychotherapy will be examined in the light of three interrelated ideas: (1) the concept of the self as a psychological structure through which self-experience assumes its characteristic quality and enduring organization, (2) the relationship between the experiential sense of self and the verbal sense of self, and (3) the intersubjective nature of self-experience. It will be proposed that the essential process of self-disclosure in psychotherapy occurs pre-reflectively and at a nonverbal level and is expressed in the enduring emotional ambience in which treatment transpires. The ambience of treatment is a product of the therapeutic dyad's unique manner of being with and handling each other over an extended period of time. Each member of the therapeutic dyad brings to the encounter his or her individualistic somato-affective presence through which each discloses some private essence of personal selfhood. Such a disclosure of self is a fundamentally intersubjective process dependent upon a capacity to evoke, register, and assimilate the self that the other is attempting to disclose. Self-disclosure as a communicative act requires a receiver as

Lawrence Josephs • Institute of Advanced Psychological Studies, Adelphi University, Garden City, New York 11530.

well as a transmitter. As each member of the therapeutic dyad engages in self-disclosure, the receiving member must discover, decipher, construct, and create a representation of the other's self from innumerable experiences of the therapeutic interaction.

For the patient, verbal self-disclosure is a crucial element of "the talking cure." Finding the right words to represent, evoke, and express the experiential self constitutes the integrative process through which the patient gains a sense of his own reality, wholeness, authenticity, and genuineness as a person. In addition to serving a communicative function in the service of psychic intimacy, the patient's verbal self-disclosure serves as a vehicle of seeing the self in perspective in listening to one's own self-perceptions said out loud. The process of self-articulation in verbal self-disclosure serves to develop a better integrated as well as a more clearly defined sense of self. Nevertheless, verbal self-disclosure is fraught with potential pitfalls to the extent that the verbal conception of self proves to be incongruent and discrepant with the experiential self. As Freud discovered, words can conceal as easily as reveal meaning. When words serve to hide the experiential self from others as well as from oneself, the verbal self can be said to be false, inauthentic, and non-genuine. The difficult task of psychotherapy is then to overcome such self-alienation in restoring the vital link between verbal self and experiential self that had been severed or perhaps never formed in the first place.

Given the double-edged nature of verbal self-disclosure, in that it conceals as it reveals, the therapist's verbal self-disclosure may be of dubious value. How can the therapist guarantee the genuineness of his verbal self-disclosure, given that his self-statements will not be subjected to the rigorous analysis, questioning, and challenging to which the patient's verbal self-reports are subjected over the course of psychotherapy? Can the therapist's self-analysis in the heat of the countertransferential moment be counted upon to ensure authenticity? Even if the therapist could ensure a congruence between his verbal self-disclosure and his experiential self as revealed to the patient in his somato-affective presence, such verbal self-disclosure may foreclose the patient's discovery of the therapist's self through the patient's own intuition based upon his experience of the therapist as a person. To the degree that the patient experiences the therapist's verbal self-disclosure as received wisdom to be taken at face value, the patient may feel that the therapist's perception of himself has more credence and takes priority over the patient's perception of the therapist.

Despite these caveats, one useful role of therapist verbal self-disclosure may be to clear up instances of misunderstanding that are inevitable over the course of psychotherapy. No matter how sincere the therapist's empathic intent, empathy remains imperfect since, after all, therapist and patient are two separate people who can never live inside each other's heads, no matter how imaginative their empathic efforts. Subsequent to a failure of empathy on the therapist's part and the misunderstanding that arises as a consequence, it may be useful for the therapist to disclose some of his thoughts and feelings so that the patient can better understand the therapist's perspective. In appreciating the therapist's perspective, the patient can better see where the therapist was coming from when his understanding was mistaken. In grasping the nature of the therapist's human fallibility and lack of omniscience, the patient is less likely to experience a misunderstanding as his responsibility alone and therefore an indication of his inadequacy in some respect.

A Developmental Analog for the Process of Self-Disclosure in Psychotherapy

Kohut (1977) in his seminal work appropriated the label "the psychology of the self" (p. xv) for his particular approach to the study of the self. Such study has a long history in psychoanalysis. Freud could be said to have been the first "self" psychologist when he used the term ego [*das ich*—literally, "the I"] as a synonym for self. Atwood and Stolorow (1984) have given one of the most lucid definitions of the self in the light of Kohut's contributions:

> The self, from the vantage point of psychoanalytic phenomenology, is a psychological structure through which self-experience acquires cohesion and continuity, and by virtue of which self-experience assumes its characteristic shape and enduring organization. (p. 34)

Self-experience refers to the immediate content of consciousness, such as: I think this; I feel this; I fantasize this, I intend this. In this instance, self-disclosure refers to revealing a particular content of consciousness. Self as a psychological structure is an enduring trait of the personality—a construction that is drawn from inference, abstraction, and generalization over time, upon the basis of innumerable instances of self-experience. The particular/momentary (i.e., self-experience) and the generalizable/enduring (i.e., self-as-structure) aspects of self are interrelated, each forming the other. The self-as-structure shapes self-experience by providing a schema through which self-experience is interpreted and assimilated. Yet each new self-experience constitutes a data base from which an evolving yet enduring representation of self is constructed. In psychotherapy, both therapist and patient are constructionists, privately constructing representations of the other through innumerable instances of mutual self-disclosure.

The sense of self originally arises in the context of the intersubjective matrix of the mother/infant dyad. Winnicott (1965) suggested: "There is no such thing as an infant; meaning, of course, that whenever one finds an infant one finds maternal care, and without maternal care there would be no infant" (p. 39). The infant, though, is not a passive participant in this process, for the infant is actively engaged in soliciting the facilitating maternal response and evoking the mother's intuition and empathy. Kohut (1971) coined the term "selfobject" to describe the role which the object (i.e., the other) assumes in regulating the sense of self so that the object is in effect a part of the self:

> The expected control over such (self-object) others is then closer to the concept of the control which a grownup expects to have over his own body and mind than to the concept of the control which he expects to have over others. (pp. 26–27)

Stern (1985) saw the mother/infant dyad as engaged in an intricate dance of mutual self-regulation through which they each discover the self of the other. Self-disclosure, then, requires a self-regulatory other whose function is to evoke, facilitate, receive, and mirror the self-disclosure, as well as one who is open to revealing the self. Much of the technique of psychotherapy is designed to facilitate the revelation of the patient's self.

Stern (1985) documented four domains of selfhood which emerge in infancy: (1) the emergent sense of self; (2) the core sense of self; (3) the subjective sense of self; and (4) the sense of a verbal self. The first three senses of self are preverbal, experiential selves, whereas the verbal self is a conceptual self, dependent upon the acquisition of language. Stern described the emergent sense of self as "the experience of organization-coming-into being" (p. 47) which characterizes the infant's sense of self in the first two months of life. The infant as well as the later adult is a constructionist, integrating and synthesizing new experiences in a process of creative discovery. If it were not for the emergent self, life would remain a disorganized and confusing array of disparate and disconnected events. In psychotherapy the patient's emergent self, usually outside of awareness, is busily collecting the manifold experiences of the treatment, gradually integrating the experiences into a coherent and meaningful whole. The therapist's role, like the mother's, is to facilitate this integrative process through the provision of what Winnicott (1965) called a "holding environment" (p. 45)—a secure, consistent, and supportive setting that allows for the unfolding of innate maturational processes, processes that reflect the infant's unique temperament.

Stern (1985) describes the core sense of self as possessing a sense of self-agency, self-coherence, self-affectivity, and self-history (p. 71). At around two to three months of age, the infant for the first time gives the impression of being a complete and integrated person in his or her own right. Yet these senses of self do not function with complete autonomy but are dependent upon the mother's facilitating responsiveness: Her enthusiastic yet non-domineering encouragement bolsters self-agency; her consistency and reliability supports self-coherence; her affective attunement and responsiveness evokes self-affectivity; and her continuity over time supports self-history. The relationship with mother becomes internalized in the form of what Stern (1985) calls "Representations of Interactions that have been Generalized (RIGS)" (p. 97). When a RIG is activated in the absence of the mother, the infant encounters an "evoked companion" (p. 111). The analog in psychotherapy is that, over time, the patient develops representations of experiences with the therapist as a self-regulating other who in absence is reconstituted as an evoked companion. Serving as a growth-promoting self-regulating other requires more than a correct technique of management: a highly personal empathic immersion in the experience of the other. Such an empathic immersion invariably expresses and reveals some private essence of the self of the self-regulatory other. Bollas (1987) suggested that each mother possesses her own particular idiom of mothering, an aesthetic of being that becomes a feature of the infant's self so that "we learn the grammar of our being before we grasp the rules of our language" (p. 36). Analogously, the therapist's self-regulatory function is mediated through his unique somato-affective presence; an individualistic sensibility that intuitively guides his aesthetic of handling and being with the patient. Thus the personal idiom of parent/therapist handling becomes translated into the internalized self-care system of the child/patient.

Between the seventh and ninth month of life, the infant develops a subjective sense of self in which it is realized that "inner subjective experiences, the 'subject matter' of the mind, are potentially shareable with someone else" (Stern, 1985, p. 24). The infant at this point can sense that others distinct from oneself possess a mind of their own in which they are capable of sharing a similar experience with the infant. This is the level of true intersubjectivity in which physical intimacy in terms of a sensitive somato-affective presence give rise to psychic intimacy in which issues of openness to disclosure versus privacy and inscrutability become relevant. At this level the infant is not only eager to share its own subjective experience but can begin to become curious as to the nature of the private subjective experience of another. Intersubjectivity at this stage is still predominantly preverbal—communication transpiring through the medium of empathic affect attunement. The implication for psychotherapy is that self-disclosure is very much mediated through the quality and intensity of spontaneous nonverbal affective responsiveness. Since spontaneous affective responsiveness is to a significant degree modulated by volitional control and therefore subject to a theory of psychotherapeutic technique, there has been much controversy as to the optimal level and quality of emotional expression which the therapist should encourage from the patient and allow for himself. A caveat, though, in terms of establishing guidelines for therapist emotional self-expression is that, however muted the intensity of affective expression, the patient is likely to register the quality of the feeling and the degree of self-inhibition in its expression. In addition, feigned affect attunement (i.e., pretending to share feelings) is likely to be registered by the patient as non-genuine. Thus, many aspects of the intersubjective affective interplay are beyond prescription.

During the second year of life the infant develops a sense of a verbal self. Through the acquisition of language, the infant acquires a greater capacity for symbolic thought. At this point the infant could be said to begin the construction of an objective self-concept in which the self is viewed from the perspective of others—possessing a unique personal name, a particular gender, and a social status within the family. Consensually validated language constitutes a common symbol system through which subjective experience can be shared verbally. Psychotherapy, as "the talking cure," has traditionally been conceptualized as a treatment for *emotional* illness through *verbal* dialogue. As language becomes more sophisticated, especially in the development of poetic devices, such as metaphor, simile, metonymy, and symbolism, language gains tremendous power to evoke vital emotional experiences. Nevertheless, language can also have a self-alienating effect when the preverbal experiential self is poorly or incompletely represented by words. After all, not everybody has a well-developed capacity for a poetic use of language, a use of language that can evoke experience that transcends the words alone. Many patients live in a concrete experiential world, rarely entering the realm of the imaginative, symbolic, or abstract (Josephs, 1989).

According to Stern (1985), "Language forces a space between interpersonal experiences as lived and as represented" (p. 182). Stern noted that the child learns very early on that one is accountable for what one says, so that what one experiences but does not say is more deniable to others, as well as to oneself. As a consequence, verbal self-disclosure is suspect, since what one says one thinks, feels, and intends may be out of touch with one's experiential self, which is denied. Whereas patient verbal self-disclosure is subject to an intensive process of exploration and analysis in the effort to link the most representative and evocative words to the patient's experiential self, the therapist's verbal self-disclosure is usually to be taken by the patient at face value, unless the roles are reversed and the patient is given the freedom to question, challenge, and analyze the therapist's verbal self-disclosure.

Implications for Psychotherapy

The implications of self psychology for self-disclosure in psychotherapy will be illustrated through a clinical vignette. A single woman in her late twenties who will be called Susan had initially sought treatment after being rejected by a man whom she hoped to marry. The rejection constituted a deep injury to her self-esteem and after about 1½ years of treatment her pride in herself had been restored. At that time she decided to remain in treatment to work on a vague sense that she lacked a depth of feeling in herself, and that even when she was aware of her feelings, it was difficult to express herself. Susan could be aptly described as "normopathic" (McDougall, 1985, p. 156), for she viewed her life as unremarkably normal, average, everyday, and uneventful. Although not particularly close to anyone, she never felt lonely, for she believed it was just a matter of time that with a little bit of luck she would find a suitable husband for herself. As a consequence of her normopathic experience of her life, she felt she had little to discuss in sessions and looked to me to inspire and guide her. When I remained passive in that regard, there were long uncomfortable silences, after which Susan would angrily complain of feeling bored with treatment. Yet when I attempted to be more active in providing her with feedback, Susan became indignant and defensive, accusing me of being overly judgmental, critical, and blaming.

In one session during which Susan complained of feeling bored and resentful in regard to her slow rate of progress, she posed the question—"Aren't you bored too?" to which I responded with the self-disclosure—"I feel frustrated." The ensuing discussion centered upon our difficulty in getting past the seeming therapeutic stalemate. As the discussion proceeded, Susan became increasingly defensive, indignant, and critical of me, as though she were under attack. I recognized that Susan had experienced my self-disclosure and the ensuing discussion as a manner of blaming her for the slow rate of progress, as though she were a willfully recalcitrant person. When I responded with an interpretation to the effect that Susan felt blamed by me, she wholeheartedly agreed and added that she had not been the one who was hypersensitive, but that I had been the one who was hypercritical. In reflecting on this incident, it occurred to me that in disclosing that I felt frustrated, I was revealing only a partial truth. It was difficult for me to acknowledge what the patient surmised, that in addition to feeling frustrated, I also felt bored with her, and blamed her for being so difficult to reach. To say that I was only frustrated and follow that up with a discussion of her difficulty expressing herself seemed to be taken as implying that I saw myself as some dedicated martyr, frustrated at not being able to help but seeing the problem as residing solely within Susan rather than in the relationship that developed as a process of mutual influence. It was to this implied aggrandizement of myself at Susan's expense that she took offense.

This vignette illustrates the double-edged nature of therapist verbal self-disclosure. If we assume that therapists rarely consciously dissimulate in their verbal self-disclosure, it can also be surmised that they rarely reveal more than a partial truth, and that what is left unsaid may be as important as what is explicitly stated. Regardless of what the therapist does or doesn't say about himself, the patient in registering the therapist's somato-affective presence is developing some representation of the therapist's experiential self to which the patient will compare any verbal self-disclosure the therapist makes. When Susan asked me if I was bored, it would have been transparently non-genuine if I denied all negative affect, as though treatment was proceeding in some interesting manner (i.e., a normopathic evasion). To have said "yes, I'm bored" would have been wounding, since, after all, Susan was fishing for some reassurance that she wasn't a totally superficial and boring person. In responding, "I feel frustrated," I was attempting to acknowledge that aspect of treatment which was an arduous task for both parties involved, yet imply that however difficult a challenge, it was not yet a hopeless situation. Nevertheless, the patient as interpreter of the therapist's experience (Hoffman, 1983) surmised that I was not only frustrated but bored and blaming as well.

It would seem that the patient may be the best spokesperson for the therapist's experiential self. After all, who can better speak for the unique idiom of the therapist's way of being as conveyed in his somato-affective presence than the patient, who has been the subject of the therapist's best efforts to establish empathic rapport? Of course, the patient is not always so articulate in describing his experience of the therapist as a person, colored as it is by his or her own fears of psychic intimacy. Much of the patient's response to the therapist's impact as a person is expressed nonverbally, outside of the patient's awareness. Thus, an important aspect of therapy is helping the patient become aware of and articulate unconscious perceptions of the therapist. In recent years this focus has been vigorously advocated by Langs (1976) and Gill (1982). Curiously, although both analysts acknowledge the importance of recognizing the plausibility of the patient's unconscious perception of the therapist, rather than view it as primarily a product of transference distortion, their attitude towards therapist verbal self-disclosure as a means of validating the patient's perception is rather conservative.

A danger of therapist verbal self-disclosure is that it may foreclose a thorough exploration of the patient's own perceptions of the therapist.

When Susan asked if the therapist was bored, the therapist could have inquired as to what about the therapist gave her the impression that he might have been bored with her and what it would mean to her if the therapist was indeed bored with her. Such a response could have helped the patient get in better touch with her own intuition and develop greater trust in her own perceptions. Foreclosing such exploration through verbal self-disclosure could readily be taken by the patient to imply that the therapist's verbal self-disclosure is to be honored as received wisdom that must be accepted at face value. In so doing, the therapist assumes an authority to define the objective nature of the interpersonal reality that implicitly devalues the patient's perception of the therapist in favor of the therapist's own self-perception. In the current example, whether I said I was frustrated, bored, challenged, stimulated, and so on would not alter one bit the validity of Susan's perception of me as bored and blaming, no matter how discrepant with my own self-perception.

Despite the potential pitfalls of therapist verbal self-disclosure, there are dangers in failing to verbally disclose the self. For example, Susan was quite sensitive to the distinction between the phrasings—"You feel I'm criticizing you" and "When I criticized you, you felt attacked." Although both statements convey a measure of empathy for her feeling criticized, the first statement could readily be construed as implying "You only imagine I'm criticizing you but in reality I'm not," whereas the second statement implies consensual validation, an acknowledgment that the therapist can entertain the view that he had indeed been critical, albeit unconsciously. For the therapist simply to explore the patient's perceptions of the therapist, while withholding comment as to whether those perceptions are congruent or incongruent with the therapist's own self-perceptions, is to treat the patient as though the patient were living in a world of illusion rather then engaged in a real relationship with a flesh-and-blood person who communicates his feelings and attitudes in innumerable nonverbal ways. For Susan, it was not enough for the therapist to empathize with her feeling blamed, for she required some validation of her sense of reality—that the therapist had actually been critical and that she had not fabricated her feelings out of some hypersensitivity to feedback. To withhold comment lends a sense of unreality to such a situation. Her question, "Are you bored too?" is a form of reality-testing, so that to fail to provide some self-disclosing response is to thwart her efforts at reality-testing.

Kohut (1984) suggested that at points of empathic failure and misunderstanding, therapist verbal self-disclosure may be useful:

> In a properly conducted analysis, the analyst takes note of the analysand's retreat, searches for any mistakes he might have made, nondefensively

> acknowledges them after he has recognized them (often with the help of the analysand). (p. 67)

Empathic failure and misunderstanding is inevitable in psychotherapy, since no therapist is omniscient. No matter the scope of the therapist's empathic comprehension, or the sincerity of the therapist's empathic intent, therapist and patient remain two distinct persons with different perspectives that can never become identical, although many connecting bridges may be formed. Although Kohut advocated acknowledging mistakes, he stopped short of recommending a disclosure of the therapist's reasoning or feelings that led to the mistake. The admission of the mistake validates the patient's sense of reality in having been misunderstood, but leaves ambiguous the intersubjective process through which the misunderstanding developed. Perhaps some disclosure of the therapist's faulty reasoning or defensiveness may help the patient grasp how the misunderstanding has come about. To fail to offer some such explanation is to leave the patient mystified as to the process through which the therapeutic dyad achieves harmony in intersubjective attunement or flounders in intersubjective misattunement. Despite the therapist's admission of making a mistake, the patient is likely to construe misunderstanding as a failing on his part as long as he lacks any clear conception of how the therapist ended up off the mark. Simply to admit mistakes remains in the absolutist psychology of right and wrong, correct and incorrect; whereas to supply the patient with some of the process behind the mistake brings the patient into the realm of relativism in which events can be seen from multiple perspectives. In the current example, for the therapist simply to have admitted having made a mistake would have reinforced the absolutist psychology of blame. Susan would have been relieved that I had accepted the blame so that she didn't have to herself; but would still be stuck in the psychology of looking for a scapegoat to be responsible for things that don't work out. Further therapist self-disclosure could be of help in determining how the therapeutic dyad came to such an impasse, allowing for a way of looking at things in which no one is to blame.

Self psychologists are sensitive to the fact that patients are often ill-prepared to consider events from any perspective external to their own, and may therefore consider it an error in technique to introduce the therapist's unique perspective. Although it is indeed crucial to demonstrate to the patient that the therapist can see things from the patient's point of view, once that fact has been established, patients are often enough curious to see things from a new vantage point. From this perspective, the therapist's verbal self-disclosure constitutes a fresh vantage point that may help the patient to see the world from multiple perspectives. When the therapist presents his verbal self-disclosure in an oracular manner suggesting omniscience, therapeutic dialogue will be stifled, but if the therapist can present his verbal self-disclosure as merely one limited perspective of one fallible human being, then the scope of the therapeutic dialogue can be expanded through the introduction of an additional perspective.

The therapist's theoretical perspective is of vital import in psychotherapy in determining the manner in which the patient's self-disclosure is registered and represented. The self that the patient discloses in psychotherapy is very much a product of the therapist's interpretive activity. In the clinical vignette, Susan's conscious self-experience is that she feels bored, is frustrated with the slow rate of progress, feels blamed by the therapist, and is indignant. These self-experiences, as particular contents of consciousness, do not reveal anything about Susan's self as an enduring psychological structure, until the therapist supplies a theory within which these self-experiences can be seen as deriving from an ongoing organization of her personality. The two major listening perspectives through which psychoanalytically oriented therapists have constructed their representations of the selves of the patients with whom they work are the archaeological mode and the empathic mode of listening (Josephs, 1988).

The archaeological mode of listening treats self-experience as a manifest content to be deconstructed into a latent content, whereas the empathic mode of listening remains within the phenomenology of the patient's self-experience. An archaeological analysis of the clinical vignette would suggest that Susan's not knowing what to discuss in sessions is an unconsciously resistant attitude that inhibits free association. Her boredom could be construed as betraying a covertly defensive, withholding, and hostile attitude for which she unconsciously expects retaliation. The projection of her unconscious persecutory anxiety gives rise to her acute sensitivity and defensiveness in regard to being blamed. Yet to interpret that her negative transference to me is a sign of the projection on to me of unacceptable aspects of herself would be experienced as a dismissal of her self-experience of being an innocent victim and as a still further example of being unfairly blamed and held responsible for something that is not her fault.

A deeper level of archaeological analysis can be derived from the theory of induced countertransference. Unconsciously, Susan could be seen as recreating an object relationship in which I am assigned a particular role—to contain aspects of herself that she finds intolerable to bear within herself. From this perspective, Susan would seem to draw me into the psychology of blame in which one party plays the critic, while the other is criticized. Her covertly withholding attitude could be seen as an unconscious provocation of my hostility, to which she then responds with self-righteous indignation.

Such a sadomasochistic power struggle would appear to recreate and mirror her childhood relationship with her mother, whom she also experienced as unfairly blaming and critical. Nevertheless, to challenge her self-perception of being an innocent victim in suggesting that she is unconsciously provocative would be experienced as blaming, of making her take responsibility for my anger and criticality, as though my negative feelings were her fault. To interpret that she is recreating her relationship with her mother might soften the blame in displacing the blame onto her mother but, since the implication is that she is identified with her mother and like her, the sense of blame remains inescapable.

In summary, the self that Susan discloses in archaeological analysis is a self in unconscious conflict, torn between an identification with a persecutory and sadistic maternal introject and a victimized, masochistic object of maternal abuse. Her conscious sense of self represents a defensive compromise formation that denies her unconscious sadomasochistic conflicts through a normopathic rationalization that justifies her alienation from others, yet blinds her to her own fears of intimacy. In treatment, whenever I failed to collude with her normopathic facade, the underlying sadomasochistic structure emerged and was externalized in the therapeutic dyad's stalemate in debating who was at fault and to blame for Susan's difficulties.

An empathic analysis of Susan's self-experience reveals a different construction of her self as an enduring psychological structure. To take a fresh look at her reported self-experiences—boredom, lack of a sense of progress, feeling blamed, feeling injured by my blame which is seen as unjust, and feeling justifiably angry with me—we can begin to explore her phenomenological sense of self. From this perspective, it could be hypothesized that there are enduring deficits in Susan's sense of a core self, especially in terms of a lack of a sense of self-agency and self-affectivity. Her boredom may reflect a lack of vitality affect. Not experiencing herself as alive, vital, involved, attached, or engaged, she experiences herself as painfully depleted and empty. She doesn't find her own inner life interesting, stimulating, enriching, spontaneous, or imaginative, so that she is chronically bored with herself. As an object to herself, she experiences herself as disengaged and lacking in feeling. Her sense of a lack of progress in therapy may be seen as reflecting a lack of a sense of self-agency. Susan experienced herself as a reactive person waiting for some external event or person to evoke a response from her. She possessed little sense of spontaneous initiative, so that she remained passive and inactive as long as there was no one to motivate and move her. As long as nothing eventful occurred in her life, nothing eventful could occur within herself. She had no sense that she could make things happen of her own volition.

Her sensitivity to criticism can be understood in terms of her lack of a sense of self-agency. Experiencing herself as a basically passive, powerless person, like a marionette on a string controlled by some external agent, it seemed incomprehensible to her to attribute intentions to herself, even unconscious intentionality, given that she experienced herself as someone lacking in intentions. Susan viewed other people as possessing complex intentions to which she reacted; but her own intentions, in her view, were no more complex than to comply with the demand characteristics of the situation in which she found herself—in other words, to meet the expectations of others. The sense of blame derived from feeling held responsible as an agent for something about herself which she experienced as outside her volitional control. Her anger and indignation were reactive affects serving to extricate herself from the humiliating sense of impotence that she experienced in being pressured to do something of which she felt incapable, that is, to be spontaneously related.

In the light of the empathic point of view, Susan's negative transference could be construed in terms of my failure as a self-regulatory other. For Susan, just being in psychotherapy in which she was expected to be reflective, introspective, and free-associate was like asking her to speak a foreign language with which she had no acquaintance and no way of gaining the necessary exposure for learning to occur. As a consequence, the therapist in the role of self-regulatory other had to supply the momentum, interest, and feelings so that Susan would feel that therapy was not a futile exercise. Whenever I failed in this function, Susan felt stuck, unable to proceed on her own steam. When I attempted to explore her lack of a sense of self-agency and self-affectivity, it was like reminding her and blaming her for some crippling defect over which she possessed little control. To discuss these perceived deficiencies was taken as an expectation that she should be able to change, and that it was readily within her power to change. Her defensiveness and indignation then seemed a wholly justified reaction to my unreasonable expectations.

Returning to the issue of patient self-disclosure, it becomes apparent that the self the patient discloses to the therapist will be very much a product of the therapist's interpretive activity. Is Susan revealing an unconscious self conflicted over sadomasochistic power struggles, or is Susan revealing an experiential self lacking in certain basic attributes, such as self-agency and self-affectivity, or both simultaneously? Of course, the self that the therapist believes the patient is disclosing is the self to which he will respond and which will guide his interventions. The patient then must learn how to contend with the therapist's view of the patient's self, especially when it is discrepant with the patient's own self-perception as it will inevitably be, given the limits of empathy. For

Susan, one arduous aspect of therapy was learning how to tolerate the psychic intimacy of opening herself up to my perceptions of her, slowly learning that in taking in some of my ego-alien views of her and making them her own she need not lose or sacrifice her enduring sense of self-sameness and self-continuity, and could perhaps enrich her sense of self in the process.

Conclusion

Self-disclosure in psychotherapy is never received wisdom whose meaning is transparent. Self-disclosure is always an intersubjective process, and the self that the discloser transmits is rarely identical with the self the listener receives, registers, and reflects back to the discloser. This discrepancy is inevitable because empathy, our only tool for grasping the self of the other, is an imperfect instrument that can aim at approximation but can never achieve absolute identity. Self-disclosure is also an intrapsychic process in which the self is disclosed as an object to oneself, in the vernacular, "getting to know oneself." The self that is disclosed as an object to oneself is also always a construction rather than a received wisdom that miraculously arises from the oracular pronouncement of the unconscious mind. In conclusion, it should be remembered that each act of self-disclosure in psychotherapy is, as well, an act of self-creation.

References

Atwood, G.G., & Stolorow, R.D. (1984). *Structures of subjectivity: Explorations in psychoanalytic phenomenology*. Hillsdale, New Jersey: Lawrence Erlbaum Associates.

Bollas, C. (1987). *The shadow of the object: Psychoanalysis of the unthought known*. New York: Columbia University Press.

Gill, M. (1982). *Analysis of transference: Vol. I*. New York: International Universities Press.

Hoffman, I. (1983). The patient as interpreter of the analyst's experience. *Contemporary Psychoanalysis, 19*, 389–422.

Josephs, L. (1988). A comparison of archaeological and empathic modes of listening. *Contemporary Psychoanalysis, 24*, 282–300.

Josephs, L. (1989). The world of the concrete: A comparative approach. *Contemporary Psychoanalysis, 25*, 477–500.

Kohut, H. (1971). *The analysis of the self: A systematic approach to the psychoanalytic treatment of narcissistic personality disorders*. New York: International Universities Press.

Kohut, H. (1977). *The restoration of the self*. New York: International Universities Press.

Kohut, H. (1984). *How does analysis cure?* Chicago: University of Chicago Press.

Langs, R. (1976). *The bipersonal field*. New York: Jason Aronson.

McDougall, J. (1985). *Theaters of the mind: Illusion and truth on the psychoanalytic stage*. New York: Basic Books.

Stern, D.N. (1985). *The interpersonal world of the infant: A view from psychoanalysis and developmental psychology*. New York: Basic Books.

Winnicott, D.W. (1968). *The maturational process and the facilitating environment*. New York: International Universities Press.

III

Therapeutic Issues

7

The Role of Implicit Communication in Therapist Self-Disclosure

Jonathan M. Jackson

We may begin by distinguishing between two different levels of therapist self-disclosure in psychoanalytically oriented psychotherapy. One is a surface or manifest level, and it refers to facts, personal data, conscious experiences of the therapist which he communicates in a variety of ways. The other is a deeper, less obvious kind of disclosure, and it concerns the communication of an individual's moral and social values, ways of relating to others, mood and disposition, intellectual acuity, esthetic tastes, etc. This second set of data comprises the kinds of knowledge one has of a person by living or working on close proximity over a long period of time. Although I will turn to a discussion of the surface level of self-disclosure first, the reader may anticipate my view of the deeper disclosures. That is, that any psychoanalytically oriented treatment must eventually turn towards a consideration of the patient's perceptions of the therapist's deep level disclosures, and that to avoid doing so denies the importance of a major capacity of the patient and a major contribution to the therapist, reciprocal aspects of the therapeutic relationship.

Traditional Views of Self-Disclosure

As a matter of technique, surface level self-disclosure has an uncertain and uncomfortable place in the more classical conceptions of

Jonathan M. Jackson • Institute of Advanced Psychological Studies, Adelphi University, Garden City, New York 11530.

psychotherapeutic work. It is not traditionally considered part of what the therapist ordinarily does or ought to do in treatment. Rather, activities such as establishing and maintaining a secure therapeutic frame (Langs, 1975), interpreting, clarifying (Strupp, 1969) and the like are considered the rightful, legitimate domain of the therapist. All these activities are focused on encouraging the production or understanding of what the patient reveals and extending the patient's self-awareness. At the same time, these therapeutic activities, focused as they are on the patient, and based on the therapist's neutral stance vis-à-vis the patient's productions, make it possible for the therapist to retain a relative degree of anonymity.

In this view, active self-disclosure by the therapist is usually seen, in contrast to the patient's disclosures, as something to be approached with caution, carrying a potential for muddying the lab of the patient's uncontaminated transference. The therapist pursues a neutral position vis-à-vis the patient's life to allow as fully as possible for a representation of conflictual material. The neutral setting is a communication from the therapist that enables the patient progressively to communicate and bring into relation to the therapist, feelings, thoughts, and memories that were previously repressed. The point of the therapist's revealing little of his attitudes or of his life is so that the patient may reveal more. According to this position, a crucial intent of the positions of neutrality and anonymity is that they will encourage an expression of the patient's experience of the therapist that has little or nothing to do with the therapist's actual behavior or attitudes. As the therapist is predominantly neutral in his dealings with the patient, the patient's attribution of a complex of motives, feelings, and thoughts to the therapist is transferred from the patient's history, from the unconscious fantasies and attitudes attached to significant people from the past.

This position, advocating the pursuit of neutrality and anonymity for the sake of the transference, has many adherents. Loewald (1960), for example, sees the analyst as a mirror who reflects the patient's unconscious back to him and who maintains his mirroring properties by being scrupulously personally neutral. The therapist is a blank slate and is advised to remain so. Thus, the therapist remains uncasted, resistant to the patient's effort to involve him in unconscious reenactment of the past. Interpretation, according to Loewald, presents the patient with his distortions in a new, objective relationship wherein the therapist's uninvolvement in the patient's drama makes him available to the patient as a voice of reality. What the therapist discloses, then, is his greater objectivity, as opposed to his subjective bias. Thus, pursuing the position of neutrality not only sets the necessary conditions for viewing the patient's experience as distorted by the past, but it also serves as a model for the patient to identify with, in the service of resolving his conflicts with self and others.

Compared with Loewald's advocacy of the therapist's neutrality, Stone (1961) relents somewhat, and allows for an attitude of benign friendliness toward the patient. The aim of this attitude, however, is consonant with Loewald's. That is, Stone wants to encourage an unfolding of the transference (motivated from persistent and unmodified wishes toward people in the past) that for some patients would be inhibited by too much silence, self-reserve, and nonresponsiveness on the part of the therapist. Benign friendliness is used to promote the patient's transference, but not to interact with it. An example of neutrality mixed with benign friendliness is seen in the advice of a colleague, who shied away from directly addressing patients by name. She argued it could imbue the transference with a warm (using first names) or cool (using last names) tone and, in so doing, interfere with revival and subsequent understanding of a patient's sense of warmth or coldness with his or her early objects. She illustrated this by citing an instance of a patient leaving a scarf behind in her waiting room at the end of a session. The therapist ran after the patient and caught her attention visually just before she passed through the elevator door, never once needing to call out the patient's name. This technique was supported by another illustrating how one may telephone a patient without addressing him or her by name either.

Kohut (1977) too is concerned with neutrality. He advocates a position of empathic involvement wherein the therapist functions as a self-object for the patient, facilitating a transference based on what the patient's developmental level requires. The therapist's personal reactions to the patient are seen as countertransferential to the extent that they veer from the patient's needs for empathic resonance and prematurely impose on the patient an awareness of the therapist as a separate person. Responding too freely out of one's personal reactions (a break in empathy vis-à-vis the patient) is traumatic because the patient is not yet able to function as a separate, differentiated self and so does not have the reciprocal capacity to treat the therapist as a separate self. Neutrality in this view is a matter of shielding the child-patient from the disruptive realities of the parent-therapist. In this sense, the therapist fosters a regressive relationship that is conceived by the therapist to be the needed restorative one, as opposed to the actual one.

Prior to Kohut, Winnicott (1965) developed the notion of holding the patient, a therapeutic function that keeps impingements from the outside environment to a minimum. Impingements refer to a class of events, including at times revelations of the therapist's personal reality, that disrupt the patient's continuity of experience and thus create dissociative trends in the personality. The therapist must remain concerned primarily with his patient's needs and respond with the correct amount or kind of environmental provision that promotes integration in the personality. Winnicott did not develop the idea of empathy as explicitly as Kohut did, perhaps because he believed it to be inherent, a natural, ordinarily available capacity in the "good-enough" therapist.

Winnicott did believe, however, and in this respect his ideas are clearly reflected in Kohut's clinical theory, that impingements were unavoidable. Thus, breaks in the holding environment ushered in breaks in the patient's continuity of experience. These breaks were undeniable, representative of the world out there, and they often provoke psychological health if properly timed and titrated. These breaks are not, however, at the center of Winnicott's or Kohut's theories. Rather, they are the facts or the realities of the world, inevitabilities to which the patient must eventually react. The therapist's role is to keep these breaks manageable for the patient.

Greenberg (1986) points out that the concept of neutrality is unpopular in many psychoanalytic circles because of its emphasis on inactivity. Unfortunately, for some therapists, inactivity is seen as the way to keep countertransference in check and thus remain nonjudgmental toward the patient's values. This concept of neutrality is rooted in the notion of the therapist who functions as an objective observer, rather than as a participant observer. Greenberg argues for a new conception of neutrality wherein the therapist's goal is to act in such a way that he encourages the patient to see him as not simply identical with transference figures. This may often entail coming out from behind anonymity, especially when the patient needs evidence to disconfirm his rigid transference experience. At the same time, the therapist cannot expect the patient openly to embrace new and mutative qualities in the therapist, and he must tolerate the patient's insistence on the "reality" of his transference. Thus, neutrality in Greenberg's view is a position somewhere between the patient's transference expectation and the reality of the therapist.

Special Events

According to the writers mentioned who represent a wide array of theoretical schools, self-disclosure is viewed as a shift away from ordinary therapeutic endeavors, to be utilized sparingly or not at all. When it cannot be avoided, self-disclosure is often seen as evidence of uncontrolled countertransference which interferes with the patient's ability to use optimally the therapeutic situation.

Weiss (1975) addresses the issue of self-disclosure as it occurs accidentally or involuntarily on the part of the therapist. Consistent with the work of Tarnower (1966) and Katz (1978) he found that special events such as chance meetings between patient and therapist, events such as the therapist's illness, etc., actually intensified rather than inhibited transference paradigms. This view contrasts starkly with the traditional one that such breaks in the therapist's neutrality and anonymity can distort or muddy the analytic work. Especially with patients who characteristically keep the transference experience pale, special events can provoke conscious awareness of previously private feelings about the therapist. Weiss includes technical errors in the class of events that are special or extraordinary, and these are caused by unchecked countertransference responses to the patient.

Viewing the therapist's pregnancy as a special event along the same line as Weiss (1975), Fenster, Phillips, and Rapaport (1986) advocate a modification in technique away from relative neutrality and toward self-disclosure at the time of the pregnancy and soon after. In their studies, they argue that the basic principles of psychoanalytic psychotherapy are not violated by the disclosures that devolve from this kind of therapist activity and, moreover, that the therapeutic process is often enhanced by such breaks in anonymity. They report that patients are often stimulated to produce previously unavailable material from their past and are enabled to create new solutions to their conflicts during their therapist's pregnancies. Perhaps mother is the necessity of invention.

Working earlier, Singer (1971) described the far-reaching effects of telling his patients of his wife's serious illness when he was forced to suddenly cancel his sessions. He observed from their reactions that disclosing this information helped them to express a capacity to be helpful and compassionate, and in so doing, made the patients' usefulness to another person become a realistic possibility perhaps for the first time. In an obvious way, Singer's move departs from the relative neutrality and anonymity of classical psychoanalysis. In so doing, Singer opened up the possibility that a legitimate goal of therapy might entail the patient's discovery of his own helpful human responsiveness. Singer's idea also goes beyond the traditional unilateral notion of the therapist being of help to the patient and allows for the patient's capacity to be of help to the therapist.

Progressive Views of Self-Disclosure

I now turn to a consideration of a deeper level of disclosure, the indirect one which entails the therapist's mode of relating to others, basic dispositions, values, and so on, which are communicated implicitly, rather than explicitly in the therapeutic situation. There are those theorists who hold that anonymity and neutrality are false issues, and that the therapist is in some respects not a blank screen, but an open book. Accordingly, self-disclosure is seen not as a discontinuous or infrequent event, but one that is continuous and common.

The origins of this position may be traced at least as far back as Ferenczi (1933/1988). Working within the theoretical framework of abreaction, he recounted how some patients, despite their reexperiencing in therapy of very intense trauma from the distant past, did not improve as expected. While some symptoms did remit, others worsened or became manifest for the first time. Unable, perhaps owing to his unceasingly optimistic outlook, to accept that his method might not be as useful as he had hoped, Ferenczi turned instead to a scrutiny of his own unconscious communications to his patients. Listening to his patients' reproaches of him as unhelpful, selfish, and cruel, Ferenczi wondered whether he was guilty of some professional hypocrisy. That is, did his promise to listen attentively and to work undauntingly mask an unconscious aversion to features of the patients' personalities? And were his patients, perceiving his unconscious withdrawal, responding to that of which he as yet was only dimly aware? Ferenczi remained concerned primarily with improving his technique to ease the way for some patients whose past experiences of hypocrisy (verbal professions of love with admixtures of physical and emotional abuse) were unwittingly repeated in the therapeutic setup. What he did not see, as it predates interpersonal notions of transference, were the broad consequences of his view of the patient as perceptive of and responsive to the therapist's unconscious communications and attitudes.

In perhaps the most fully elaborated presentation of the idea of the patient perceiving the therapist without the latter intentionally disclosing anything, Hoffman (1983) challenges what he calls the "naive patient" fallacy. The fallacy is

> ...the notion that the patient, insofar as he is rational, takes the analyst's behavior at face value even while his own is scrutinized for the most subtle indications of unspoken or unconscious meanings. (p. 395)

In Hoffman's view, and he cites the work of Gill (1982), Racker (1968), and Levenson (1981) as supportive of his central notions, the patient is engaged in interpretive activity just as the therapist is. Hoffman posits two ideas that form the basis for this conclusion. According to one idea, the patient senses that the therapist's behavior is at best only partially indicative of the therapist's entire experience. Thus, the patient is in an ambiguous situation regarding the entirety of who the therapist is, and the patient's interpretative activity is necessary in order to construct a relatively full and meaningful picture of what is on the therapist's mind. Hoffman holds that while the picture of the therapist that the patient construes may be accurate or not, there is no final expert on hand to judge. The patient's picture of the therapist is an inference born partly out of fact (the therapist's behavior) and partly out of (the patient's selective attention or transference inclinations), and therapy concerns itself with a full understanding of these two constituents of experience.

According to Hoffman's second idea about the patient's basis for constructing the therapist's inner reality, the patient senses that his behavior influences the therapist's personal experience and activities as a therapist. Put more simply, the patient knows he creates an atmosphere by virtue of his being persistently and potently who he is, and that he inducts the therapist into an emotional field of his own creation.

Thus, in this view, there are personal contributions made by each participant. On the patient's part, he fleshes out the skeleton of the therapist's anonymity and neutrality by constructing a full picture, and he must interpret to do this. One source of his interpretations is certain to be his past relationships with significant others. In this way the patient casts the therapist in a drama from the past. The therapist, if he is willing to recognize his delimited hold on his anonymity and neutrality, can experience experimentally these roles and respond with interpretations. Thus, the therapeutic relationship is an intimacy realized by virtue of the patient's transference and the therapist's willingness to respond. The patient intuits that the therapist's responsiveness (or lack thereof) indicates something important about the therapist's personal experience of the patient. And the patient interprets this experience as being based in part on the therapist's past relationships, moods, disposition, and so forth.

The blank screen concept, unlike the above notions of interactional and implicit self-disclosure, sees the therapist as becoming known to the patient only through discrete, intentionally orchestrated or accidental incidents. This concept in turn is rooted in a fallacy about the patient's inability to be perceptive about the therapist as long as the therapist does not actively disclose information about himself. Even to use the term self-disclosure implies that what is known to the patient about the therapist is limited to what the therapist decides to disclose, or to accidental breaks in neutrality. This is a variant of the "naive patient" fallacy, holding that what the patient knows about the therapist is controlled by the therapist's outward behavior, and that what the patient otherwise presumes to know about the therapist is transference distortion, subject to therapeutic scrutiny.

Characteristics of Neutrality-Seeking Therapists

If we examine the consequences of the traditional versus the progressive views of self-disclosure a bit further, we are left with another conclusion. The underlying assumption behind the traditional therapist's position is that he knows the reality, both in terms of what the patient really needs (e.g., Kohut and Winnicott) and in terms of who the therapist really is (e.g., Loewald, Stone) behind the screen. Thus, these therapists presume they are in possession of a better grasp of reality and a healthier psyche than their patients, capabilities that their patients strive to attain. Proponents of neutrality who regard the therapist as the one who decides when and in what form self-disclosure is an appropriate deviation from the blank screen position, assume characteristically what could be termed an authoritarian stance vis-à-vis the patient. (See Hirsch, 1981, for a full discussion of this issue.) Thus, it is the therapist's choice whether and to what extent to disclose. The therapist is dispassionate in his craft, not polarized, not ordinarily susceptible to being pulled or coerced into enacting a role that complements the patient's mind-set, having been inoculated against these enticements by virtue of his training. He may be empathic toward the patient's efforts to pull him into the action, but is supposed to remain nonporous as a matter of technical necessity. An arbiter of reality, the traditional therapist might disclose the truth to confirm the patient's sense of reality, to confer on to it truth value, or else to designate it as false. Patients too may accept or even prefer an impersonally neutral therapist, idealizable, hierarchically superior because he holds the truth. This is evident when, for example, a patient addresses the therapist as a representative of the profession, an expert or a keeper of knowledge as opposed to an individual with these or those particular qualities, these or those personal strengths or weaknesses.

Paradoxically, those therapists who in their endeavor to downplay authoritarian and hierarchical disparities between themselves and their patient, frequently disclose personal facts, feelings, thoughts, etc., also imply that their patients are naive. This is because in the view of these therapists, the patient does not recognize his ability to understand who the therapist is and must rely on the therapist's disclosures for a glimpse behind the veil of anonymity. Although the thrust of liberal doses of therapist self-disclosure comes out of the tradition of humanism (see, for example, Jourard, 1971) it too often appears a gesture in which the therapist emerges from his usual or expected position of neutrality and anonymity.

What I am suggesting, too, is that the progressive therapist preserves his neutrality and anonymity not in order to allow the transference distortions to unfold unimpeded and uncontaminated by the therapist; but to allow for the possibility that the patient will come to his senses and know what he is as yet unwilling or unable to know. Erich Fromm (1951) believed dreams were the place where patients were less inhibited about what they knew and that dream images often represented knowledge that was disavowed in waking life. For Fromm, Hoffman, and a group of psychoanalytic psychotherapists I have labeled as progressive, insight is a discovering of one's own ability to know. Further, knowledge is not so much disclosed by the therapist, but recovered by the patients.

References

Fenster, S., Phillips, S., & Rapaport. (1986). *The therapist's pregnancy: Intrusion in the analytic space*. Hillsdale, NJ: The Analytic Press.

Ferenczi, S. (1988). Confusion of tongues between adults and the child: The language of tenderness and of passion. *Contemporary Psychoanalysis, 24*, 196–206. (Originally published 1933.)

Fromm, E. (1951). *The forgotten language*. New York: Grove Press.

Gill, M.M. (1982). *Analysis of transference I: Theory and technique*. New York: International Universities Press.

Greenberg, J. (1986). Theoretical models and the analyst's neutrality. *Contemporary Psychoanalysis, 22*, 87–106.

Hirsch, I. (1981). Authoritarian aspects of the therapeutic relationship. *Review of Existential Psychology and Psychiatry, 17*, 105–133.

Hoffman, I.Z. (1983). The patient as interpreter of the analyst's experience. *Contemporary Psychoanalysis, 19*, 389–422.

Jourard, S.M. (1971). *The transparent self*. New York: Van Nostrand Reinhold.

Katz, J. (1978). A psychoanalyst's anonymity: Fiddler behind the couch. *Bulletin of the Menninger Clinic 42*, 520–524. New York: International Universities Press.

Kohut, H. (1977). *The restoration of the self*. New York: International Universities Press.

Langs, R. (1975). The therapeutic relationship and deviations in technique. *International Journal of Psychoanalytic Psychotherapy, 4*, 106–141.

Levenson, E. (1981). Facts or fantasies: The nature of psychoanalytic data. *Contemporary Psychoanalysis, 17*, 486–500.

Loewald, H. (1960). On the therapeutic action of psychoanalysis. *International Journal of Psychoanalysis 41*, 16–33.

Racker, H. (1968). *Transference and countertransference*. New York: International Universities Press.

Singer, E. (1971). The patient aids the analyst: Some clinical and theoretical observations. In B. Landis and E.S. Tauber (Eds.), *In the name of life—Essays in honor of Erich Fromm*, New York: Holt, Rinehart and Winston.

Stone, L. (1961). *The psychoanalytic situation*. New York: International Universities Press.

Strupp, H. (1969). Psychoanalytic psychotherapy and research. In L.D. Eron and R. Callahan (Eds.). *The relation of theory to practice in psychotherapy*. Chicago: Aldine Publishing.

Tarnower, W. (1966). Extra-analytic contacts between the psychoanalyst and the patient. *The Psychoanalytic Quarterly, 35*, 399–413.

Weiss, E. (1975). The effect on the transference of special events occurring during psychoanalysis. *International Journal of Psychoanalysis, 56*, 69–75.
Winnicott, D.W. (1965). *Maturational processing and the facilitating environment*. New York: International Universities Press.

8

Transference, Countertransference, and Therapeutic Efficacy in Relation to Self-Disclosure by the Analyst

Esther Menaker

Very little has been written in the psychoanalytic literature about self-disclosure—that is, self-disclosure by the analyst. In fact there is no such category in the Grinstein *Index of Psychoanalytic Writings*. This is not surprising since the very essence of the philosophy of classical psychoanalytic technique rests on the premise that the "cure" for the patient depends on the creation of a "transference neurosis" within the context of the psychoanalytic situation; and this in turn depends on the neutrality of the analyst. Neutrality in this case means a minimum of self-revelation: no disclosure of opinions, values, or advice; no sharing of personal experiences of biographical facts. The analyst is to remain a nonperson in the name of fostering the development of the transference—that projection onto the person of the analyst of each individual's specific way of loving—or hating—which is the legacy of constitution and early childhood experience (Freud, 1953). In the face of a person's search for psychological help the therapist, according to classical psychoanalytic theory, is to remain *neutral*, that is, not interact with the patient in any way other than to foster the uncovering of unconscious impulses and to communicate such insights to the patient. This procedure is founded on the premise that help or cure for the patient is

Esther Menaker • Postdoctoral Program for Training in Psychoanalysis and Psychotherapy, Department of Psychology, New York University, New York, New York 10003, and Private Practice, 20 West 77 Street, New York, New York 10024.

based on the lifting of the repression of unwelcome impulses—that is, that the making conscious of previously unconscious wishes would effect change in an individual's personality. This premise is in turn based on another preceding premise, namely, that neuroses or disturbances in personality functioning are caused by repression of impulses, especially sexual impulses. Neither premise, while describing some truth about personality functioning, has been found empirically to be the exclusive cause of neurosis or of disorders of the personality. It should follow, then, that in the name of therapeutic efficacy, the *cultivation* of the transference is unproductive. The emphasis is upon the word "cultivation," for it is indeed impossible to prevent the development of transference phenomena in any human interaction between two people, be it in ordinary life or in the therapeutic situation. The way of loving or hating which is so much a product of past experience becomes an intrinsic part of an individual's personality and is bound to express itself in psychoanalysis as well as in life in general. Freud was aware that transference phenomena take place in life as well as in psychoanalysis; but he wanted an intensification of transference feelings for the analytic situation and to this end he advocated the neutrality of the analyst.

Many years ago, a patient whom I shall call Ruth, came to me because her relationships with men were never consummated in a permanent relationship of any kind. She would have wished to be married or at least to live with a man in a constant, companionable relationship. But she always seemed to fall in love either with married or inappropriate men; or to be unable to find men to whom she might be attracted. She was a woman of about forty, not particularly attractive physically, but she had a fine character, was highly intelligent, and had a lively, outgoing personality that made up for her deficits in the realm of beauty. She described her needs and wishes to me very clearly in our first meeting, realizing fully that her social difficulties with men had to do with inner conflicts of which she was not fully aware. As we concluded our arrangements for her therapeutic work with me, I experienced an impulse to tell her something of my life.

I was about 65 at this juncture. It was about a year after the death of my husband, when I began to live with an elderly man who had been a mutual friend of ours many years ago in our student days in Vienna. We had re-met, were both free, were attracted to each other, and were unusually compatible. We decided to join our lives; and since I had a large apartment, he moved in with me. My office and home were combined; and patients, as they waited for me in a small anteroom near the front door, occasionally saw family members coming in or out of the apartment. I knew that sooner or later someone would see my new "roommate" entering or leaving the house. Contrary to classical psychoanalytic policy practiced by most of my colleagues in order—supposedly—not to interfere with transference reactions, I wanted no unknowns, no mysteries about the major biographical facts and events of my life. I told Ruth about my life arrangements of that time. Her reaction is extremely important. After having listened intently, she turned to me and said: "Then there's hope for me." "Yes, of course," I replied.

As I look back on the fact that I followed my impulse to reveal the nature of my personal life at the time, if only in broad generalities, I wonder what impelled me to follow my inclination—an inclination so opposed to the therapeutic philosophy in which I had originally been trained. Yet even that statement is not entirely accurate, for in my second analysis with Willi Hoffer during my psychoanalytic student days in Vienna, he himself was changing his personal life situation. He had been divorced, and when I began my analysis with him, was living alone and working in an apartment from which he was about to move. When he gave me his new address, I asked about the reason for the move. He told me that he was to be married soon and that he and his wife were to move into the new apartment. He even told me who his new wife was, Hedwig Schaxel—a nonmedical analyst who was a member of the Vienna Psychoanalytic Society and a person whom I had seen at meetings.

I expressed surprise at this forthright answer to my question, for I had been indoctrinated to believe that any personal revelations on the part of the analyst would interfere with the purity of the transference reactions. "But," said Dr. Hoffer, "I believe that a patient has the right to know the basic biographical facts of his or her analyst's life: whether he or she is married or single, whether he has children and what his educational and psychoanalytic training consisted of." He presented this as if he considered the biographical facts to be in the nature of credentials whose meaning would differ for individual prospective patients, but whose reality would give individuals the opportunity to make choices. The simplicity and honesty of his remarks pleased me, and had the therapeutic effect of creating trust. I never had the opportunity to discuss with Dr. Hoffer the extent to which his modifications of standard psychoanalytic procedure were a part of a thought-out therapeutic philosophy or derived naturally from his broad empirical experience with human reactions which he was willing to affirm and take at face value. It is significant that he never wrote on this theme; and that, in fact, most classical analysts are timid about revealing what they regard as "transgressions" of accepted procedure.

For me, the experience with Willi Hoffer liberated me at that time [described in my memoir (Menaker, 1989)] from any tendency toward an absolute faith in the validity of psychoanalytic theory and its technical practices. Undoubtedly in my interaction with the patient described, the nature of my analysis with Dr. Hoffer and his lack of fear of self-disclosure (at therapeutically appropriate times; he had told me incidents of his childhood, about his warm relationship with his father, a country doctor, whom he often accompanied on home visits to his patients) reenforced my own inclination to share my life situation with my patient. But to what end, one might ask? Not only to create an honest atmosphere in which to conduct her analysis—although I consider this extremely important—but also to make clear to her, longing for a relationship with a man, that even at my age this was possible.

Her answer about hope for herself confirms the effectiveness of my self-disclosure. A number of years later she did indeed meet a man within her professional circle with whom she fell in love and with whom she has established a permanent and compatible relationship. Obviously it was not merely my remarks about myself that enabled her to establish a good relationship with a man. Much analytic work took place in the intervening years. She learned a great deal that had been unknown to her before. Her overattachment, yet ambivalence, to a father who was inclined to be grandiose, and the way in which this affected her life became clear, and her identification with him diminished. She came to be less critical and more appreciative of a mother whom she had formerly regarded with predominantly hostile feelings. Such insights played a major role in the changes that took place in her character and in her behavior.

However, it seems important to emphasize that the analysis took place in an atmosphere of nonjudgmental dialogue about shared experiences. We had much in common: our values and our familial background were similar. Our parents were professional people of Russian origin. I understood the idiosyncrasies of that culture and could often respond to her anecdotes with similar ones from my own background. This created a powerful bond between us. Some might be inclined to say that the special circumstances that derived from certain actual similarities in our emotional experiences invalidate the assumption that self-disclosure is of great importance. On the contrary: what is in this case an *actual* similarity points to the importance of finding and expressing in the interaction with patients those human commonalities which exist for all of us, and to convey in these interchanges an affirmation of our common human heritage and an expression of hope that the realization of the patient's goals for his or her life—for which treatment was sought in the first place—will be fulfilled.

Does such an exchange of experience and emotion between patient and therapist preclude the development of the transference that is, in the thinking of the classical analyst, the sine qua non of the psychoanalytic undertaking? I think not, for the simple reason that transference reactions occur constantly in all our life situations, as I have already remarked, and as Freud himself stated. We carry with us the baggage of our past which influences all our perceptions. It used to be called, in academic psychological circles, our apperceptive background. The imprint of past experience influences our perception of present-day events, including the perception of people and their interaction with us. Furthermore, the self-disclosure of the analyst is not—nor should it be—a contrived technique calculated to further the therapeutic process. The analyst unavoidably reveals him or herself in the course of interacting with the patient through appearance, voice tone, way of expressing herself, gait and body stance, to mention only a few of the cues that we all pick up in the course of any human interaction. But self-disclosure of the analyst in the analytic situation, as I understand it, is more than that. It is a spontaneous empathic response to the patient's communication by sharing an analogous feeling or experience in the life of the analyst. The purpose of the disclosure is to underscore for the patient the fact that the analyst has understood the import of the communication and that he or she affirms the patient's reality. Sometimes, of course, such an interaction goes awry. The analyst may not have understood, or not have understood fully. But no matter; for the very willingness to share experiences on the part of the analyst creates an atmosphere congenial to dialogue; and in the course of the subsequent interchange greater understanding and trust is inevitably achieved and a closer bond between the two participating individuals is created.

The fostering of an understanding bond between patient and therapist in the name of arriving at a *mutually acceptable* understanding of the patient's reality is, of course, the opposite of the Freudian approach, which seeks to uncover a reality unknown to the patient—the repressed and therefore unconscious, unacceptable instinctual impulses which are seen as the cause of neurosis or of neurotic symptoms. A major vehicle for this archaeological task is the analysis of the transference: that projection of the patient's inner emotional life, complete with distortions, upon the relatively nonparticipating personality of the analyst. Thus a "truth" is arrived at that supposedly reflects hitherto unknown feelings, wishes, and impulses. Once such previously unconscious impulses are brought into awareness, they exist in the domain of the ego and can be volitionally accepted or rejected, acted upon or not. The possibility of choice has become part of the patient's psychological life. The premise that underlies this approach to therapy is that the curative factor in the analytic situation is the uncovering of the unconscious (largely through free association, the analysis of dreams and fantasies, and the analysis of the transference), making it known to the patient and helping him or her to work through and assimilate the newly acquired knowledge. The "real" or "actual" relationship of the patient to the analyst is rarely of any consequence, since the analyst is viewed as an outside observer, not as a participant in a relationship. This is the model in broad strokes of the classical Freudian philosophy of therapy. It is based primarily on a theory of conflict in which human development takes place primarily as a struggle between drives that seek pleasure (the release of tension) and superego constraints that represent the demands of society.

A different view of development leads to a very different theory of therapy—one in which the active role of the analyst plays a crucial part, and in which the element of self-disclosure may contribute to the outcome. It is in the approach of self psychology as it was begun by Heinz Kohut that the patient's relationship to and interaction with the analyst is decisive for change and/or cure. The analyst's way of observing as a self psychologist differs from that of the Freudian analyst. For Kohut advocates what he terms an introspective, empathic stance. In following this directive the analyst is an active participant in the interchange with the patient, observing the patient not as an object to be comprehended from a distance outside oneself, but as someone whose emotions one can take in even to the extent of momentarily losing oneself and merging with the patient. It is through such empathy that the self-psychologist hopes to make good those deficits in the patient's development that are responsible for the maladaptations and unhappiness that brought him or her to seek psychotherapeutic treatment. Self psychology rarely speaks of neurosis or of conflict, but rather of arrests or deficits in an individual's development due to familial experiences that failed to provide adequate nourishment for the child's developing self. A major aspect of the analyst's task is to provide that nourishment.

The rudiments of self-structure are given from the beginning of life in the very nature of a child's constitution—in the way of responding to the environment, the sensitivity to stimuli, and the reactivity of the nervous system, for example. There are great individual differences in the basic psychobiologic nature of individuals, for each person is unique. Yet this uniqueness is further augmented by the specific nature of the familial experience in the course of which the structure of the self is laid down through processes of internalization. The child takes into him- or herself the parents' very way of being: first the external traits—the way of speaking, of walking, of gesturing; then the more internal—the way of thinking, of relating to others, of feeling about oneself. Thus the self of the child is structured.

Of course, the child is not a duplicate of his/her parents, for the identifications have been added to the initial predispositions and a new and unique personality has been structured through his amalgamation, as well as through the internalization of experiences and contacts with individuals outside the family. Often identifications are rejected. Particular aspects of a parent's character or behavior are found objectionable. Often, as therapists, we hear, for example, from young women: "I never wanted to be like my mother," or "I have made up my mind that I would never treat my child as my mother treated me." But all too often the rejected identification is repressed only to appear in some distorted form when the child-rearing situation becomes a reality. Whether identifications are successfully assimilated into the self-structure or are repressed, or are rejected out of hand, or are simply absent, leaving large vacancies in the self, is determined by the nature of the parent–child bond during the phases of development. Successful internalizations that lead ultimately to a cohesive self-structure take place in a familial atmosphere of love, of relatedness, of parental affirmation of the child. It is loving respect for the growing, striving self of the developing child that forms the nourishing soil for the integration of a self in the growing individual—a self that can relate well to others, make emotional commitments in close relationships, and enjoy a secure sense of self-esteem.

One day a psychologically sophisticated middle-aged man whom I shall call Karl, who had been in treatment at various times in his life, and with me for more than a year, came to his session in a discouraged mood. He had been looking back on the history of his emotional life and realized that he had never been able to make a commitment to a woman that had any degree of permanency. He had had two unsuccessful marriages and his current relationship was one to which he felt he could be loyal only in a limited way. He wished very much to be able to love fully enough to commit himself to a marriage. He feared that it would always be this way, for while his various therapies in the course of the years had provided him with considerable insight into the psychodynamics of the emotional interactions among family members, they had not been able to help him toward a full love relationship.

Knowing a little about the emotional limitations in his relationship to his mother, and suspecting that there might still be aspects of this relationship of which he was unaware, I began asking him about his mother in greater detail. My patient began to describe a person who was timid, uncertain, and unassertive in her relationship to individuals outside the home, and who was unfocused and detached in her relationships within the family. She sounded unformed in her own personality structure and unable to be totally committed to relationships—to her children, to her husband, and to those outside the family.

It suddenly struck me that my patient's inability to commit himself to a relationship signaled a profound and completely unconscious identification with a similar inability in his mother—one that he had incorporated and that became a profound imprint that determined the nature of his relationships to women. I communicated to him my *hypothesis* that his own limitations in his ability to become attached in a profound way to women *might* be the result of an identification with his mother—with her inability to relate to others—in fact, with her detachment and isolation.

I emphasize the word "hypothesis" because the manner in which an insight is conveyed is of great importance, especially in relation to the issue of self-disclosure. To hand down interpretations as absolute truth is to present oneself as an autocratic therapist, even as an autocratic individual. The authoritarian stance vis-à-vis the patient is, to some degree, the psychoanalytic legacy of its historical origins in hypnosis, although, even in this connection, psychoanalysis distinguishes between the authoritarian and the persuasive maternal type of approach in hypnosis. If, on the other hand, one is engaged as a therapist in a dialogue with a patient—a dialogue that seeks to explore possible explanations for a patient's character structure or behavior—in an egalitarian atmosphere, one wins the patient's trust and reveals oneself as an empathic person capable of precisely that kind of relatedness which the patient lacked in the course of development.

My conjecture about my patient's possible identification with a withdrawn mother made a profound impression upon him. He could scarcely believe that in the many years of therapy that he had experienced, the possibility of this aspect of his personality development had never been unearthed. He seemed relieved by the insight—by the knowledge that he had been a victim of an unconscious unwelcome introject that was his mother's way of relating to others. He was imbued with some faith that this introject could be exorcised. He could become his own person and discover his own way of loving.

Karl began his treatment with me in the reserved and somewhat distant manner to which he was accustomed from previous therapies. Gradually he began to respond to my somewhat casual manner. In the beginning I noticed his surprise if I shared some of my experiences and reactions with him. For example, we might recently have heard the same concert, or have gone to the same art gallery. It would not be unusual for me not only to hear about his reactions with interest, but to share my own with him; I recall clearly an occasion when we spoke about an exhibition of primitive art that he particularly enjoyed. It happened that I had found this art form somewhat uncanny and I described to him my hypersensitivity to any quality of eerieness in works of art or even sometimes in natural scenes. I told him of a childhood experience when, upon returning from school one afternoon, I had come unexpectedly upon a reproduction of the Mona Lisa. The picture which had just been given to my mother by a neighbor was standing against a wall waiting to be hung. I had been frightened by her strange enigmatic smile and ran screaming down the hall to ask my mother: "Who is that Indian down the hall?" Even as an adult and even after having seen the original, I have never succeeded in feeling comfortable with da Vinci's supposed masterpiece.

Such small vignettes out of my own life, particularly out of my childhood that revealed my own emotions gradually helped Karl to experience his own feelings in a less muted form. My disclosures also enabled him to perceive and experience me as a real person with strengths and weaknesses, with tastes and values that sometimes coincided with his own, but were sometimes quite different. What is therapeutically important is that my revealed authenticity helped him to delineate and define his own.

But what of the transference, that supposedly therapeutic vehicle through the analysis of which memories are to be recovered, repressions lifted, insight gained? The transference both in life and in the therapeutic situation, since it is an individual's way of relating to others, occurs inevitably. Yet the classic analytic situation, by virtue of the analyst's lack of participation, intensifies and distorts the projection of the patient's emotions onto the person of the analyst. I am reminded in this connection of a film that grew out of Brazelton's infant research which I had the good fortune to have seen in 1977.

The researchers were studying mother–infant interaction. One frame showed an infant of about nine months sitting in his high chair, expectantly awaiting the arrival of his mother. When she entered the room, smiling, cooing, and expressing her pleasure in being with him, the little boy smiled, made gleeful sounds and body movements which he could scarcely contain for sheer joy. The same child on another occasion in which the setup was the same was confronted by his mother, not with a smiling face but with a "dead" face in which no emotion was expressed. The disappointed and frustrated child tried in every way—by cooing and smiling himself, and by physically reaching out toward his mother—to elicit a response from her. It was all to no avail. She remained stony-faced. Finally, in frustration, the child began to cry, and what began as a cry that expressed need, longing, disappointment, and anxiety at being thus abandoned, turned into a cry of rage.

In the psychoanalytic situation, a similar scenario is recreated: the childhood situation of the patient in which "The inevitable hierarchy of the parent as protector but inevitably as final authority on the one hand and dependent child on the other is repeated in the authoritative position of the analyst and the inevitably submissive position of the patient"

(Menaker, 1988). Furthermore, the objective neutral stance and noninteracting posture of the analyst which is recommended for classic psychoanalytic procedure is a contrived technique that artificially induces extreme emotions in the transference—usually, and ultimately, rage—which are then interpreted as products of the patient's neurosis. They are in fact normal reactions to needlessly created frustrations in a situation in which one individual is asking another to be of help.

A patient's reaction of anger to the unempathic, detached behavior of the analyst is not necessarily a regression to the infantile reaction to frustration which I have just cited in my description of the film on the infant research study. The parallel between the "dead" face of the mother and the unresponsive so-called neutral stance of the analyst illustrates the normal human need for social interaction.

The issue of self-disclosure on the part of the analyst is ultimately bound up, as we have already seen, with the problem of the transference, which in turn reflects the analyst's theory of neurosis, as well as the very philosophy of cure. To my mind, we are confronted here with two separate views of neurosis and therefore with two different conceptions of therapy. I would like to emphasize the existence of two distinct vantage points, both of which can play a role in the actual treatment of a particular individual, but which are philosophically separate.

If, with Freud, we view neurosis as the result of the repression of unacceptable sexual impulses which have been banished from consciousness but which, from their existence in the realm of the unconscious, continue to exert a deleterious effect on the personality of the neurotic individual, then the goal of treatment becomes the lifting of repression. It is important in psychoanalytic treatment to bring the repressed impulses into awareness so that they can exist in the domain of the ego and can thus be controlled by the ego. The use of free association and the analysis of an intensified transference to the analyst thus become the essential hallmarks of a classical psychoanalysis.

Freud attributes the intensification of the transference to the factor of abstinence, i.e., the absence of the gratification of impulses. It is precisely the lack of reciprocity in the classical analytic situation that causes the libido to leave the world of reality, to regress to earlier stages of libido development, and thus to reanimate the internalized imagoes of early childhood toward which the impulses were originally directed. To justify or rationalize this regression, the patient in the psychoanalytic situation distorts by a process of projection his or her perception of the analyst to achieve a correspondence between reality and the infantile imagoes that reside in the unconscious. Making this process of distortion conscious for the patient constitutes a major therapeutic goal of the analytic process.

The fact that the analyst is an objective observer, rather than a participant, that there is no reciprocity in the relationship accounts for the intensification of the patient's need for response—much as the infant's response described above. The regression, the infantile response is induced by the analytic situation and the analyst's technique of non-participation. For the classic analyst, the return to the past is considered of primary importance for the patient's cure or betterment. The transference phenomenon becomes a vehicle for unveiling what psychoanalysis considers a convincing return to the infantile past that is supposedly at the core of the patient's neurosis.

However, a different view of the genesis of neurosis would lead of necessity to a modification, if not a complete change, in psychoanalytic procedure. It is to Heinz Kohut that we owe a different perspective on the origins of personality disturbances. For him there was a major line of human development that differed from the development of the libidinal stages which Freud had hypothesized. This was the development of the self. The rudimentary self which is given at birth, develops further as the child grows through processes of internalization—namely, through the internalization not only of parental imagoes but of those parental attitudes toward the child that were experienced in the interaction between the child and the parents. Kohut's emphasis in evaluating emotional disturbances was heavily weighted in the direction of a concern with self-esteem. Self-esteem in turn depends on the nutrients for self-development which the child receives from the parents in the form of mirroring or the opportunity for idealization.

For example, the pleasure that a child perceives in his mother's face as she enjoys his or her activity, his accomplishments, in fact, his very being, is internalized and becomes his own image of himself in which he can take pleasure; his self-esteem is nourished and becomes secure. In addition, if a parent—often the father—furthers the child's idealization of him (or her), the growing self of the child is given another opportunity through an internalization of the ideal to support his growing self and thus to achieve a good sense of self-esteem.

In familial situations that provide only a dearth of the nourishment needed for the growth of a healthy, cohesive, and integrated self, the child suffers emotional damage which is manifest in behavioral and psychological maladaptation. Most often the result of such deficits is a loss of self-esteem. This is true not only for narcissistic personality disorders, as Kohut thought at first, but for all those disturbances of personality that come to the attention of the psychoanalyst. The analyst's therapeutic task then, according to Kohut, is not *primarily* to uncover unconscious impulses and make them accessible to the conscious personality of the patient in the name of resolving conflict, but rather to strengthen the self by making good those emotional deficits of the patient's childhood that resulted in his or her failure to form a securely consolidated self. This is achieved through the analyst's clear affirmation of the *person* of the patient.

Otto Rank, who can be considered a forerunner of self psychology and who thought that neurotics suffered from an inhibition in the function of "willing," due to a failure on the part of parents to accept the child's will, also emphasizes the therapeutic effect of affirmation—in his own terms, affirming the patient's will. Above all the analyst must not further damage the patient's already fragile self-esteem. This can easily happen if the analyst presents a cold, distant, authoritarian stance. One of the dangers in the classic approach is precisely that the observing objective (neutral) stance of the analyst can too easily become an attitude of detachment, which inevitably lowers the patient's self-esteem. The empathic stance of the psychoanalytic self psychologist, because it is participatory, lends itself to interaction between patient and therapist in which the therapist becomes the self-object for the structuring of the patient's self. In the empathic mode, the purity of the transference, be it mirroring or idealizing, need not be threatened, as in the case of traditional analysis, by the active participation of the analyst. It is the fact of participation in the relationship to the patient that opens the way for self-disclosure by the analyst.

When the analyst reveals something about him or herself—about his life or experience—at a time and in a context that is appropriate relative to the patient's communication, it becomes an echo, or an elaboration on the echo, of the patient's own experience, and thus serves to cement a bond between the patient and the analyst, inhibiting processes of projection and fostering identification. The analyst, since he or she functions as a self-object for the patient, becomes authentic, and thereby better serves to sustain and further the structuring of the patient's growing self. I would like to emphasize the factor of the authenticity of the therapist in the treatment situation; for whatever the nature of a particular human interaction—be it between parent and child, teacher and pupil, friend and friend, or analyst and patient—when the "other" is felt as authentic, the delineation of the self is thereby furthered: differences and similarities come into sharper relief and the self, as well as the capacity for mature relatedness, is enhanced.

Self-disclosure cannot of course be random. It must be sensitively attuned to the needs of the therapy; that is, to the particular needs of the patient's developing self.

The question of countertransference is bound to arise in connection with self-disclosure: does the analyst have an emotional need to reveal himself or herself to the patient; and if the answer is yes, does this invalidate the procedure? Since we are speaking of an intense emotional interaction between two individuals who undoubtedly have an effect on one another, the answer to the first question may be affirmative. But if the need is not quantitatively excessive, there is no reason to fear that it will interfere with the patient's analysis. In an empathic atmosphere, the needs of each individual as they interact with one another can be met within limits. However, the patient's need for self-development in the therapy must be of primary concern and the therapist must try to judge when self-disclosure is productive and when it could become an obstacle to the goal of treatment. In general, when self-disclosures are honestly motivated by the analyst's desire to be helpful, even if they misfire because of a failure in perfect empathic understanding, they can be used productively in the analysis to demonstrate convincingly for the patient the struggle between expectation and disappointment.

In conclusion, it would seem that self-disclosure lends itself much more naturally to the empathic introspective stance of psychoanalytic self psychology than to rigidly traditional psychoanalytic procedures. There also remains the important question of the relation between theory and technique. I have sketched the differences between the Freudian and the Kohutian theory: the emphasis upon the repression of libido, in the one case, and, in the other, that of the role of the developing self and the deficits that may accrue to it. From these divergent positions concerning the *genesis* of neurosis emerge the different technical procedures: that of the "neutral" stance in classical psychoanalysis and that of the empathic introspection of the self psychologist. The important issue is whether psychoanalysis will continue to see itself as an already defined system of theory and practice—the practice of which inevitably reinforces the theory, e.g., the neutral stance actually *eliciting* the extent of the distortions in the transference—or whether psychoanalysis will come to see itself as a theory open to being modified by clinical experience. The issue of self-disclosure and its efficacy is one such testing ground.

References

Brazelton, T.B. (1977). Demonstration at NPAP's celebration of the twenty-fifth anniversary of their acquisition of the *Psychoanalytic Review*.

Freud, S. (1953). Dynamics of the transference. *Collected Papers* Vol. II, London: Hogarth Press.

Menaker, E. (1988). Pitfalls of the transference. Paper delivered at the Adelphi University Conference, *How people change: Inside and outside therapy*. October 1, 1988. (in press.)

Menaker, E. (1989). *Appointment in Vienna*. New York: St. Martin's Press.

9

Self-Disclosure and the Nonwhite Ethnic Minority Patient

Adelbert H. Jenkins

In this chapter I will concentrate selectively on certain issues involved in self-disclosure in psychodynamic therapy with nonwhite ethnic minority people. It will be my basic position here that psychotherapy with ethnic minorities can draw on principles and concepts that are applicable to people generally. However, adaptations in conceptualization and technique must be made for the important variations in class and culture that exist in this country. Ordinarily the term "minority" in the United States is applied to people of African-American, Asian-American, Hispanic American, and Native American or Indian descent. It is of course not possible to do justice here to the range of issues that are pertinent to these groups on so fundamental a concept as self-disclosure in therapy.

I will approach this material by limiting the discussion to a few topics relevant to the theme of this chapter. I will be writing from my greater knowledge of the literature on African-Americans, although I will attempt to formulate what I have to say so as to make it broadly relevant to nonwhite American groups. I will have in mind here the more frequent context in which the therapist is white, although of course much of this discussion will apply to nonwhite minority therapists working with nonwhite clients as well. [For more detailed discussions of specific groups, the reader is referred to the considerable amount of emerging literature on psychotherapy with nonwhite minorities, some of which is cited in the References at the end of this chapter. Such edited

Adelbert H. Jenkins • Department of Psychology, New York University, New York, New York 10003.

collections as those by Comas-Diaz & Griffith (1988); Dudley & Rawlins (1985); McGoldrick, Pearce, & Giordano (1982); and Pederson (1985) are good examples of this work.]

The Racial Context of American Society

Before proceeding to a discussion of factors that enhance self-disclosure with the nonwhite ethnic minority client, we should note that it may not be clear to some readers what the need is for a special chapter on this topic. In attempting to answer this question we would have to confront the dilemma posed by the very term "minority." While such a term does properly characterize the political and social status to which these people have been relegated, for the most part the usefulness of the label "minority" stops there. Obviously there are considerable between-group differences in the history and culture of these people and much within-group variability among the individuals in these groups. In actuality, the labeling of particular sets of people as "minorities" tells us more about the dominant society that has coined the term than about the people to whom it is applied.

Historically, Americans of European background came to the new world with religious and cultural traditions that gave strong emotionally laden connotations to the concept "white." The fantasies Europeans developed about the darker-skinned people they came across in Africa, Asia, and the Americas, helped them define their own sense of self (Jordan, 1968). Thus, minorities have become the "Other," a dialectic pole of self and identity for white Americans. American society has needed to maintain its denigrated image of these Others in order to sustain an acceptable sense of itself (Kovel, 1984). It has resisted allowing colored minorities to rise too high in social status because that would change some of the terms of self-definition for the dominant group.

These issues are relevant to our discussion here because mental health service in general and psychotherapy in particular have been carried out within this highly biased historical and social context (Thomas & Sillen, 1972). Americans—including mental health workers—are heirs to this way of looking at people of color, and the personal and institutional practices flowing from such attitudes continue to have a pervasive effect on personal and social life in this country. Though nonwhite ethnic minorities have some of the familiar human problems of living and, in addition, have had the special psychological stresses of adapting to mainstream American society, it is not surprising that they have not as readily availed themselves of traditional mental health services.

If any client or patient (in this chapter I will use these two terms interchangeably to describe the person seeking psychotherapy) is to be helped (s)he must be enabled to talk freely and disclose or reveal aspects of the self that may be seldom discussed or even thought about, but which represent important limitations to that person's functioning. With the minority client, even where the therapist gives evidence of being well-meaning, (s)he may very well be seen as representing a social structure that has been oppressive and judgmental and that seeks continually to work to its own advantage at the expense of the minority individual (Bulhan, 1985). Thus, the American racial context puts an added burden on the already difficult processes involved in self-disclosure. Nevertheless, it is this writer's view that psychotherapy in cross-ethnic situations can be useful to nonwhite minority clients and the problems that impede such work can be overcome. With these thoughts in mind I will focus the discussion on two issues: (1) engaging the minority client in therapy; and (2) addressing language factors in the cross-ethnic psychotherapy situation.

Engaging the Minority Client in Psychotherapy

The Problem of Attrition

Discussion about self-disclosure with the minority client is academic if that person does not remain in therapy. An important indication of the fact that minority patients are wary about engaging in therapy is the high attrition rate from psychotherapy for those minority persons who seek therapy (Sue, 1977) and an underutilization rate for some minority groups (Sue & Sue, 1987). In efforts to account for these phenomena some writers have suggested that there are natural potential pitfalls in interview contexts where the ethnic background or social class of therapist and client differ, especially where the therapist is white in these dyads (Banks, Berenson, & Carkhuff, 1967; Carkhuff & Pierce, 1967; Plasky & Lorion, 1984). For a time it was being suggested that perhaps therapies emphasizing self-exploration were not appropriate for the presumably nonverbal and nonreflective person of working or lower-class minority background. (See Smith & Dejoie-Smith, 1984, for a review of some of this literature.) However, other writers have suggested, more wisely, I think, that if one is prepared to understand the nature of the processes that go on in relationships where racial backgrounds differ, a workable alliance can be established (Comas-Diaz, 1988; Gardner, 1971; Jones, 1978; Sue & Zane, 1987).

Cultural Paranoia

Those writing about work with black clients have frequently spoken about the reticent and rather suspicious manner with which these clients relate to mental health workers (Block, 1981). Ridley (1984) writing about the "nondisclosing black client" points out the appropriateness for black people of a kind of "cultural paranoia" (Grier & Cobbs, 1968), a wariness regarding the behavior and motivations of white people. He suggests that for the therapist working with a black client, the dynamics of self-disclosure involve recognizing the difference for a given client between "functional paranoia," based on maladaptive personal reactions not related to race, and cultural paranoia. A "healthy cultural paranoiac"—low on functional paranoia and high on cultural paranoia—is more likely to be disclosive to a black therapist and nondisclosive to a white therapist, in this view. A "functional paranoiac"—low on cultural paranoia and high on nonracially based paranoid reactions—would be nondisclosing to either a black or a white therapist. Ridley goes on to suggest different strategies for addressing the client within this conception.

Managing the Early Sessions

Credibility

As problems of attrition with nonwhite ethnic minority clients are likely to be most acute early in the therapy encounter, what happens in the initial sessions is crucial. Gibbs (1985) and Griffith and Jones (1979) have suggested that one has the best chance of preventing premature termination in therapy with the minority client if one works actively and tactfully to engage the client from the very beginning of the contact. Sue and Zane (1987) indicate that the therapist must be able early on to establish his/her "credibility" and fulfill the client's expectation that (s)he is going to get something from the experience.

The client may begin to self-disclose on the basis of a therapist's "ascribed credibility," credit granted immediately based on his/her age, training, gender, and perhaps ethnic background if it matches that of the client. But the therapist must quickly move beyond this to work toward an "achieved credibility" by showing skill in dealing with the client. This accrues as the therapist is able to conceptualize the problem in a way that is compatible with the client's belief system and helps the client work toward goals and new ways of responding that are compatible with the client's culture. Thus, to take an obvious example, in working with a client from a traditional Asian-American background, it is probably well to be quite cautious about advocating frank expression of aggression to one's in-laws living in a traditionally structured family setting.

Sue and Zane (1987) suggest that another tradition from the Asian culture, that of gift-giving, may be broadly relevant with minority clients. Such "gifts" do not refer to tangible material objects, of course, but rather to such things as relief from negative feeling states; cognitive clarification—providing some initial enlightenment about what seems a hopelessly muddled situation; and "normalization," a sense that the problem, though having features unique to the client, is like those that other people have. Such interventions made early in the contact help the client feel more like pursuing the difficult process of self-revelation and self-exploration.

The Interpersonal Phase

Gibbs (1985) conceptualizes the dynamics in those early sessions in more detail. She argues that black clients tend to take an "interpersonal" stance in the psychotherapy initially rather than an "instrumental" stance to the treatment process. This interpersonal phase, which probably lasts no more than two or three sessions, is one in which the client is at first more attuned to the nature of the interaction with the therapist than to the particulars of the presenting problem. Until (s)he is satisfied with regard to the therapist's ability to be respectful of his/her ethnic sensitivities, the client will be minimally self-disclosing. Gibbs describes a sequence of several "microstages" in which the client assesses the therapist's ability to interact in a truly egalitarian way. If the therapist handles the stages of this phase appropriately, an alliance develops which enables the client to move into the more task-oriented, "instrumental" phase, in which the client begins to work on the more personality-based problem that initiated the search for help. It is at this point that the client becomes more genuinely self-disclosing. If the therapist does not respond appropriately, the client may well leave within two or three sessions. This perspective can probably be taken to have application to clients from varying nonwhite groups.

"Agency" in the Minority Client

The Gibbs perspective is consistent with the idea that the minority client, though troubled, and in some sense "demoralized" (Frank, 1973, p. 314) as (s)he comes to therapy, nevertheless attempts to take an active and purposeful role in the therapy situation. To some degree, these are aspects of the exercise of "psychological agency" that minority people use generally to maintain a viable sense of self as they negotiate life in a hostile society.

As I have suggested elsewhere (Jenkins, 1982, 1989) the term "psychological agency" characterizes a broadly human capacity which minorities have used to survive in America. This perspective draws on a specific and well-articulated approach to humanistic psychology (Rychlak, 1988). Key principles in this approach are: (1) subjectively held intentions and purposes are a primary though not exclusive motivating factor in human behavior; (2) "dialectical" thinking, the ability to fashion alternative conceptions of life circumstances is often used by people to circumvent negative situations; and (3) human mentality is actively structuring as it approaches experience and "constructs" the "reality" it considers to be meaningful. This framework is further enriched by including the notion that a lifelong striving for effective and competent interaction with the environment characterizes human behavior (White, 1963). Through the exercise of these features of psychological agency, many nonwhite ethnic minorities have survived their oppressive experience in America by bringing to life conceptions of their competence that have been at (dialectical) variance with the judgments that the majority society has made of them.

Agency and the Sense of Self

One way of describing the subjective sense of this agency in the person is by the concept of "self." From this introspective view, self is the sense of orientation or identity that guides a person's life choices. The notion of self also embodies the sense of authorship of one's thoughts and actions. Much of an individual's activity in life is oriented toward maintaining a sense of competence or self-esteem (White, 1963; Basch, 1988). Of course psychodynamic theory holds that important aspects of an individual's agency are not in awareness, and some initiatives that (s)he seeks to carry out stem from unconscious thoughts and feelings that are maladaptive in their effect. One of the fundamental purposes of enhancing self-disclosure in therapy is to help individuals become more aware of the disavowed scope of their agency and thus gain more control of their lives (Schafer, 1978, p. 180). This is as true for the nonwhite minority individual as for anyone. Persons who are freer from emotional disabilities are more able to act in the world and join with others to bring about social justice.

Racism and ethnic prejudice are assaults on these healthy self processes. The average ethnic minority person is able to withstand the buffeting of a hostile society, at some cost in personal energy, by pursuing competence strivings. Basch (1980), writing from the perspective of modern self psychology in psychoanalysis, argues that patients coming to psychotherapy bring the hope that they will be able to further the development of important aspects of their self-esteem that were hampered in the course of their living. Unconsciously they hope to be able to use the therapist as a kind of "selfobject" (Kohut, 1977), a person who will respond in ways that meet the specific needs of the developmentally weakened self. As noted, when the minority person acknowledges the need for psychological help, before (s)he can make use of the therapist in this way, (s)he must try and be certain of what kinds of attitudes the therapist brings from the larger society.

The added distrust that the minority client brings is not necessarily "resistance" generated by the processes of the "instrumental" phase (Gibbs, 1985; Jenkins, 1985). The minority client's special scrutiny of the therapist early in therapy and his/her concerns about the therapist's credibility involve some of the same processes of self-enhancement and self-assertiveness (s)he has had to use to adapt to the larger society. Research suggests that poor and minority clients are very sensitive to the presence or absence of "egalitarian" attitudes in the therapist (Lerner, 1972; Ross, 1983). Clearly the therapist's task is to be open to this scrutinizing activity if (s)he is to be taken as an ally in the minority client's efforts to remobilize his/her effectiveness.

Language and Psychotherapy

A more specific set of concerns with respect to self-disclosure by minority clients derives from the importance of language in psychotherapy. Levenson (1983, p. 143) suggests that, in general, the patient coming into psychotherapy may be described as suffering from a kind of "semiotic defect" in which, as a result of a history of distorted communication patterns with significant others, (s)he is unable effectively to symbolize in words the meaning of important aspects of past and present experience. From this writer's perspective, such a defect constrains the individual's exercise of his/her agency.

In focusing on the centrality of the construction and communication of meaning in psychotherapy, Levenson knowingly touches on an issue that is at the core of being human. Developing the capacity for language during growth gives the individual a powerful tool for fashioning the self. In all cultures, language is a preeminent means for shaping and framing intentions, and hence is at the heart of the exercise of one's agency and effectiveness in the world. It is also critical to the sense of being a participant in an ethnic heritage. To speak a language, said the psychiatrist Frantz Fanon (1967), "means above all to assume a culture"

(p. 17). Language processes are at the heart of the therapeutic enterprise, of course, and almost by definition are fundamental to issues related to self-disclosure.

The Therapist's Skill: "Linguistic Competence"

The importance of language in psychotherapy poses a particular kind of challenge to the dynamic therapist with any patient. In addition to creating a genuinely accepting atmosphere, the therapist's task is to understand the cognitive and, especially, the affective meaning embedded in the patient's speech. Psychodynamic theorists believe that this requires exercising the therapist's empathic abilities (Korchin, 1976, chap. 7; Jones, 1985). From Marshall Edelson's perspective (1975), such a skill depends to an important degree on the therapist's "linguistic competence": "the internalized knowledge of language that is possessed without conscious awareness of it or even the ability to explicate it..." (p. 27). This is so even where therapist and patient are from the same language community.

A further particular challenge for the psychodynamic therapist stems from what I would call the "dialectic" quality of human symbolizing capacities (Jenkins, 1988; Rychlak, 1979). Here this refers to the fact that people (often unconsciously) intend to convey alternative, even opposite, meanings with the same word or image, thus giving a rich complexity to verbal productions and fantasy life. This makes a patient's statements about a particular problem ambiguous on the surface. (This was nicely exemplified by the patient of hysterical character makeup who entered this writer's office in her overcoat one cold winter day. Seeing the window temporarily open so as to air out the overheated room, she stated firmly, "I'm not getting *undressed* until you close that window!") The therapist's task is to help the patient to "disambiguate" his/her utterances so that (s)he can get better control over what is being experienced (Edelson, 1975). Edelson continues this line of thought:

> What we call "intuition" in the psychoanalytic process may be an end product of the psychoanalyst's disciplined preconscious decision to permit himself to hear all the possible meanings of the analysand's language, no matter what particular meaning seems dictated by an immediate context. (p. 23)

Sociolinguistic Issues in Psychotherapy

Because language issues are important to self-disclosure, problems are likely to arise where patient and therapist do not share the same communicative style. The language disparity could occur either at the level of dialect differences or in differences in the mother tongue that each has learned to speak. As Russell (1988) notes in his excellent recent review of issues related to language and psychotherapy, language differences can affect the client's perception of the similarity between the therapist and patient, and this in turn can affect the patient's readiness to self-disclose, or even remain in therapy. The therapist's linguistic style can also affect his/her credibility in the patient's eyes (Russell, 1988). Although manifest structural differences in language between speakers can obviously complicate the communication process, perhaps even more important are the "sociolinguistic" aspects of speech in the therapy situation. Such concerns have to do with language "as a social and cultural phenomenon" (Trudgill, 1974, p. 32).

Language as Status Marker

One of the problems for the self-disclosure process in psychotherapy is that, in the larger society, speech differences are habitually used as a status marker for separating people into categories of worth (Trudgill, 1974; Williams, 1970). In our society, the prevailing view tends to be that all language forms that deviate from the standard represent language *deficits*—a failure to have learned to speak properly. Even more, those who speak a nonstandard dialect are seen as being inferior and not fully civilized. Fanon (1967) takes note of this in his caustic comments about the French attitudes toward colonials:

> The Negro of the Antilles will be proportionately whiter—that is, he will come closer to being a real human being—in direct ratio to his mastery of the French language. (p. 18)
>
> Yes, I must take great pains with my speech, because I shall be more or less judged by it. With great contempt they will say of me, "He doesn't even know how to speak French." (p. 20)

Such a way of thinking certainly characterizes the predominantly monolingual mainstream American society. It is a part of that biased milieu mentioned earlier in this paper that can affect the quality of the therapeutic interaction.

Suitability for Therapy

One of the effects on therapy of pejorative attitudes toward language difference is that it probably contributes to the tendency to judge the speaker with a different language background as being more disordered and/or generally less suitable for the expressive psychotherapies (Geller, 1988). Apart from there being little empirical evidence to support this notion, it seems wrong in principle. Recognizing that language is crucial to the full development of a person in any cultural setting, to treat some groups of people as if words don't ordinarily mean much to them is almost to consider them less than human. As Marshall Edelson (1971) notes, "a scarcity of language resources... [and the] inability to symbolize emotional, physiological, and sensory experience is not incidental to psychological illness but may in fact doom an individual to it" (p. 119). To deny a person the opportunity to overcome personal "semiotic defects" (Levenson, 1983) within his/her own idiom in therapy would perhaps be tantamount to abandoning the patient "to a life of sleepwalking in a twilight zone of quasi-consciousness, in which he [would have to] depend for relief of his pain solely upon the efficient manipulation of his body and his environment" (Edelson, 1971, p. 119).

Russell (1988) suggests that while many therapists are able to ward off the blatant American stereotypes associated with ethnic characteristics of nonwhite persons, particularly if these clients are standard English (SE) speakers, these therapists are much more vulnerable to the culture's attitudes toward people whose dialect is not standard. Thus, Russell asserts that no matter how well-meaning the therapist is, unless (s)he has considerable experience with a *nonclinical* sample of the language group from which a given client comes, the chances are great that the clinician will misconceptualize the nonstandard English (NSE) speaking client. Russell suggests that, among other things, the therapist should be ready to call on a knowledgeable consultant in working with such persons. (The need for such help is particularly likely when the clients are depressed, acting-out, lower-class black male adolescents, an especially resistive and nondisclosing group (Gibbs, 1988; Paster, 1985).

Self-Disclosure to Oneself

It is not only that subtly pejorative attitudes on the therapist's part stifle revelation to another person; an important *intrapersonal* process is shut off as well. Self-disclosure involves not only communication between persons, it involves the individual's disclosing hidden or unarticulated aspects of experience to himself/herself. Citing a clinical example, Basch (1988) reports having commented to a patient who described himself as not being "much of a talker," that the problem wasn't so much his inability to talk to other people. The primary difficulty was "that you can't talk things over with yourself inside your head. Without words, it's hard to think things through, to consider different possibilities" (p. 230). The opportunity to develop new labels and new constructions of past and current experience allows the person a changed way of "coming at" the world.

Some Dynamics of Language Difference in Therapy

That which smothers open communication strikes at the very heart of the healing process in therapy. This is made even more complex where there are issues of language difference between therapist and patient. Some writers suggest that such issues have implication for technique in the therapy situation.

The "Language Barrier"

Clinical experience with bilingual patients suggests that when psychotherapy is conducted in the language in which the patient is less fluent, the person's ability to express affect is often hindered by a kind of "language barrier" (Marcos & Urcuyo, 1979). In such circumstances, the patient may show considerable emotional detachment from material being discussed, leading to a kind of vagueness in the affective experiences described, and an inability to benefit from catharsis and abreaction in therapy. Marcos postulates that, for one thing, a person speaking the language in which (s)he is less proficient, tends to go through a special encoding and translation process which focuses the person more on *how* (s)he is speaking rather than on *what* (s)he is saying. The speaker becomes more concentrated on the cognitive and linguistic aspects of the communication, to the detriment of the affect involved (Marcos, 1976; Marcos & Urcuyo, 1979).

Rozensky and Gomez (1983) point also to the fact that the speaker's subordinate language is usually learned at a later stage in personality development than is the first language or the "mother tongue." Thus many important developmental experiences are not as readily available to the patient in verbal form when the therapy is conducted in the patient's second language. From a psychodynamic perspective, "Therapy which uses the second tongue as the main form of communication may suppress the mother tongue and the affective experiences tied to it" (p. 154). Thus, when warded-off material emerges in therapy, it "may not accurately reflect the experiential aspects of the original events" (p. 155).

Some bilingual persons have native proficiency in both languages. Even here there can be language-related problems in the therapy. Where these persons have learned each language in a different cultural context, they may "operate parallel encoding mechanisms, each with its own stream of associations between message words and events in the ideational system" (Marcos & Urcuyo, 1979, p. 334). This separation in the patient's intrapsychic experience may extend to the point of a rather deep-seated duality in the sense of self, and such patients may "feel and perceive themselves as two different persons according to the language that they speak" (p. 335). These patients do not necessarily come into therapy for identity conflicts related to language, but as therapy progresses, problems come to light that sometimes reveal a number of concerns regarding ethnicity and acculturation.

Bidialectic Speakers and "Code Switching"

Nonwhite minorities in the U.S. often come from bidialectic, if not bilingual, social backgrounds and contexts. That is, even if they have a workable command of SE for use in more formal social situations or with relative strangers, they may use a nonstandard dialect or their "mother tongue" in informal or more intimate situations (Gumperz & Hernandez-Chavez, 1972; Kernan, 1971; Russell, 1988). In linguistic terms, they may engage in "code switching" in their daily lives. Jenkins (1982, Chapter 4) has suggested that in spite of its controversial status Black Nonstandard English or "Black English" is a means that African-American individuals have of "coming home" to their own culture, as it were, even though they may be full participants in many aspects of the broad American social scene. The command of the dialect is a way of keeping alive the ethnic roots that have nurtured them.

Ideally, as clients delve into unresolved conflictual issues in therapy, they would feel comfortable in expressing themselves in NSE to capture the full impact of a feeling or experience they are struggling with. However, Russell (1988) asserts that this development in therapy does not necessarily come easily, even once the client has moved into the "instrumental" phase of therapy (Gibbs, 1985). Clients who are comfortable in both SE and NSE, and accustomed to using SE in more formal situations, are prone to match the therapist's SE style. Such formality is likely to lead to greater restriction of personal information and lowered emotional expressiveness on the client's part. Russell suggests that to circumvent this, the therapist might explore with the patient who the people are with whom the patient shares more intimate information, and what the context is in which (s)he does so. This discussion should also begin to include exploration of the differences the client feels in talking with the therapist about intimate things. From these kinds of efforts an atmosphere ideally develops in which the patient begins to feel encouraged to use in therapy the style that allows greater self-disclosure and thus enhances the processes that are fundamental to successful self-exploration.

Language Switching

In some instances, with bilingual patients, the use of "language switching" is advocated, that is, explicitly encouraging the client to discuss or label in the mother tongue a troubling conflict that emerges in therapy (Marcos & Urcuyo, 1979; Rozensky & Gomez, 1983). Such a strategy can presumably help clients overcome the detachment in their description of emotional experiences, or facilitate gaining access to early developmental issues that may be central to a key conflict. Rozensky and Gomez (1983) present several illustrative case examples. Even when the therapist does not share the patient's bilinguality, encouraging the client to describe the essence of an experience or feeling in the mother tongue and then discussing the meaning with the therapist may open new avenues of self-exploration and even be enhancing to the relationship.

It is acknowledged that selective use of this technique is called for in the context of an evaluation of the patient's language status. At times it may be more adaptive to encourage the patient to use the second language to defend against being overwhelmed by an affective issue (Marcos & Urcuyo, 1979; Rozensky & Gomez, 1983). The degree to which the client's language status affects the ability to gain access to his/her emotionality in therapy in the second language depends on a variety of factors, such as the relative extent to which each language is used in the patient's daily life; the age at which the second language was acquired; and how emotionally expressive each of the two languages is (Rozensky & Gomez, 1983).

The overall point here is that with many nonwhite ethnic minority patients there will be the likelihood of some language-related dynamics both from the patient's as well as the therapist's side that will affect the atmosphere for self-disclosure. A patient's NSE dialect or native tongue is an important tool of self-assertion and an important aspect of self-identification. The therapist's sensitivity to that language is a concrete example of wanting to understand the patient on his/her "own terms." Russell (1988) goes so far as to suggest that

> Many of the typical problems identified in work with low-income and minority clients (not being verbal, failing to self-disclose, and looking for quick solutions and direction as opposed to introspection) can at least be partially explained by language-related dynamics. (p. 64)

Therapist Self-Disclosure

Much of the discussion in this chapter has pointed implicitly to the complementary issue regarding self-disclosure, namely self-revelation by the therapist. Again, much could be said about this topic, but we will have to confine ourselves to a few points here. Humanistic therapists write of the need for "genuineness" in the therapeutic encounter, which could include disclosure by the therapist of personal feelings or history

(Rogers, 1957). Traditional psychodynamic therapists are likely to be more reticent about frank self-revelation. As an "interpersonal paradigm" (Gill, 1983) begins to gain more support from various quarters within the psychodynamic perspective (Levenson, 1983; Luborsky, 1984; Strupp & Binder, 1984), it is becoming clearer that it is impossible for the therapist not to disclose aspects of himself/herself, even while attempting to be neutral.

Harking back to our earlier discussion in this chapter regarding the person as active agent, we must recognize that the observation process in any interpersonal situation is a two-way street. The patient is actively observing the therapist and bringing to this observation his/her typical way of constructing images of other people and relationships. Levenson (1983) cites an example from Ralph Greenson:

> a patient points out that when he expresses opinions that match the therapist's, he gets marginal cues of approval; when he doesn't, he is subjected to masked hostile analysis. He documents this position with examples. The therapist, decently and honestly, [confirms this blind spot]. (p. 86)

While the patient's sensitivity to the subtly authoritarian quality in this relationship stemmed from his own personality dispositions, these characterological problems were played out in the context of actual contributions from the therapist.

The "Contextual Unit"

In this regard the particular focus on transference taken by the psychoanalyst Evelyne Schwaber is relevant. In her writing she criticizes the traditional tendency of therapists to respond to transference material as if it came *only* from the patient's dynamics. Such a stance allows the therapist to overlook his/her contribution to the interpersonal field in which the therapy takes place. She proposes instead that the participants in therapy are best seen as making up a "contextual unit" in which each one's experience of the reality in that system comes from how each one views (that is, makes mental constructs of) the participation of the other, as well as from what each brings to it in terms of personality dispositions. From this view Schwaber (1983) notes that her therapeutic stance is a mode of listening that "is characterized by my sustained effort to seek out my place in the patient's experience, as part of the context that is perceived or felt" (p. 523). This means that the therapist cannot consider herself/himself to be outside the contextual unit that is the therapy situation, because his/her inevitable participation determines the very nature of it.

This adds a particular emphasis to the earlier discussion of how minority patients in particular see it as a matter of self-preservation to assess their therapist's cultural attitudes and flexibility (Gibbs, 1985; Jenkins, 1985). Thus, a particular challenge for the therapist with the minority client is to become aware of—that is, to disclose to oneself—and master those negative attitudes that are very likely to carry over from the larger social milieu. Various writers have suggested ways that therapists can monitor themselves and continue their education (for example, Acosta, Yamamoto, & Evans, 1982; Cheek, 1976; Russell, 1988; Smith, Burlew, Mosley, & Whitney, 1978).

Conclusion

I have proposed here that enhancing self-disclosure in therapy with the nonwhite ethnic minority client requires first that the therapist be fully conscious of the ongoing racial context in which (s)he and the patient live. It requires the therapist's recognition that (s)he is in some way affected by this atmosphere and brings that to the treatment situation.

I have also proposed that we must add to the usual, too-simple view of the minority patient as only a victim, facing the double jeopardy of social oppression and personal psychopathology. The nonwhite ethnic minority client, like all people, is an agent seeking to further a sense of competence in life. Minority patients in the interests of survival bring the same carefully evaluative attitudes to therapy that they have used historically to adapt to institutions in this society. The effective therapist must be open from the beginning to the special scrutiny of his/her egalitarianism. (S)he must also be prepared to develop a special sensitivity to the dynamics of language use in the therapy situation. I believe that there is no question that dynamic psychotherapy relevant to the patient's personal needs and ethnocultural heritage can be empowering for minority clients. As Lerner (1974) notes:

> Generic psychotherapy is fully compatible with social change because it is an attempt to restore personal power—self-understanding, self-control, self-direction, and self-esteem—through the development of an honest, empathic egalitarian relationship with another human being. (p. 53)

I believe also that such a process can occur in cross-ethnic therapy situations if a skilled therapist is honest and open with himself/herself and prepared to learn.

References

Acosta, F.X., Yamamoto, J., & Evans, L.A. (1982). *Effective psychotherapy for low-income and minority patients*. New York: Plenum.

Banks, G., Berenson, B.G., & Carkhuff, R.R. (1967). The effects of counselor race and training upon the counseling process with Negro clients in initial interviews. *Journal of Clinical Psychology, 23*, 70–72.

Basch, M.F. (1980). *Doing psychotherapy*. New York: Basic Books.

Basch, M.F. (1988). *Understanding psychotherapy: The science behind the art*. New York: Basic Books.

Block, C.B. (1981). Black Americans and the cross-cultural counseling and psychotherapy experience. In A.J. Marsella & P.B. Pedersen (Eds.), *Cross-cultural counseling and psychotherapy* (pp. 177–194). Elmsford, NY: Pergamon.

Bulhan, H.A. (1985). *Frantz Fanon and the psychology of oppression*. New York: Plenum.

Carkhuff, R.R., & Pierce, R. (1967). Differential effects of therapist race and social class upon patient depth of self-exploration in the initial clinical interview. *Journal of Consulting Psychology, 31*, 632–634.

Cheek, D.K. (1976). *Assertive black...puzzled white*. San Luis Obispo, CA: Impact.

Comas-Diaz, L. (1988). Cross-cultural mental health treatment. In L. Comas-Diaz & E.E.H. Griffiths (Eds.), *Clinical guidelines in cross-cultural mental health* (pp. 335–361). New York: Wiley.

Comas-Diaz, L., & Griffiths, E.E.H. (Eds.). (1988). *Clinical guidelines in cross-cultural mental health*. New York: Wiley.

Dudley, R., & Rawlins, M. (Eds.). (1985). Special issue: Psychotherapy with ethnic minorities. *Psychotherapy: Theory, Research, Practice, Training, 22*, No. 2 (Supp.).

Edelson, M. (1971). *The idea of a mental illness*. New Haven: Yale University Press.

Edelson, M. (1975). *Language and interpretation in psychoanalysis*. New Haven: Yale University Press.

Fanon, F. (1967). *Black skin, white masks*. New York: Grove.

Frank, J.D. (1973). *Persuasion and healing: A comparative study of psychotherapy* (2nd ed.). Baltimore: Johns Hopkins University Press.

Gardner, LaM. H. (1971). The therapeutic relationship under varying conditions of race. *Psychotherapy: Theory, Research and Practice, 8*, 78–87.

Geller, J.D. (1988). Racial bias in the evaluation of patients for psychotherapy. In L. Comas-Diaz & E.E.H. Griffiths (Eds.), *Clinical guidelines in cross-cultural mental health* (pp. 112–134). New York: Wiley.

Gibbs, J.T. (1985). Treatment relationships with black clients: Interpersonal vs. instrumental strategies. In *Advances in clinical social work practice*. Silver Spring, MD: National Assoc. of Social Workers, Inc.

Gibbs, J.T. (Ed.). (1988). *Young, black, and male in America*. Dover, MA: Auburn House.

Gill, M.M. (1983). The interpersonal paradigm and the degree of the therapist's involvement. *Contemporary Psychoanalysis, 19*, 200–237.

Grier, W.H., & Cobbs, P.M. (1968). *Black rage*. New York: Basic Books.

Griffith, M.S., & Jones, E.E. (1979). Race and psychotherapy: Changing perspectives. In J.H. Masserman (Ed.), *Current psychiatric therapies*, Vol. 18 (pp. 225–235). New York: Grune & Stratton.

Gumperz, J.J., & Hernandez-Chavez, E. (1972). Bilingualism, bidialectalism, and classroom interaction. In C.B. Cazden, V.P. John & D. Hymes (Eds.). *Functions of language in the classroom* (pp. 84–108). New York: Teachers College Press.

Jenkins, A.H. (1982). *The psychology of the Afro-American: A humanistic approach*. Elmsford, NY: Pergamon.

Jenkins, A.H. (1985). Attending to self-activity in the Afro-American client. *Psychotherapy: Theory, Research, Practice, Training, 22*, (2 S), 335–341.

Jenkins, A.H. (1988). *Contributions of a rigorous humanism to psychoanalytic theory*. Paper presented at American Psychological Assn. meeting, Atlanta, Ga.

Jenkins, A.H. (1989). Psychological agency: A crucial concept for minorities. *Theoretical and Philosophical Psychology, 9*, 4–11.

Jones, E.E. (1978). Effects of race on psychotherapy process and outcome: An exploratory investigation. *Psychotherapy: Theory, Research and Practice, 15,* 226–236.
Jones, E.E. (1985). Psychotherapy and counseling with black clients. In P. Pedersen (Ed.), *Handbook of Cross-cultural counseling and therapy.* Westport, CT.: Greenwood.
Jordan, W. (1968). *White over black.* Chapel Hill: University of North Carolina Press.
Kernan, C.M. (1971). Language behavior in a black urban community. *Monographs of the Language-Behavior Research Laboratory,* University of California, Berkeley, No. 2.
Kohut, H. (1977). *The restoration of the self.* New York: International Universities Press.
Korchin, S.J. (1976). *Modern clinical psychology.* New York: Basic Books.
Kovel, J. (1984). *White racism: A psychohistory* (2nd ed.). New York: Columbia University Press.
Lerner, B. (1972). *Therapy in the ghetto: Political impotence and personal disintegration.* Baltimore: Johns Hopkins University Press.
Lerner, B. (1974). Is psychotherapy relevant to the needs of the poor? In D.A. Evans & W.L. Claiborn (Eds.), *Mental health issues and the urban poor* (pp. 49–54). Elmsford, N.Y.: Pergamon.
Levenson, E.A. (1983). *The ambiguity of change: An inquiry into the nature of psychoanalytic reality.* New York: Basic Books.
Luborsky, L. (1984). *Principles of psychoanalytic psychotherapy: A manual for supportive-expressive treatment.* New York: Basic Books.
Marcos, L.R. (1976). Bilinguals in psychotherapy: Language as an emotional barrier. *American Journal of Psychotherapy, 30,* 552–560.
Marcos, L.R., & Urcuyo, L. (1979). Dynamic psychotherapy with the bilingual patient. *American Journal of Psychotherapy, 33,* 331–338.
McGoldrick, M., Pearce, J.K., & Giordano, J. (Eds.). (1982). *Ethnicity and family therapy.* New York: Guilford.
Paster, V.S. (1985). Adapting psychotherapy for the depressed, unacculturated, acting-out, black male adolescent. *Psychotherapy: Theory, Research, Practice, Training, 22,* (2 S), 408–417.
Pedersen, P. (Ed.). (1985). *Handbook of cross-cultural counseling and therapy.* Westport, CT: Greenwood.
Plasky, P., & Lorion, R.P. (1984). Demographic parameters of self-disclosure to psychotherapists and others. *Psychotherapy: Theory, Research, Practice, Training, 21,* 483–490.
Ridley, C.R. (1984). Clinical treatment of the nondisclosing black client: A therapeutic paradox. *American Psychologist, 39,* 1234–1244.
Rogers, C.R. (1957). The necessary and sufficient conditions of therapeutic personality change. *Journal of Consulting Psychology, 21,* 95–103.
Ross, S. (1983). Variables associated with dropping out of therapy. (Doctoral dissertation, New York University, 1983). *Dissertation Abstracts International, 44,* 616B.
Rozensky, R.H., & Gomez, M.Y. (1983). Language switching in psychotherapy with bilinguals: Two problems, two models, and case examples. *Psychotherapy: Theory, Research and Practice, 20,* 152–160.
Russell, D.M. (1988). Language and psychotherapy: The influence of nonstandard English in clinical practice. In L. Comas-Diaz & E.E.H. Griffiths (Eds.), *Clinical guidelines in cross-cultural mental health* (pp. 33–68). New York: Wiley.
Rychlak, J.F. (1979). *Discovering free will and personal responsibility.* New York: Oxford University Press.
Rychlak, J.F. (1988). *The psychology of rigorous humanism* (2nd ed.). New York: New York University Press.
Schafer, R. (1978). *Language and insight: The Sigmund Freud Memorial Lectures 1975–1976, University College London.* New Haven, Conn. and London: Yale University Press.
Schwaber, E.A. (1983). A particular perspective on psychoanalytic listening. *Psychoanalytic Study of the Child, 38,* 519–546.

Smith, M., & Dejoie-Smith, M. (1984). Behavior therapy for nonwhite, non-YAVIS clients: Myth or panacea? *Psychotherapy: Theory, Research, Practice, Training, 21*, 524–529.

Smith, W.D., Burlew, A.K., Mosley, M.H., & Whitney, W.M. (1978). *Minority issues in mental health*. Reading, MA: Addison-Wesley.

Strupp, H.H., & Binder, J.L. (1984). *Psychotherapy in a new key: A guide to time-limited dynamic psychotherapy*. New York: Basic Books.

Sue, S. (1977). Community mental health services to minority groups: Some optimism, some pessimism. *American Psychologist, 32*, 616–624.

Sue, D., & Sue, S. (1987). Cultural factors in the clinical assessment of Asian Americans. *Journal of Consulting & Clinical Psychology, 55*, 479–487.

Sue, S., & Zane, N. (1987). The role of culture and cultural techniques in psychotherapy: A critique and reformulation. *American Psychologist, 42*, 37–45.

Thomas, A., & Sillen, S. (1972). *Racism and psychiatry*. New York: Brunner/Mazel.

Trudgill, P. (1974). *Sociolinguistics: An introduction*. Harmondsworth, England: Penguin Books.

White, R.W. (1963). Ego and reality in psychoanalytic theory. *Psychological Issues, 3*, (11).

Williams, F. (1970). Language, attitude, and social change. In F. Williams (Ed.), *Language and poverty* (pp. 380–399). Chicago: Markham.

10

Feminist Therapy Perspectives on Self-Disclosure

Laura S. Brown and Lenore E. A. Walker

Introduction

Unlike many other theories of psychotherapy, feminist therapy theory has from its inception promulgated the idea that self-disclosure by the therapist may be a valuable part of the therapy process (Greenspan, 1986). This concept appears in some of the earliest literature addressing the nature of the client–therapist relationship in feminist therapy (Mander & Rush, 1974; Lerman, 1976; Rawlings & Carter, 1977), and has continued to form a core of the feminist therapy mandate to empower clients, as well as heal their wounds. Guidelines for the use of self-disclosure can be found in the Ethical Code of the Feminist Therapy Institute (FTI), which specifically refers to ethical ways in which self-disclosure can and should be used by a therapist (Feminist Therapy Ethical Code, 1987), and discussion of the implementation of this code and its norms is ongoing (Lerman & Porter, 1990). This proactive embrace of self-disclosure is unique among theories of psychotherapy, and reflects certain core tenets of feminist therapy theory regarding the relationship of client and therapist and the role of the therapist in the healing process.

In this chapter, we will review those aspects of feminist therapy theory that tend to support the use of self-disclosure in therapy, discuss the development of that theory, including some of the early difficulties

Laura S. Brown • 4527 First Avenue NE, Seattle, Washington 98105. **Lenore E. A. Walker** • Walker and Associates, 50 South Steele Street, Suite 850, Denver, Colorado 80209.

encountered in the use of self-disclosure, and then explore ways in which feminist therapists use self-disclosure as a part of their work. In reviewing this history, it is important to remember that feminist therapy is a grassroots phenomenon with no single acknowledged founder or leader. It grew out of critiques by the feminist movement of the 1960s and early 1970s in the United States, which pointed out that the goals of traditional psychotherapy appeared to promote women's adjustment to an oppressive status quo rather than supporting women's struggles toward equality (Chesler, 1972; Weisstein, 1970).

Initially, feminist therapy was primarily a philosophy by which therapy was approached rather than a prescription of techniques, although certain norms were implied. The acceptance and, some would say, the implied prescription of self-disclosure so as to create a "consciousness-raising group of two" (Maracek & Kravetz, 1977) was one of the hallmarks of this "first generation" philosophy of feminist therapy. By the early 1980s, feminist therapy began to integrate into its core those modifications to traditional systems that had been made by feminist practitioners of various standard approaches to psychotherapy. This "second generation" of feminist therapy theory created variations on the model for self-disclosure and debates about its use, but retained the notion that therapist self-disclosure and the active use of self by the therapist were essential elements of feminist therapy practice (Douglas & Walker, 1988; Ballou & Gabalac, 1985; Sturdivant, 1980). Work is currently in progress on the development of a cohesive model of feminist therapy, and all indications are that self-disclosure will continue to hold a central place in what might be called the "third generation" of feminist therapy (Dutton-Douglas & Walker, 1989; Lerman & Porter, 1990).

A Brief Review of Self-Disclosure in Feminist Therapy Theory

Feminist therapy as a concept arose from the second wave of the North American women's movement in the late 1960s and early 1970s. It was spread by word of mouth throughout Europe and South America, and its worldwide practice was well established by the time of the 1985 Nairobi Conference marking the end of the UN Decade for Women (Gore & Walker, 1986). Feminist therapy as practiced reflects the norms and modes of mental health care delivery that predominate in a given cultural or social context. However, certain tenets appear to be core and to transcend cultural differences.

During the initial development of feminist therapy theorizing, psychotherapists who were also feminists began to apply the political critique of sexism found in other cultural institutions to the institution of psychotherapy. Data had begun to grow demonstrating the negative impact of sexism and sexist practices on women's mental health (Walker, 1984a; Reiker & Carmen, 1984; Chesler, 1972). In addition, feminists in general targeted psychotherapy as one of those institutions of modern culture that attempted to impose social controls on women's freedom of action and self-definition by defining a rigid feminine gender role as the only path for "normalcy" or "mental health" for women.

Such critiques resonated for many women, and in fact found empirical validation soon after being raised in the work of Broverman and her colleagues, which demonstrated the presence of a double and lesser standard of mental health for women (Broverman, Broverman, Clarkson, Rosencrantz, & Vogel, 1970). Other critiques exposed how labeling women as psychologically "ill" was used as a strategy for maintaining women in their prescribed social roles (Chesler, 1972), and sexist bias within the practice of psychotherapy was described (Report of the Task Force, 1975). Although almost two decades have passed since these criticisms were first raised, current data suggests that gender bias still remains a problematic and present factor in the practice of traditional psychotherapies (Rosencrantz, Delorey, & Broverman, 1985; Rosewater & Walker, 1985; Ballou & Gabalac, 1985).

Seizing upon these criticisms, early feminist therapists attempted to integrate this political analysis into their work with clients. Such political analysis included the compilation of individual women's stories with the goal of extracting a common theme that could be used to help clients comprehend the roots and impact of their oppression. This feminist notion that "the personal is political" grew from the consciousness-raising process in which women joined together to share personal stories in a nontherapeutic context of mutual self-help and support.

Because of the blurred boundaries between feminist therapy as it was first practiced and consciousness-raising, which was an explicitly political rather than therapeutic approach to women's lives and problems, some early feminist thinkers felt that therapy of any sort would undermine political analysis and growth, and could not avoid some of the problems inherent in the psychotherapy process per se (Wycoff, 1977). This criticism that any therapy, even feminist therapy, is overly embedded in traditional and masculinist social status quos is still held by some feminist philosophers (Hoagland, 1988; Dykewomon, 1988; Raymond, 1986). Others have attempted to reconcile these tensions by overtly integrating political action into therapeutic work (Pheterson, 1988). However, many other feminists, desiring a psychotherapeutic experience for themselves, have felt that a feminist therapy perspective, in which attention was paid to social and contextual factors, was valuable and worth developing. Much of the initial work of feminist therapists centers on sorting out the differences between problems of living that are common to the experience of being a particular gender, race, class, or sexual orientation, as opposed to problems that are still current evidence of individual personal problems.

The first generation of feminist therapists also struggled with the questions of whether and to what degree biology as versus social context contributed to the development of personality. The initial resolution of this question within feminist therapy was to assume social construction of gendered behavior until and unless more convincing evidence could be marshaled for a biological explanation. Since the sexist bias of the life sciences in the formulation and interpretation of research questions has been well-documented (Bleier, 1984), most feminist therapists would agree that while there is most likely an interactive relationship between nature and nurture in the development of gendered behavior, the meaning and contribution of biology cannot be well understood at this time because of this bias in the biological literature and its impact on the nature of empiricism and scientific inquiry.

Although feminist therapy does not, as previously mentioned, have a founder or official spokesperson, most feminist therapists would probably agree with certain basic definitions of feminist therapy (Greenspan, 1983; Rosewater, 1988; Brown & Liss-Levinson, 1981; Cammaert & Larsen, 1989; Dutton-Douglas & Walker, 1989; Gilbert, 1980). Such definitions emphasize that the absence of equality between women and men in social, political, economic, educational, and other spheres requires that therapists take a stance of political action and advocacy, and that such a stance be explicitly integrated into the work of therapy. This proactive advocacy model differentiates *feminist* therapy from *nonsexist* therapy, an approach that simply acknowledges that such inequalities exist (Rawlings & Carter, 1977). The modal definition of feminist therapy includes norms for practice. These include the importance of developing an egalitarian relationship between client and therapist as a model for the overall development of such relationships in the client's life and the rendering of close attention to the impact of all the various forms of oppression and discrimination experienced by clients, including but not limited to racism, classism, heterosexism, homophobia, ageism, able-bodiedism, and fat oppression. Another important modal value of feminist therapy has been that of analysis of the power imbalance inherent in the psychotherapeutic relationship, and a focus on empowering clients to define the meanings of their own lives. Feminist therapists have paid particular attention to the impact of high base-rate phenomena in women's lives, such as violence in the home, and have noted how the common female experience of being harmed and betrayed by one on whom you are dependent and whom you love (e.g., incestuous fathers, battering partners) implies careful attention to the arrangement of power and dependency in the psychotherapeutic relationship. Feminist therapists have attempted to develop strategies for reducing rather than reinforcing the power imbalance. Therapist self-disclosure has been such a strategy in a relationship of inherently unequal power such as psychotherapy.

The corrective experience, as conceptualized from a feminist therapy framework, has included the therapist's ability to aid her client in expanding her/his vision of the alternatives available so that she/he can make informed choices rather than nonconsciously acquiescing to the norms of sexist stereotypes (Bem & Bem, 1976). Change is construed as occurring in all domains, e.g., cognitive, affective, and behavioral, and a variety of techniques have been integrated into feminist therapy practice to provide the opportunity for such changes. Bibliotherapy, body work, dream analysis, political analysis, skill enhancement, cognitive restructuring and reframing, desensitization, assertion training, gestalt awareness techniques, and various approaches to affective catharsis have all found a place in the work of feminist therapists (Dutton-Douglas & Walker, 1989; Rosewater & Walker, 1985).

In picking and choosing different techniques from among already extant therapies, first generation feminist therapy developed as a hybrid. However, each of these approaches, often developing initially in ignorance of others, has maintained the convergence on those modal principles of feminist therapy described, and resemble one another closely enough to be all included under the rubric of feminist therapy. While some groups of feminist therapists have concentrated on mainstreaming its perspective into traditional approaches to psychotherapy, (cf. the work of the Stone Center group of authors) others have aimed at creating a system separate and unique from the mainstream (Brown, 1988a). Second and third generation feminist therapy includes both these perspectives (Dutton-Douglas & Walker, 1988).

Self-Disclosure in Feminist Therapy Theory

Among one of the primary critiques leveled by feminists against psychotherapy, as it has been traditionally practiced, is the nature of the power imbalance between therapist and client. Therapists, who have traditionally mostly been men, treat clients, who have been predominantly women, from behind the cloak of anonymity and authoritarian expertise. This heritage from the psychoanalytic roots of therapy practice encourages therapists to retain power and take control of the therapy session. The male therapist, with his role-assigned expertise, often feels free to make pronouncements and prescriptions to his female clients about how best to lead their lives. Although therapists are professionally socialized to see themselves as anonymous and value-free, making only such behavioral prescriptions or interpretations as are clearly in the client's best interests, the data from research on sexism in psychotherapy shows that therapists in actuality promote a very particular value system, one that reflects an androcentric norm (Chesler, 1972; Report of the Task Force, 1975; Rawlings & Carter, 1975). One of the earliest goals of feminist therapy has been to attempt the rebalancing of power in psychotherapy. This is accomplished by attending to those elements of the therapy process that enhance the power differential, then moving to modify or eliminate them. Self-disclosure, which makes the therapist's values known and available for scrutiny and discussion by the client, is but one of several methods initially used to accomplish this rebalancing (Greenspan, 1986).

Given the core principle of feminist therapy that the therapy relationship should be an egalitarian one, in which the values of the therapist are clearly delineated so that the client is freer to reject or accept them in a conscious fashion, several strategies became popular in first generation feminist therapy practice. First names have been used by both therapist and client, rather than having the therapist called by the honorific "Dr. X," while the client is referred to by her first name. This change acknowledges the equal value of each partner in the therapy process, and particularly is meant to underscore the importance of the client's contribution to therapy rather than minimizing the value of the therapist's contribution. The client has been defined as fully expert regarding her own needs and values as the therapist, with the therapist's expertise more narrowly defined in terms of specific knowledge and skills that are useful in facilitating the client's goals. Although on occasion either therapist or client carried this equalizing process to extremes in which the therapist's knowledge was so devalued as to undermine any therapeutic movement at all, in general this move away from an authoritarian model for therapists models a challenge to therapist power and was taken up by other systems of psychotherapy during the 1970s.

Formal diagnosis was initially eschewed as unnecessarily stigmatizing and as serving only to create distance between therapist and client (Rawlings & Carter, 1977). The process of diagnosis and assessment as traditionally practiced encouraged therapists to think and talk about their clients in a particularistic language, not readily understood by the client; the metamessage of such diagnostic thinking was to create a separate species of humans, called by their various diagnostic categories, from whom therapists maintained emotional and social distance. The methods by which formal psychiatric diagnoses were developed were also problematic in being themselves biased by sexist and other oppressive perspectives (Kaplan, 1983; Caplan, 1984; Rothblum, Solomon, & Albee, 1986). While feminist therapists have begun to reevaluate the use of diagnosis in their practice, particularly in light of recent movements towards even more sexist diagnostic categories in the latest revision of the Diagnostic and Statistical Manual III (1987), this reevaluation has focused on ways in which diagnosis becomes a dialogue between client and therapist with the client empowered to better understand the social and cultural roots of her/his distress (Brown, 1986, 1988b; Walker, 1986, 1988). Feminist therapists would argue that in order to participate in this egalitarian approach to diagnosis, a certain degree of therapist self-disclosure is required, both to clarify how the therapist developed her/his perspectives, and to model more openness by the client in sharing information for the diagnostic process. Thus, the therapist must disclose how she/he has developed her/his hypotheses about the client, what theories she/he references, and how she/he has included or discarded particular diagnostic ideas, rather than appealing to authority in imposing a diagnosis.

The Nature of Self-Disclosure in Feminist Therapy

Feminist therapists are encouraged to disclose to their client their personal values and biases, usually verbally, (although some feminist therapists also utilize written information to aid in the retention of such data) as part of the development of the therapeutic relationship (Mander & Rush, 1974; Wycoff, 1977; Greenspan, 1983; Brown & Liss-Levinson, 1981). To facilitate this process, feminist therapists have developed guidelines for clients about how to elicit such information and strategies for challenging therapists who are unwilling to be forthcoming. Such feminist psychology organizations as the Division of Psychology of Women of the American Psychological Association (APA), APA's Committee on Women in Psychology (CWP), and the Association for Women in Psychology (AWP) have participated in jointly preparing, publishing and distributing consumer rights pamphlets aimed at women psychotherapy clients (Women and Psychotherapy, 1985; If Sex Enters, 1987).

Consumer rights have thus been one factor motivating the use of at least some degree of self-disclosure as a norm in feminist therapy. If the therapist did not disclose information such as her/his views on highly charged and value-laden topics, e.g., nonmonogamous relationships, reproductive rights, women working outside the home, or lesbianism, then how was the client to know whether the therapist would offer (as would be hoped) nonsexist and unbiased support should these issues arise? Clients were also encouraged by feminist therapy consumer guidelines to find therapists who matched them on such variables as ethnicity, class background, sexual orientation, or political values, not all of which are apparent simply from visual inspection of the therapist. For clients to obtain such information with which to make decisions about seeing a particular practitioner, therapists were required to disclose a large amount of what had previously been considered personal and off-limits data about themselves.

A second goal for self-disclosure in feminist therapy was to facilitate the therapist's serving as a role model for her clients (a supposition which underlies the suggestion that clients find therapists who matched them demographically). In our own participation in the consciousness-raising group process of the late 1960s and early 1970s, feminist therapists had discovered that many of what had seemed private and unique concerns were in fact issues that most other women had faced and dealt with. Many feminist self-help groups were an outgrowth of this realization. The sharing of experiences between women feels so liberating, as well as healing, that the spirit of consciousness-raising groups pervaded early feminist therapy theorizing. As described earlier, individual feminist therapy has been construed as potentially being a consciousness-raising group of two (Kravetz, 1976). When the therapist self-disclosed and shared her personal vulnerabilities and solutions with the client, she validated the client's realities, letting the latter know that she/he was not alone nor pathological in her/his dilemmas. The therapist would become more real, more human. Symbolic or transferential aspects of the therapy process were downplayed or devalued in this first-generation approach to self-disclosure (Brown, 1984a; Greenspan, 1986). However, problems soon began to arise with this strategy, which will be more fully discussed at a later point.

One outgrowth of this devaluation of the transferential aspects of the therapist–client relationship was a series of experiments by feminist therapists in modifying the meaning of dual relationships so as to encompass ethically what appeared to be often unavoidable overlap between the personal and social lives of feminist clients and feminist therapists (Berman, 1985). Feminist therapists recognized that feminist communities functioned as psychological small towns; the probability became high that clients and therapists would encounter one another at political gatherings, women's cultural events, and even in social settings in the homes of mutual acquaintances (Brown, 1987a, 1990). Feminist therapists' personal behaviors and political beliefs may thus be disclosed to clients by demonstration or reputation within a community (Brown, 1984b). It quickly became apparent to many feminist therapists that it was impossible to create any semblance of anonymity in their work, and that the real self of the therapist would always be integrated into any symbolic representations that the client might develop.

If a particular feminist therapist is well-known and her opinions represented by the media when she is called upon as an expert in her field, she also self-discloses; at times, this can lead to distortions of the therapist's actual beliefs that must then be clarified with clients. Additionally, such self-disclosure means that the therapist may be known, occasionally inaccurately, to potential clients; without the therapist's making overt self-disclosures, clients enter treatment with knowledge of who the therapist is (both authors of this chapter, for example, have had new clients inform us that we were chosen after reading one of our published works). Often, particular issues provoke controversy within feminist communities (e.g., pornography, surrogate motherhood). When a feminist therapist is known to espouse one among many diverse positions on such an issue as the result of her own active participation in the feminist political discourse, she also self-discloses, whether she chooses to do so actively in a therapy session or not. Such political activity is considered ethically imperative for feminist therapists (Feminist Therapy Ethical Code, 1987); consequently, no matter how low the level of exposure that a particular feminist therapist might choose to express her political activism, it will lead to some degree of self-disclosure by implication.

Finally, the use of self-disclosure in feminist therapy was fueled by reaction against the overly distant, pseudo-anonymous style of orthodox psychoanalysis, which was the highest-status and often primary therapy modality being practiced during the period in which feminist therapy began to develop. Feminist therapists have continued over time to be critical of an overly distant style on the part of androcentrically trained therapists (Jordan, Surrey, & Kaplan, 1983; Greenspan, 1986).

In fact, some recent authors (Lerman & Porter, 1990) have suggested that being overly distant may be as damaging and thus ethically problematic in therapy as is an overt violation of a boundary under the guise of "closeness." Many early feminist therapy writings contain first-person accounts of frustration and struggles against the wall of a silent male analyst (Chesler, 1972; Report of the Task Force, 1975; Mander & Rush, 1974; Greenspan, 1983). Since criticism of other aspects of psychoanalytic theory and practice is also a common aspect of first generation feminist therapy writings, it should not be surprising to find that one remedy suggested for transforming therapy to a more human exchange was the encouragement of personal openness and genuineness on the part of the therapist. In this regard, early feminist therapy thinking was also strongly influenced by the work of Rogers (1951, 1961) and Perls (1971) regarding the value of the use of self by the therapist. The humanistic psychology movement of the 1970s had a profound impact on the training of many current feminist therapists, and a relationship between feminist therapy and other theories emphasizing personal growth and valuing wholeness is still quite common.

Several early feminist therapy writers also promulgated a perspective on therapy in which the therapist was more of a "facilitator," and less a therapist. This can particularly be found in the work of Wycoff (1976, 1977) and other writers who worked within the context of the Berkeley Radical Psychiatry movement of the early 1970s (Steiner, Wycoff, Goldstine, Lariviere, Schwebel, & Marcus, 1975). This school of thought, which began as an offshoot of Transactional Analysis, underplayed the special role of the therapist, and discouraged individual psychotherapy in favor of "problem-solving groups," in which all, including the facilitator, would work together as co-equals to deal with whatever issues group members would bring up. In such a context, which can still be found in the form of women's self-help groups, self-disclosure by the therapist/facilitator was a given, since she was expected to be a participant in the group herself, and to share in the process of personal and political analysis that took place.

All of these factors combined to create an implicit norm among feminist therapists that it was therapeutic to share our own experiences with our clients when the latter came to similar developmental milestones or crises. While most feminist therapists were able to integrate this use of self-disclosure into their work in a way that continued to be respectful of the needs and boundaries of the client, some problems arose early on that point out how self-disclosure, while continuing to be useful, must be applied in a very specific and thoughtful way rather than generally and across the board.

Problems in the Use of Self-Disclosure in Feminist Therapy

Perhaps the most common problem that arose among feminist therapists who were using self-disclosure as a therapeutic technique was the way in which it risked a blurring and obscuring of boundaries between the roles of client and therapist. Some therapists found themselves, under the guise of using self-disclosure to help the client, taking the therapy hour to discuss and deal with their own personal problems, thus engaging in what feminist therapists would consider unethical and potentially damaging role reversals. Such therapists were often substituting their own needs for supervision, consultation, or personal therapy with "mutual consciousness-raising" with clients. Some more naive therapists equated the concept of "egalitarian" relationships in therapy with "equal" relationships, attempting to establish a symmetry that was not present and could not be therapeutic, creating confusions between friendship and psychotherapy (Hoagland, 1988). "Empowering the client" by making her into the therapist's confidant was one particularly potentially harmful misapplication of the feminist therapy principles regarding self-disclosure.

Because self-disclosure was allowed and, to a certain degree, encouraged among therapists who often had no training or role models for effecting this behavior appropriately, it became difficult for some feminist therapists to allow themselves their own personal boundaries and privacy, and not to self-disclose at the client's request when it felt uncomfortable, unwise, or countertherapeutic to do so. This was often the case when the clients themselves were members of the feminist political community, and consequently invested in the belief that the therapist's views on all issues should be known so that that client could feel completely mirrored and validated.

Additionally, the small-community aspect of feminist therapy work often meant that the therapist's own joys and griefs would be known to clients; when a particular therapist prefers that she process her own pains in the privacy of friendship networks, therapy, or consultation, such a desire for boundaries should not be seen as running counter to the feminist therapy norm of self-disclosure, particularly since a client's request for more information may in fact be a thinly disguised wish for reassurance that the therapist will still be present for the client while processing her own issues. Each of the current authors has had the experience of having personally painful events occur in ways that made them known to parts of our client network, and has found that often what is most essential to actively self-disclose to clients at such times (given that the noncontrolled self-disclosure that we described has already occurred without our intent to share) is our ongoing commitment to self-care, which will *not* include processing the problem with our clients nor leaning on them for support in our own times of need. This modeling of self-care and the choice of appropriate sources of emotional support, can, however, be a useful application of self-disclosure, particularly with women clients who are themselves in caretaker roles.

It is not unusual for meetings of feminist therapists to be filled with conversations about difficult decisions in boundary management, especially with clients who are part of the feminist political community. Therapists discuss feeling trapped when queried by clients who are political activists, in particular when the latter represent viewpoints different from our own. This can be especially challenging when clients present with strong tendencies towards splitting and severe narcissistic wounds that demand constant mirroring and validation. Feminist therapists can often feel caught between the perceived "imperative" to self-disclose upon request, and our own needs to maintain privacy and exercise clinical judgment. Learning to create this balance has characterized much of the work done in the second and third generations of feminist therapy theory development (Brown, 1987a).

Another problem that arose early in the development of feminist therapy with the use of self-disclosure was that it encouraged therapists to overgeneralize from their own experiences, and potentially discount and devalue differences between the needs, skills, and resources of client and therapist. This problem takes on particular significance when client and therapist differ on such important variables as race, class, sexual orientation, age, and other factors that tend to affect a person's degree of personal safety and cultural privilege. As was pointed out in an earlier paper by one of the authors (Brown, 1988a), using the personal as a heuristic for generating strategies to share with your clients may be fine as long as you are generalizing to other members of your own group. Even with a perfect match on all overt variables, however, there will be ways to deal with a problem other than those used by the therapist. After all, another central tenet of feminist therapy has been to empower clients to explore all possible alternatives so as to make an informed choice. Thus the therapist must support the client in finding her/his own way, at her/his own pace, without undue pressure to follow the therapist's path via intrusive self-disclosures. The gratuitous assumptions of early feminism that all women's experiences would be similar ignored the very real differences among women (Kanuha, 1990).

Self-disclosing the strategies used by an upper middle-class, highly educated heterosexual white woman to a client who has only female gender in common with the therapist ignores both the very real differences in access to resources available to the therapist, as well as obscuring the unique and rich possibilities for productive coping that might be culture, class, or social-group specific. Even when the therapist herself was a member of one minority group, her strategies might not be appropriate or useful for members of a different minority group (Greene, 1986). Self-disclosure, then, could offer an overly simplistic way of creating a false sense of empathy and connection between culturally different clients and therapists. This glossing over of differences during the first generation of feminist therapy had the effect of alienating some working-class, ethnic, and sexual minority clients (Cardea, 1985; Kanuha, 1990).

A final problem with the use of self-disclosure in feminist therapy has to do with the motivations for its use. In theory, self-disclosure occurs to empower the client. It demystifies the person of the therapist and makes her more human, reducing the "us vs. them" quality of the interaction, and underscores the impact of the therapist's personhood on the interaction rather than her formal training. Although the potential danger here is that the therapist's personality becomes more important than her skills, thus increasing the risk of a cult developing around a particular therapist (Brown, 1990b), in the best of all worlds it allows the client to experience therapy as an interchange between two humans rather than between "expert" and "patient." Self-disclosure can decrease the isolation of the client, allowing her to see how her problems have been encountered even by her therapist. In theory, self-disclosure is one response that a feminist therapist can make to the client's needs for sisterhood and solidarity.

In practice, however, self-disclosure can become distorted into a strategy for the therapist to reduce her *own* isolation. Hill (1990) has pointed out that therapists (feminist as well as otherwise) often engage in low-level violations of their clients' boundaries by self-disclosing at inappropriate times in order to meet their own needs for emotional intimacy, contact, nurturance, and validation. Those feminist therapists who themselves feel marginal (Coffman, 1988) may have an even more difficult challenge in selecting appropriate times for self-disclosure with the client's needs as sole or primary.

As Hill points out, feminist therapists may be particularly vulnerable in this regard because of our commitment to appear as genuine human beings rather than as mystified therapy goddesses. If we are steadfast in our commitment, we may lose some of the usual intangible rewards of the work of therapy, e.g., feeling oneself glowingly responsible for the client's progress or savoring the role of expert and guide. On occasion, the tension generated by balancing genuineness with respect for the client's boundaries and a focus on the client's wants and needs may be the catalyst for inappropriate self-disclosures, statements that serve primarily to soothe the therapist rather than enlighten or empower the client. One client, speaking of another feminist therapist with whom she had chosen to terminate treatment reported that she had decided to stop because she was tired of hearing about how the therapist had dealt with their many shared issues. "I wanted the time and space to talk about *my* experiences, and didn't want to hear about what she had done. After a while it stopped being helpful and started feeling selfish."

In this and other similar cases the therapist may be substituting self-disclosure and the use of personal experience for reliance on appropriate training and consultation, access to information, or therapy expertise. It is thus noteworthy that the Feminist Therapy Ethics Code requires attention to consultation, supervision, ongoing training, and self-care as ethical imperatives, along with the appropriate use of self-disclosure. As feminist therapy has developed, we have found that preventing distress in the therapist appears to be one of the most efficacious strategies for continuing to work in an empowering rather than authoritarian manner.

Many of these problems with the use of self-disclosure occurred in the early period of feminist therapy, before we had developed clear models for its use, and at times when training and experience were undervalued. The problems that we have discussed tend currently to arise when a given feminist therapist is either inexperienced, poorly trained, or lacking in appropriate resources for self-care. It is not the permission to self-disclose, but rather inadequate preparation on the part of the therapist to use self-disclosure that accounts for such problems. In fact, when self-disclosure is both professionally ego-syntonic, and modeled appropriately in training, consultation, and supervision, it is more likely to be used in an effective and clearly therapeutic manner than when it is perceived by the therapist as an error or a rebellion against training.

Current Applications of Self-Disclosure in Feminist Therapy

One of the most enduring aspects of self-disclosure in feminist therapy has been the consumer education model used by most feminist therapists in initiating work with new clients. Such self-disclosure typically includes, although is not limited to, information about the therapist's values and therapeutic orientation, and the outline and rationale of the course of treatment to be pursued. Mutual goal-setting as well as open discussion about therapeutic techniques that the therapist can be expected to use are also often included in initial sessions. Feminist therapists are more likely to discuss the question of diagnosis with the client and work cooperatively to choose the appropriate category, rather than simply imposing a diagnostic label. Feminist therapists are also likely to educate the client about how the diagnosis will be used. A number of feminist therapists routinely share written information with clients about their rights as consumers of psychotherapy, and may have written or oral contracts with the client, presaging recent developments in some states which now require that all therapists share such information. It is not unusual for feminist therapists to frame an initial session as a mutual decision-making interview, often conducted at a reduced fee. During this initial session, the client is actively encouraged to ask both personal and professional questions about the therapist in order to make as informed as possible a decision about working with this particular therapist. This session also offers the therapist the opportunity to clarify what her limits are regarding the sharing of information (e.g., "I will gladly share my views on a particular topic, e.g., non-monogamy, but I will not be willing to share details of how I integrate them into my personal life"), modeling the ability of both parties to have their boundaries respected while maintaining an atmosphere of openness and flexibility.

It has been the experience of feminist therapists that this consumer-rights orientation to the use of self-disclosure in the therapist selection process makes a powerful initial statement to clients about the nature of the psychotherapy relationship. Therapy is framed as being simultaneously healing/protective and empowering. Clients comment that they feel safer and more trusting of a therapist who is willing to be forthcoming, and who, in essence, models that sharing some type of personal information is a risk worth taking. There is also an immediate sense of boundaries being valued, and thus an awareness that the client's needs to control the pacing of the process will be respected. Clients often comment that even though they may have had no questions to ask of their therapist at an initial encounter, they felt less frightened about starting therapy because they knew that the permission to ask was present.

The original feminist therapy notion that self-disclosure by the therapist would create an atmosphere of shared value and expertise has, with some modifications, proved to be of use as well. Feminist therapists have become more sensitive to the wide varieties of female experience and to the ways in which we differ from our women clients; this has allowed us to fine-tune our use of self-disclosure. But the overt permission for the therapist to self-disclose or for the client to request information has been useful for coping with unusual occurrences in the lives of either therapist or client, or with those situations in which the therapist's style or practice setting calls for more personal information to be shared.

For example, one author (Walker) is frequently involved in media interviews, and often travels away from her therapy practice to testify in forensic settings, usually in highly publicized cases of battered women who kill in self-defense. Her clients may need to know literally where she is on a given day, and to have sufficient information about her public work to feel comfortable sharing her in this way. Some clients need the reassurance that their problems are not seen by her as trivial when contrasted with the dramatic issues they see her dealing with in the media and out of town. The other author (Brown) has developed a neurological impairment that leaves her unable to talk without mechanical assistance for several months during each year. During the period of time in which her condition was quite audibly developing and being diagnosed, her clients felt free to ask the questions they needed in order to feel secure in their therapist's availability, and certain that the therapist was pursuing appropriate medical intervention. Yet they knew that the therapist would not intrude that information into the relationship, but rather would make it available upon request.

While these examples may seem highly unusual, in fact it is our experience that most therapists are likely to have events occur in their nontherapy lives that visibly leak into their practice. Rather than promoting a game of hide-and-seek between client and therapist, the feminist therapy model gives clear guidelines about the appropriateness of self-disclosure, as well as giving the therapist the message that she/he will need to plan in advance with how to disclose when such inevitable events as birth, death, illness, or personal transformation of some kind occur.

Since many of the clients who seek feminist therapy are victims/survivors of violent or otherwise dysfunctional families in which problems were never discussed in an open manner, and in which secrets were kept, even though people could sense that something serious was wrong, the therapists' willingness and comfort in providing information about their own situations serves as an opportunity to process old pain about secrets and the denial of one's perceptions. The timing of dealing with issues such as these in the life of the therapist needs to be carefully evaluated with regard to each client. The therapist does not disclose ad libitum, but rather to those clients who inquire or who appear to need to know, and only the information that is appropriate for the particular client-therapist dyad at that point in time. In some cases when the client has a history of needing explicit support to ask for clarification, having already discussed with the therapist at the inception of treatment that asking is acceptable and will be responded to in a genuine and positive manner can be an essential element in the client's ability to ask, and the therapist may refresh this permission by clarifying that this may be one of the times when the client has questions they wish to raise.

Such a reliance on the client's initiation of the request for more information rather than simply providing it to her is one of the major transitions in the use of self-disclosure that we have seen occur over the two decades of feminist therapy practice, a change that brings the practice even closer to the norm of empowering the client. Now, rather than the therapist deciding what part of her experiences the client should hear, the client is given encouragement and permission to ask for information as she/he perceives the need for it, but also the same support to not receive it. This makes the act of self-disclosure less likely to be an engagement in narcissistic self-indulgence on the part of the therapist, and further empowers clients by giving them a chance to practice skills to ask for what is needed. Feminist therapy thus also has become more clearly differentiated from consciousness-raising per se; while each remains a political act and integrates political analysis, feminist therapy has more concretely claimed the territory of healing, with political advocacy work seen as less immediately and directly central to the work of feminist therapists in the therapy hour. Feminist therapists continue to share information and resources with clients, but in a manner that is more respectful of what the client wishes to know. The asymmetry of the relationship and the distinction between egalitarian and genuinely equal is explicitly acknowledged, while the commitment to openness is retained.

Conclusion

Women have, in the past two decades, reclaimed and recreated their ancient role and work as healers through the development of feminist therapy. Being a feminist therapist requires special training in feminist techniques and philosophy and a grounding in the new feminist scholarship on the psychology of women. It also leads to a connection to a larger spiritual movement which emphasizes the interrelatedness between women's mental and physical health. Our growing awareness of the extent to which women, people of color, other oppressed groups, and the very planet itself have been violated by patriarchal power and attempts to impose control makes this feminist political perspective crucial if we are to develop the long-term strength and strategies to heal these wounds and return power to those who have been violated (Spretnak, 1982; Greenspan, 1988). Our belief, consonant with that of most feminist therapists, is that the basic tenets of feminist therapy are, at their core, those which are necessary for good therapy, in which there is both closeness and empathy, yet respect for boundaries and human diversity. The use of self-disclosure has been a primary technique utilized by feminist therapists in building a feminist, egalitarian, and genuinely healing approach to psychotherapy.

References

Ballou, M., & Gabalac, N. (1985). *A feminist position on mental health*. Springfield, IL: Charles C. Thomas.

Bem, S. & Bem, D. (1976). Case study of a non-conscious ideology: Training the woman to know her place: In S. Cox (Ed.), *Female psychology: The emerging self*. Chicago: SRA.

Berman, J.S. (1985). Ethical feminist perspectives on dual relationships with clients. In L.B. Rosewater & L.E.A. Walker (Eds.), *Handbook of feminist therapy: Women's issues in psychotherapy*. New York: Springer.

Bleier, R. (1984). *Science and gender*. New York: Pergamon.

Broverman, I.K., Broverman, D., Clarkson, F., Rosencrantz, P., & Vogel, S. (1970). Sex-role stereotypes and clinical judgments of mental health. *Journal of Consulting and Clinical Psychology, 34*, 1–7.

Brown, L.S., & Liss-Levinson, N. (1981). Feminist therapy. In R. Corsini (Ed.) *Handbook of innovative psychotherapies*. New York: Wiley.

Brown, L.S. (1984a). Finding new language: Getting beyond analytic verbal shorthand in feminist therapy. *Women and Therapy, 3*, 73–80.

Brown, L.S. (1984b). The lesbian-feminist therapist and her community. *Psychotherapy in private practice, 2*, 9–16.

Brown, L.S. (1986). Diagnosis and the zeitgeist: The politics of masochism in the DSM-III-R. In R. Garfinkel, (Chair), *The politics of diagnosis: Feminist psychology and the DSM-III-R*. Symposium presented at the 94th Annual Convention of the American Psychological Association, Washington, D.C., Aug.

Brown, L.S. (1987a). Learning to think about ethics: A guide for the perplexed lesbian feminist therapist. Keynote address presented at a conference, *Boundary dilemmas in the client–therapist relationship: A working conference for lesbian therapists*. Los Angeles, CA, Jan.

Brown, L.S. (1987b). Beyond "Thou shalt not": Developing conceptual framework for ethical decision-making. In L. Garnets, (Chair), *Ethical and boundary dilemmas for lesbian and gay psychotherapists*, Symposium presented to the 95th Annual Convention of the American Psychological Association, New York, Aug.

Brown, L.S. (1988a). *The meaning of a multi-cultural perspective for theory-building in feminist therapy*. Presented at the Seventh Advanced Feminist Therapy Institute, Seattle, WA, May.

Brown, L.S. (1988b). *Feminist therapy perspectives on psychodiagnosis: Beyond DSM and ICD*. Keynote address presented at the First International Congress on Mental Health Care for Women, Amsterdam, The Netherlands, Dec.

Brown, L.S. (1990a). Structuring the business of feminist therapy responsibility. In H. Lerman & N. Porter (Eds.), *Ethics in psychotherapy: Feminist perspectives*. New York: Springer.

Brown, L.S. (1990b). Confronting ethically problematic behaviors in feminist therapy colleagues. In H. Lerman & N. Porter (Eds.) *Ethics in psychotherapy: Feminist perspectives* New York: Springer.

Caplan, P.J. (1984). The myth of women's masochism. *American Psychologist, 39*, 130–139.

Cammaert, L., & Larsen, C. (1989). Feminist frameworks of psychotherapy. In M.A. Dutton-Douglas & L.E.A. Walker (Eds.), *Feminist psychotherapies: Integrations of therapeutic and feminist systems*. Norwood NJ: Ablex Publishing.

Cardea, C. (1985). The lesbian revolution and the 50-minute hour: A working-class look at therapy and the movement. *Lesbian Ethics, 1*, 46–68.

Chesler, P. (1972). *Women and madness*. New York: Doubleday.

Coffman, S. (1988). *Developing a feminist model for clinical consultation: Combining diversity and commonality*. Presented at the Seventh Advanced Feminist Therapy Institute, Seattle, WA, May.

Diagnostic and statistical manual of mental disorders, III, revised. (1987). American Psychiatric Association, Washington, D.C.

Dutton-Douglas, M.A., & Walker, L.E.A. (1989). *Feminist psychotherapies: Integrations of therapeutic and feminist systems*. Norwood NJ: Ablex Publishing.

Dykewomon, E. (Ed.) (1988). Surviving psychiatric assault. *Sinister Wisdom, 36*.

Feminist therapy ethical code. (1987). Feminist Therapy Institute, Denver CO: Author.
Gilbert, L.A. (1980). Feminist therapy. In A. Brodsky & R. Hare-Mustin (Eds.), *Women and psychotherapy: An assessment of research and practice.* New York: Guilford.
Gore, S., & Walker, L.E.A. (1986). *International women's mental health agenda: Modifications from the UN End of the Decade Meeting in Nairobi, Kenya.* Symposium presented at the National Conference of the Association for Women in Psychology, Oakland, CA, Mar.
Greene, B. (1986). When the therapist is white and the patient is Black: Considerations for psychotherapy in the feminist heterosexual and lesbian communities. *Women and Therapy, 5,* 41–46.
Greenspan, M. (1983). *A new approach to women and therapy.* New York: McGraw-Hill.
Greenspan, M. (1986). Should therapists be personal? Self-disclosure and therapeutic difference in feminist therapy. *Women and Therapy, 5,* 5–17.
Greenspan, M. (1988). *Creating a political spiritual model for feminist therapy.* Keynote address presented at the First International Congress on Mental Health Care for Women, Amsterdam, The Netherlands, Dec.
Hill, M. (1990). On creating a theory of feminist therapy. In L.S. Brown & M.P.P. Root (Eds.). *Diversity and complexity in feminist therapy.* New York: Haworth Press.
Hoagland, S.L. (1988). *Lesbian ethics: Toward new values.* Palo Alto, CA: Institute of Lesbian Studies.
If sex enters into the psychotherapy relationship. (1987). Committee on Women in Psychology. Washington, D.C.: American Psychological Association.
Jordan, J.V., Surrey, J.L., & Kaplan, A.G. (1983). *Women and empathy: Implications for psychological development and psychotherapy.* Wellesley, Mass: Stone Center for Developmental Studies and Services.
Kanuha, V. (1990). The importance of an integrated analysis of oppression in feminist therapy. In H. Lerman & N. Porter (Eds.), *Ethics in psychotherapy: Feminist perspectives.* New York: Springer.
Kaplan, M. (1983). A woman's view of the DSM-III. *American Psychologist, 38,* 786–792.
Kravetz, D. (1976). Consciousness-raising groups and group psychotherapy: Alternative mental health resources for women. *Psychotherapy: Theory, Research, Practice, 13,* 66–71.
Lerman, H. (1976). What happens in feminist therapy. In S. Cox (Ed.) *Female psychology: The emerging self.* Chicago: SRA.
Lerman, H., & Porter, N. (Eds.). (1990). *Ethics in psychotherapy: Feminist perspectives.* New York: Springer.
Mander, A.V., & Rush, A.K. (1974). *Feminism as therapy.* San Francisco: Random House/Bookworks.
Maracek, J., & Kravetz, D. (1977). Women and mental health: A review of feminist change efforts. *Psychiatry, 40,* 323–329.
Perls, F.S. (1971). *Gestalt therapy verbatim.* New York: Bantam.
Pheterson, G. (1988). *From the therapeutic to the political stage: Psychological disciplines in feminist thought and action.* Keynote address presented at the First International Congress on Mental Health Care for Women, Amsterdam, The Netherlands, Dec.
Rawlings, E., & Carter, D. (Eds.) (1977). *Psychotherapy for women: Treatment toward equality.* Springfield Ill: Charles C. Thomas.
Raymond, J. (1986). *A passion for friends: Toward a philosophy of female affection.* Boston: Beacon Press.
Reiker, P.P., & Carmen, E.D. (Eds.). (1984). *The gender gap in psychotherapy: Social realities and psychological processes.* New York: Plenum.
Report of the task force on sex bias and sex-role stereotyping in psychotherapy. (1975). American Psychological Association Task Force. *American Psychologist, 30,* 1169–1175.
Rogers, C.R. (1951). *Client-centered therapy.* Boston: Houghton Mifflin.
Rogers, C.R. (1961). *On becoming a person.* Boston: Houghton Mifflin.

Rosencrantz, P.S., Delorey, C., & Broverman, I.K. (1985). *One half a generation later: sex-role stereotypes revisited*. Paper presented at the 93rd Annual Convention of the American Psychological Association, Los Angeles, CA, Aug.

Rosewater, L.B. (1989). Feminist therapies with women. In M.A. Dutton-Douglas & L.E.A. Walker (Eds.), *Feminist psychotherapies: Integrations of therapeutic and feminist systems*. Norwood, NJ: Ablex.

Rosewater, L.B. & Walker, L.E.A. (Eds.) (1985). *Handbook of feminist therapy: Women's issues in psychotherapy*. New York: Springer.

Rothblum, E.D., Solomon, L., & Albee, G. (1986). A sociopolitical perspective of DSM-III. In T. Millon & G. Klerman (Eds.), *Contemporary directions in psychopathology: Toward the DSM-IV*. New York: Guilford.

Spretnak, C. (Ed.). (1982). *The politics of women's spirituality*. New York: Anchor/Doubleday.

Steiner, C., Wycoff, H., Goldstine, D., Lariviere, P., Schwebel, R., & Marcus, J. (1975). *Readings in radical psychiatry*. New York: Grove Press.

Sturdivant, S. (1980). *Therapy with women: A feminist philosophy of treatment*. New York: Springer.

Walker, L.E.A. (Ed.) (1984a). *Women and mental health policy*. Beverly Hills, CA: Sage.

Walker, L.E.A. (1984b). Battered women, psychology and public policy. *American Psychologist, 29*, 1178.

Walker, L.E.A. (1986). Diagnosis and politics: Abuse disorders. In R. Garfinkel (Chair) *The politics of diagnosis: Feminist therapy and the DSM-III-R*. Symposium presented at the 94th Annual Convention of the American Psychological Association, Washington, D.C., Aug.

Walker, L.E.A. (1988). *Diagnostic systems (DSM-III) and violence against women*. Keynote address presented at the First International Congress on Mental Health Care for Women, Amsterdam, The Netherlands, Dec.

Weisstein, N. (1970). Kinder, kuche, kirche as scientific law: Psychology constructs the female. In R. Morgan (Ed.), *Sisterhood is powerful*. New York: Vintage.

Women and psychotherapy: A consumer handbook. (Rev. ed.). (1985). Committee on Women in Psychology. Washington, D.C.

Wycoff, H. (Ed.). (1976). *Love, therapy and politics: Issues in radical therapy—The first year*. New York: Grove Press.

Wycoff, H. (1977). *Solving women's problems through awareness, action, and contact*. New York: Grove Press.

IV

Therapeutic Modalities

11

Self-Disclosure and Psychotherapy with Children and Adolescents

Nicholas Papouchis

Introduction

The focus of this chapter is a discussion of the concept of self-disclosure as it applies to therapeutic work with adolescents and children. This begins with a brief discussion of the relevance of self-disclosure in psychotherapeutic work with adults, in order to demonstrate the importance of using a developmental perspective in understanding this phenomenon in work with a younger population. It will also briefly review the positions taken by different analytic schools of thought regarding the therapist's self-disclosure in work with adult patients.

In the discussion that follows, the terms analyst and psychotherapist will be used interchangeably, although the author acknowledges that there are technical differences between the two.

The Concept of Self-Disclosure

In our interactions with other people we reveal ourselves in many ways. The tone of our voice, the way in which we position our body, our ability to make eye contact, the distance we maintain when talking to one another all reveal something about us. Many of these behaviors are automatic and outside of conscious awareness. By contrast, in the

Nicholas Papouchis • Program in Clinical Psychology, Long Island University, Brooklyn Center, Brooklyn, New York 11201.

traditional psychotherapeutic situation with adults, verbal communication between the participants is the major form of interaction. Therapist and patient reveal themselves primarily through the verbal interactions that take place in the therapeutic setting. Seen in this context, self-disclosure has been equated with verbal disclosure. This definition has also been restricted to verbal information intentionally revealed by one person to the other.

The concept of self-disclosure and its impact on the therapeutic process has been discussed most thoroughly in the work of Jourard (1964, 1968, 1971), who argued in favor of the reciprocal nature of self-disclosure. He maintained that self-disclosure on the part of one participant in an interaction had a dyadic effect, in that increased openness on the part of one individual led to increased openness on the part of the other. When applied to psychotherapy, advocates of the existential position espoused by Jourard (1971) have argued that the therapist's self-disclosures serve a critical function in building the therapeutic relationship. The patient's increased ability to be genuine and self-disclosing was thus seen to be a direct result of the therapist's behavior. Similarly, Truax and Carkhuff (1965), working in a Rogerian tradition, have demonstrated that the greater the therapist's openness, the more likely the patient will be to become self-disclosing.

While there has been general agreement about what it means for the patient or client to be self-disclosing, it has not been equally clear which of the therapist's verbal responses should be characterized as self-disclosing. However, it has been generally agreed that self-disclosing responses reflect some intimate aspect of the therapist's experience that is revealed verbally to the patient (Chelune, 1975; Cozby, 1973; Jourard, 1968, 1971; Truax & Carkhuff, 1965). Thus, in response to the patient's thoughts and behaviors as they unfold in the therapeutic interaction, the therapist may reveal some personal reaction to the patient's verbalizations, or reveal something about his (the therapist's) life experiences outside the therapeutic situation. While both classes of events may be described as self-disclosure, it is important to distinguish between them, since they are likely to have a differential impact on the therapeutic process.

McCarthy and Betz (1978) proposed two types of therapist self-disclosures. The first, defined as "self-involving disclosures," involved those statements that were direct expressions of the therapist's feelings or reactions to the statements and behaviors of the patient. The second, "self-disclosing statements," referred to the past history or personal experiences of the therapist. Subsequently, Nilsson, Strassberg, and Bannon (1979) defined two categories of therapist self-disclosure. "Interpersonal" self-disclosures referred to personal feelings about the patient's problems or the therapeutic relationship, while "intrapersonal" self-disclosures referred to statements about the therapist's life outside the therapeutic relationship. The terms used in this latter definition seem less awkward and confusing than the one offered by McCarthy and Betz. In the discussion that follows we will use the terms "interpersonal" or "intrapersonal" self-disclosures to refer to the two classes of therapist self-revelations.

Self-Disclosure in Psychoanalytic Psychotherapy with Adults

Increased self-disclosure on the part of the adult patient has been seen by practitioners of psychoanalytic psychotherapy as a sign of therapeutic progress. The progressive self-exploration in which adult patients examine their motives, relationships with others, fears, and life choices, as well as their belief systems and values, has traditionally been viewed as a fundamental aspect of the process of increased engagement in psychotherapy. Clinicians have typically described patients as demonstrating "greater insight" into the sources of their emotional difficulties or as having a "greater awareness" of themselves, when they have wanted to indicate how well the therapeutic work was progressing. Similarly, they have used the adult patients' ability to speak more openly about their emotional experiences, whether they are painful or humiliating, as a barometer of therapeutic progress and as a sign of a more trusting, viable therapeutic alliance. Thus, the adult patients' ability to become increasingly self-disclosing, to reveal more intimate and important details of themselves to the therapist and significant others, has been a widely accepted tenet of psychotherapeutic work. Empirical work (Truax & Carkhuff, 1965) evaluating the outcome of the psychotherapeutic process has also supported the belief that the greater the degree of self-exploration, the greater the potential for constructive personality change in that patient.

Psychoanalytic clinicians, depending upon their particular theoretical orientation, give different weight to the therapist's self-disclosures. The classical psychoanalytic position in working with adult patients has argued that the therapist's behavior should be characterized by neutrality and abstinence (Freud, 1912, 1914; Langs, 1978). Psychoanalytic practitioners working from this vantage point have considered self-revealing comments on the part of the therapist as therapeutic errors and a sign of countertransferential difficulties.

The psychoanalytic position of therapeutic neutrality stemmed from Freud's (1912) recommendation that "the doctor should be opaque to his patients, and like a mirror, should show them nothing but what is shown to him." This facilitated the projection of the patient's inner life onto the person of the therapist (analyst), and contributed to the development of the transference neurosis. The resolution of the resulting psychic conflict was achieved through the process of the analyst's interpretations, which led to insight and "working through." However, some respected psychoanalytic practitioners (Stone, 1961; Greenson, 1969) have indicated that there are situations that call for information about the therapist as a person. Similarly, Schafer (1983), in describing the classical analyst's empathic stance, noted that "there is always room in the analytic work for courtesy, cordiality, gentleness, sincere empathic participation and comment, and other such personal, though not socially intimate, modes of relationship." While Schafer was describing the analyst's departures from a position of neutrality, his remarks are equally applicable to the question of self-disclosure.

In spite of these attempts to articulate the classical analyst's empathic response to the patient, the emphasis on interpretation as the major agent of therapeutic change has led most psychoanalysts working with adults to pay insufficient attention to the relational issues that contribute to therapeutic change. In the discussion that follows I will refer to these relational aspects of the therapeutic relationship as the interpersonal-object relationship between therapist and patient. This term is intended to capture both the style of relating and the inner psychological makeup of both participants. I believe that this term encompasses more than what Greenson and Wexler (1969) meant by the term "real relationship."

In the last 20 years, clinicians working with adult patients within the classical tradition have begun to emphasize the reality aspects of the therapeutic relationship. Greenson and Wexler's (1969) description of the importance of the "real relationship" in therapy underscored the contribution of the therapist's personality to the therapeutic alliance. They noted that the rules of abstinence can be adhered to all too literally. They suggested that the analyst feel free to offer an expression of compassion or concern, or even an admission of technical error, when appropriate. In the language of the present discussion, they encouraged "interpersonal" self-disclosure on the part of the classical analyst. Similarly, psychoanalytic clinicians working with more severely disturbed patients have emphasized the importance of modifying the therapist's neutral stance in working with more disturbed patients whose lack of psychic organization left them unable to tolerate the therapist's distance. (Arieti, 1974; Meissner, 1986; Pine, 1985; Winnicott, 1965). Their recommendations underscored the importance of the interpersonal-object relationship between therapist and patient as the foundation that facilitated the development of the therapeutic alliance, and which provided, to use Winnicott's term (1965), a "holding environment" for the difficult psychotherapeutic process which ensued.

The interpersonal-object relationship in psychotherapy and psychoanalysis is important for all patients, not simply more disturbed patients. Most clinicians fondly remember many of the interpersonal attributes of their own analysts. They also vividly remember the poignant moments when the analyst revealed himself in a moment of particularly intimate relatedness.

Other therapeutic positions have lent further support to the argument of the therapist's interpersonal-object relational importance. The work of the British Object Relations School, particularly the seminal contributions of Fairbairn (1952), Guntrip (1971), and Winnicott (1965), have all emphasized the importance of the real relationship between therapist and patient. Each has cogently argued for the importance of the new object-relational experience the adult patient has with his analyst. From their perspective, the psychotherapeutic experience is not simply a reliving of the patient's old object relationships. It is more accurately conceptualized as a reworking of the old conflicts in the safety of a new growth-producing relationship, which allows for a new experience that had not been previously possible. In this context, selective "interpersonal" self-disclosure on the part of the analyst facilitates the interpersonal-object relationship that develops by helping more clearly to define the analyst as a new object.

Sullivan's (1953) interpersonal theory has also underlined the therapist's continued and repeated personal contribution to the therapeutic interaction. His conceptualization of the therapist's role has been succinctly captured in his description of the therapist's involvement as one of "participant observation." In the interpersonal model one cannot participate without revealing some aspect of the self (often quite directly), and one cannot observe the therapeutic interaction without observing some aspect of the self in interaction.

What I wish to highlight here is Sullivan's view of the analyst as an ongoing contributor to the patient's experience. This does not mean that the interpersonal analyst is by definition interactive. That is more a matter of personal style. I am also not suggesting that the interpersonal analyst be more self-disclosing. That too is a matter of individual style, and not theoretical orientation. In fact, from this author's interpersonal perspective, "intrapersonal" self-disclosures, that is, statements about the analyst's personal life outside the treatment relationship, are rarely indicated, and very likely to be signs of countertransference difficulties to be examined. I include here the analyst's responses to the seemingly innocuous impersonal questions that patients ask as well. Further, I would argue that in psychotherapy with adult patients the therapist should not make more than infrequent, selective use of "interpersonal" self-disclosure. More than this dilutes the meaning of these interventions, and interferes with the analyst's ability to help the patient differentiate his transferential distortions from the analyst's behavior.

Self-disclosure on the part of the analyst would seem to be intimately related to his conception of countertransference. The classical analytic position has traditionally viewed countertransference as an unwanted contribution of the analyst's unresolved psychic conflicts (Marshall, 1988). More recently within this tradition (Renik, 1986), there has been an increasing tendency to see countertransference as a useful tool, although there is still controversy as to how it should be used. Thus, while acknowledged as an important aspect of the therapeutic process, its disclosure in the therapeutic interaction has not been widely accepted. In contrast, the interpersonal analytic position espoused by Epstein and Feiner (1979) and Marshall and Marshall (1988), among others, has more consistently argued for the use of countertransference feelings as internal cues to the patient's experience, and supported the selective disclosure of these feelings to the patient. Springmann (1986), for example, has argued that the understanding of client-induced countertransference is an integral part of psychotherapy and that it should be revealed to the patient at the appropriate times. To the extent that "interpersonal" self-disclosure may be seen as following from the analyst's view of the meaning of his countertransference to the patient, it is clear from the above discussion that analysts of the interpersonal school are less likely to be hesitant to discuss their reactions to the patient.

In sum, it is this author's position that self-disclosure on the part of the therapist has been accepted as an integral part of the therapeutic relationship by all schools of psychoanalytic thought. Each of the schools, however, has different theoretical conceptions as to how the issues of self-disclosure are to be viewed, the conditions under which they come about, and how they are to be addressed. The major question that will continue to be addressed in work with adults is to what extent and under what conditions should the adult psychotherapist be self-disclosing. With this brief summary as a point of contrast, let us now turn to the issue of self-disclosure with adolescents and children.

Self-Disclosure with Children and Adolescents: A Developmental Perspective

Self-Disclosure in Psychotherapy with Children

The issue of self-disclosure must be viewed from a different vantage point when we work therapeutically with adolescents and children.

Here the developmental tasks and needs of our younger patients are an important determinant in understanding how the phenomenon of self-disclosure manifests itself in both patient and therapist. For example, it is not always possible, nor even desirable, for our younger patients to be self-disclosing in the way that our adult patients are. Latency-age children express themselves symbolically through activity as well as through language. Thus, the child therapist, working with his patient in a combination of verbal and play therapy, looks for the resolution of psychic conflicts in the child's play, and in descriptions of his behavior from teachers and parents, rather than solely through the child's verbal productions. Premature verbal disclosure of psychic conflict, even when possible, may tax the child's developing ego resources and impede rather than facilitate future ego development.

The child therapist must be aware of the developmental tasks that the latency age child faces. Each of these tasks requires the child's increasing ego mastery of the issues he is faced with. Therapeutic efforts are directed toward the removal of the obstacles that interfere with mastery of these tasks, and facilitating the child's development through periods of disequilibrium as these tasks are mastered (Pine, 1985). The child therapist, aware of the ways in which his child patient's premature self-disclosures may represent a threat to a developing sense of self, and the child's ego resources, modifies the degree to which the child's self-discovery proceeds.

Let us articulate some of the important tasks of the latency period before proceeding further:

1. Increasing independence from parents, including opportunities for other objects of authority with whom to identify.
2. The development of peer relations, including the mastery of issues of competition and cooperation in work and play.
3. Increased ego functioning manifested in greater defensive control over instinctual life, adaptation to reality, and the capacity for intellectual mastery of school-based learning.

To illustrate the importance of this knowledge in working with children, let us specify the age of a hypothetical patient as six years old. The child at this age, early in latency, is concerned with repression of preoedipal issues, and is struggling with the mastery of his inner life (Bornstein, 1951). Premature self-disclosure of sexual or aggressive material thus represents a threat to the child's developing psychic equilibrium. Further, the child, at this age, may be using language which is still too intimately tied to emotional experience. Words may be experienced as equivalent to the actions they describe. From this perspective, the therapist's insistence on continued exploration of dynamic issues represents a distinct threat to the child, and is to be carefully avoided.

The Therapist's Role and the Issue of Self-Disclosure with Children

Anna Freud has emphasized how the child's developing object relationships demand that the child therapist or analyst must be anything but impersonal or shadowy (1976). The latency-age child, like the adolescent, still has his original objects present. The parents exist, not only in fantasy, as they do with adult patients, but continue to determine the child's gratifications and disappointments in his everyday life. Thus, the analyst enters the therapeutic relationship as a new object and the developing interpersonal-object relationship that ensues contributes significantly to the child's development.

In contrast to Melanie Klein's position regarding the interpretation of transference, Anna Freud (1976) argues that the behavior of the analyst of children is not solely intended to produce a transference that can be interpreted. Instead, she notes that the person of the analyst is of great interest to the child, whom he (the child) endows with a variety of attractive and interesting qualities. Further, the analyst's educational efforts, and setting of limits informs the child what the analyst sanctions or disapproves of. Thus, as with the adolescent therapist, the child therapist reveals himself, and his belief system in his efforts at education or limit setting. These behaviors are invariably self-disclosing.

Other child therapists (Ross, 1964; Ginott, 1964) have also pointed out that the child's questions must be responded to differently than an adult's. Children's questions are often centered on trying to find their place in the world, and who belongs where. The therapist who deflects their questions by interpreting the unconscious reasons for their asking, demonstrates a lack of interest in these concerns, and may interfere with the child's ability to master reality. Although it is useful to give the child an opportunity to explore their fantasies about the way they "would like things to be," the therapist should also respond to questions in a manner that is simple and direct (Ross, 1964).

Similarly, the therapist who intersperses his interpretative inquiries about the meaning of a child's curiosity about the therapist with some brief and general answers to the child's questions, addresses both the unconscious and reality-oriented meaning of the child's concerns (Ginott, 1964). As the treatment relationship develops, the therapist may also be able to respond directly to the child's inquiries about his mood. To the extent that the therapist comfortably responds to direct questions about countertransferential responses that are evident in the analyst's behavior, he enhances the child's faith in the therapist's reliability, and helps the child to realize that some temporary problem in the relationship does not interfere with the core of the interpersonal-object relationship between them (Colm, 1964). These self-disclosures also support the child's developing ability to experience feelings of ambivalence toward the significant people in his life. It should also be emphasized here, that those feelings which the analyst experiences as the result of unresolved inner conflicts are not part of the self-disclosure.

Let us turn next to the issues of self-disclosure in therapeutic work with adolescents. Issues of self-disclosure with this population become more complex because of the complexity of the developmental tasks which the adolescent faces.

Self-Disclosure and the Adolescent Patient

The early adolescent patient, unlike the latency age child, has developed the capacity to represent psychic issues symbolically in a verbal manner. Yet, he may be equally unprepared to be verbally self-disclosing. The emergence of drive activity at puberty, the dramatic physical changes that ensue, and the confused, and at times embarrassed sense of inner states of feeling often make the early adolescent acutely sensitive to what is private and what is public. Adolescents are also acutely sensitive to issues which threaten their desire for autonomy, and which reawaken dependent wishes for support from parents. It is often not until mid-to-late adolescence when ego functioning and the capacity for formal operational thought (Flavell, 1963) have developed sufficiently, that adolescents feel some sense of mastery over their inner life. At this time in development, interpersonal skills have developed to the point where heterosexual relationships have begun. The adolescent has begun to develop some confidence in his sexual identity and more intimate verbal self-disclosure may become possible without representing a threat to their sense of self.

Even at this point in the adolescent's development, he is rarely able to approximate the sustained self-examination that one sees with adult patients. The therapist who naively follows an adolescent's open self-revealing discussion in a therapy session, without being aware of the threat that this material presents to the patient, is often surprised when his adolescent patient misses the next session. Or, if the material has been too threatening, the patient decides to terminate therapy. This can often happen without the adolescent appearing to be aware of how threatening the experience of self-disclosure was. From this developmental perspective, it is important for the therapist to know that verbal self-disclosure on the part of his younger patient may not always be a sign of therapeutic progress, but rather may represent a danger that threatens to disrupt a developing therapeutic alliance.

> John, an articulate 16-year-old adolescent, had spent the previous session describing with considerable clarity how he felt his father was competing with him, and favored his younger brother. He began the next session by

saying that he had thought about discontinuing therapy, but he wasn't sure why. When his therapist pointed out to him that he had talked a great deal about angry feelings toward his father in the previous session, he responded by saying that he had felt guilty about complaining so angrily, but had not connected these guilty feelings with his thoughts of stopping therapy. The therapist then slowly began to help John face and accept the anger which he avoided in a number of other interpersonal situations.

The therapist often helps the adolescent patient by indicating that there are some things "that may be too upsetting to talk about right now." Or that the ability to understand the nature of what they are feeling may proceed at a slower pace. This is not to say that the adolescent therapist should help the patient avoid self-disclosing. Instead, the therapist monitors the impact of all self-disclosures on the patient's attitudes toward therapy.

Before proceeding to a discussion of the therapist's self-disclosure with adolescents, it will be helpful to review briefly some of the major developmental tasks of adolescence. Blos (1979) has described the period of adolescence as "the second separation-individuation process." Among the major developmental tasks of this developmental period are:

1. Intrapsychic separation from the family of origin.
2. Mastery of the biological event of puberty with the necessary changes in ego functioning, and the initial mastery and acceptance of sexuality.
3. The intimately related tasks of the development of a sense of identity and an ego-ideal.

The therapist working intensively with adolescents will invariably be forced to help his adolescent patient deal with all these issues. More often than not, they are going on simultaneously, and the therapist has to choose which of them to work on at that moment. This usually depends upon which of the issues is highest on the adolescent's list of psychic priorities. The therapist often finds himself helping his patient deal with feeling overwhelmed, while respectfully encouraging his patient's developing ability to cope with the concrete problem at hand. Similarly, the therapist may deliberately not interpret what he knows to be a deeply conflictual issue, in favor of supporting the adolescent's resourceful autonomous coping with that issue. This is not to say that the adolescent therapist avoids the interpretation of conflictual material. Rather, that his primary focus is more likely to be on the interpretation of defenses against affects which interfere with ego development (Meeks, 1986).

Sam, a depressed 17-year-old boy, was constantly fighting with his parents. Many of his disputes were with his mother to whom he had a decidedly erotic attachment. His fights were thus designed to distance him from an attachment which he felt to be both overwhelming and highly sexualized. Interpretive work was directed toward understanding how his fights were designed to ward off a feeling of powerlessness, and avoided any reference to sexual feelings.

The Therapist's Self-Disclosure with Adolescents

The therapist who works with adolescents is invariably more self-disclosing than the therapist working with adults. The intrapsychic separation from parents that adolescents have begun at puberty leads them to seek out new adult objects with whom to identify. At the same time, the adolescents' intense discomfort and mistrust of any dependent relationship with adults requires a different therapeutic stance on the part of the therapist. Their need is for an adult who can understand them on their terms without losing their status as an adult. Simultaneously, that adult (the therapist) has to demonstrate continuously that he is interested in helping the adolescent establish his autonomy, not in recreating the adolescent's dependent relationship with the parents. The therapist, often sought out as an alternative adult model to the parents, must be prepared to be subjected to careful scrutiny from his adolescent patient who evaluates and questions his behavior with an intensity not found in the adult or child patient.

The adolescent who comes to psychotherapy suspicious of adults, and resistant to treatment, is likely to become increasingly wary of the therapist who avoids direct questions and relies on technical skills to avoid inquiries about herself. In contrast, the therapist who treats the adolescent's questions respectfully and thoughtfully and without undue anxiety, demonstrates to the adolescent that the therapy office is a place where honesty and frankness are valued. These conditions make the interpersonal-object relationship between therapist and adolescent a critical factor in the therapeutic process. To use Bowlby's (1969) language, the developing attachment to the therapist makes the understanding of the analysis of transference possible.

One of the effects of the therapeutic interactions that follow is that the therapist employs a style of relating that is likely to result in more "interpersonal" self-disclosure than is usually found in work with children and adults. This does not mean that the therapist of adolescents abandons his interpretive stance, or that the therapist is excessively self-disclosing. In fact, the therapist's more interpersonal, interactive style is likely to enhance the impact of interpretations when they are offered, and to facilitate identification with the therapist's analytic posture toward the patient's problems. The therapist's empathic understanding of the adolescent's developmental tasks and the difficulties they entail make him a more attractive attachment figure. The person of the adolescent therapist is also available for the adolescent to discuss ideas with, disagree and argue with, and to accept support from, since that support need not threaten the adolescents' fragile sense of autonomy.

Adatto (1966) has used the term "special friend" to describe the nature of the relationship between adolescent and therapist described above. Clinicians have often described the relationship as avuncular, to characterize the important interpersonal-object relationship that develops between them. Let me also emphasize that the therapist does not offer himself as a replacement for the lost relationship with the parents. To the contrary, the therapist should actively interpret his adolescent patient's efforts to place him in a parental role (Meeks, 1986). Instead, the therapist, depending upon the age of the adolescent, is a trusted adult who stands somewhere between the adolescent's struggle to hold onto wishes to remain a child, and his drive to become an autonomous individual on the way to adulthood.

To do this the therapist must present himself as an authentic, caring presence with whom both aspects of the struggle for autonomy may be discussed without unduly threatening the adolescent's self-esteem. When the therapist offers evasive responses to direct questions, refuses to help solve real problems in the life of the adolescent, or continues to insist on focusing only on the unconscious meaning of the adolescent's statements, the adolescent's resistance stiffens and the development of a therapeutic alliance is impeded. Instead, the therapist who demonstrates his support for the adolescent's interest in expanding his ego's mastery of both his inner life and reality, and his efforts to develop a sense of identity, can become a trusted ally. From this perspective, "interpersonal" self-disclosing statements from the therapist help to demonstrate to the adolescent that he or she is to be trusted.

We are taught that with adult patients all questions about the therapist are grist for the mill. In contrast, with adolescents and children, one is more likely to respond directly to questions that do not seem to be related to dynamic issues. Thus, the therapist who answers an early adolescent's question as to whether they (the therapist) had hobbies as a teenager, is more likely to be trusted than the therapist who feels compelled to "analyze" all such questions. Similarly, the therapist who directly and comfortably answers an adolescent patient's question about his life, and then inquires about the nature of the adolescent's curiosity in this area, is more likely to facilitate true self-examination in his adolescent patient, than the therapist who carefully works at showing the patient that his questions have dynamic significance.

Sheila, a 17-year-old black adolescent, had recently been discharged from the hospital, and was living again in a foster home. Several months later, during one of her outpatient visits, as she talked with an air of casualness about her relationship with her parents, she noticed that her therapist had tears in his eyes. After summoning her courage, she asked the therapist why he seemed to be crying. He replied simply that her description of her life had made him sad. She then began to weep openly, and reported later that it was one of the few times she had been able to cry about the fact that her mother had been in a mental hospital most of her life, and that she rarely saw her alcoholic father. From that time on, she called her therapist the "feeling doctor."

The Therapeutic Alliance and Self-Disclosure

From the outset of the treatment, the therapist's style of relating to the adolescent patient is one of the most important factors in engaging the patient and facilitating the development of a therapeutic alliance (Adatto, 1966; Kessler, 1979; Papouchis, 1982). Many authors (Holmes, 1964; Meeks, 1985; Weiner, 1970) have argued that a natural, informal style combined with the readiness and willingness to participate actively and directly (to be willing to be "interpersonally" self-disclosing) in therapeutic interactions contributes to the adolescent's ability to trust the therapist. Please note that I am not speaking here of a pseudo-easygoing, artificial role adopted by the therapist to convince his adolescent patient that he can be trusted. The adolescent's sensitivity to such a manipulative stance would in all likelihood doom the therapy from the outset. Both Anthony (1969) and Meeks (1986) have spoken to the countertransference dangers that work with adolescents involves. I am referring instead to someone whose style is genuinely natural; who is not assuming a therapeutic stance in order to seduce the adolescent into a treatment relationship. I would also like to add, as I have stated elsewhere (Papouchis, 1982), that this style of relating cuts across a variety of personality types, and many analysts who are thoughtful and quiet when working with adults, are quite comfortable interacting spontaneously and directly with their adolescent patients.

Perhaps this style of relating is most comfortable to clinicians working from within a developmental perspective. As Pine (1985) has argued, research and knowledge of developmental issues may effect the practice of psychoanalysis and psychotherapy by influencing the language that the analyst uses in speaking to the patient. Or it may help him (the analyst) more precisely to describe the phenomena to which that language refers. In either case, it seems clear that a language and style of communication close to the adolescent patient's concrete experience is likely to be maximally evocative.

In describing the adolescent therapist's style of relating, Meeks (1985), Holmes (1964), and Weiner (1970) have argued that authenticity and genuineness on the therapist's part lead to the therapist revealing more of himself or herself in the therapeutic interactions. It is difficult to be direct and spontaneous without being in a position where the therapeutic interactions require greater degrees of self-disclosures on the part of the therapist. The therapist of the adolescent thus consistently reveals more of himself than he would to his adult or child patient.

Holmes (1964) has characterized this style of interacting as one which involves "abnormal candor." He notes that:

> The therapist reveals much of his personality for two reasons: (1) he can't hide it from the adolescent anyway; and (2) there is no good reason to try to hide it even if it were possible. The adolescent is able to tell too much about us even when it is our intention to tell him nothing at all. Our efforts to operate as emotional technicians of some sort are transparent to him; they only increase his embarrassment and uneasiness in a situation that is already strained at best. A conversational style which would appear to the average adult to be one of "abnormal candor" contributes much to the atmosphere in which the adolescent can work best. This will do far more than an explanation of the "basic rule" toward making it possible for him to let us know what is going on in his mind. He will approach the work of therapy according to his therapist's lead. (p. 103)

As indicated above, one way to conceptualize this type of interaction is to understand it as one that is developmentally appropriate to the needs of the patient. The directedness of expression and style of relating employed by the therapist have the effect of meeting the adolescent in a communicative domain that is familiar to him and which encourages his view of the therapist as a potential ally.

The Adolescent Therapist as an Object of Identification

Adolescents are intensely curious about the way the adult world works. In fact, although they are often among the most outspoken critics of the existing social order, they are also anxious to find their place in it and search for adult models with whom to identify (Meeks, 1986). Curious about the world, anxious to find concrete solutions to problems with which they are faced, they often look to these adult models and to the person of their therapist for information about how to deal with these issues. Thus, the therapist's attitude about the issue or his stance about the importance of the problem quietly influences the adolescent's perspective on a particular issue. Beyond the implicit questions, there are also the less frequent explicit questions about how the therapist would deal with these issues. The selected "interpersonal" and less common "intrapersonal" self-disclosures thus help the adolescents to cope with their confusion about the issues at hand.

Jim, an articulate, 17-year-old high school senior, was quite depressed about a love relationship he was having. His parents had told him that he should forget about the relationship with this younger girl. However, he was unable to do so and continued to pine for her. His therapist, instead of analyzing his inability to do so, said simply. "In my day, the pain you are feeling over this relationship was thought of as one of the painful introductions to adulthood." Jim relaxed noticeably and in subsequent sessions was able to begin to talk about how difficult it had always been for him to end relationships with people, no matter how problematic they were.

In this manner, self-disclosure contributes to the adolescent's identification with aspects of the therapist's personality or attitude about the world (Adatto, 1966; Hendrick, 1988; Giovacchini, 1974; Papouchis, 1982). Selected aspects of the therapist's personality are then available to contribute to the development of the adolescent's ego ideal. Self-disclosure also prevents the exaggerated idealizations that may develop from the adolescent's projection of omnipotence onto the therapist. This is not to say that some degree of idealization is not an inevitable aspect of the therapeutic process. Rather, I would argue that it is important to avoid the excessive idealization that may interfere with an adolescent's ability to experiment with problem solving because of his mistaken belief in the existence of a "right" answer to a problem. It is essential therefore that the therapist convey to his patient that his way of solving a particular problem or way of looking at a particular issue is only one of a number of possible alternatives. It is equally important that the therapist emphasize that the point of view he presently adopts is one that developed after considerable reexamination over some period of time. The absence of omnipotence in the therapist's stance thus offers the adolescent the opportunity to identify selectively with some of the therapist's ways of coping with the world, and enhances the adolescent's ego functioning, without undermining his autonomy or self-esteem.

To do this the therapist must also respectfully encourage and acknowledge the adolescent's unique and often creative ways of coping with the world. While the adolescent may look to the therapist to help fill the void created by his intrapsychic disengagement from his parents, he is not looking for parental substitutes with whom he can recreate the same dependent relationship. Unlike the parent, the therapist must demonstrate to the adolescent that he does not have a narcissistic investment in the adolescent's following his advice or way of seeing things, and respects the adolescent's differences of opinion.

It is critical that the therapist demonstrate this by a willingness to let the adolescent work things out on his own. Unlike the concerned but controlling parent who must "help" the adolescent work out their problems, the effective therapist of adolescents acknowledges that there are a number of different ways to solve problems, and respects the fact that the adolescent's task is to discover those that work most effectively for him.

It is equally important that the therapist's comfort with self-disclosure involves a willingness to examine her own beliefs as they come under scrutiny, especially to acknowledge when those beliefs might be wrong. Authentic self-disclosure that leads to greater interpersonal intimacy and promotes therapeutic progress thus involves a readiness to acknowledge mistakes, and to listen with respect to the opinion of the adolescent with whom one is working (Giovacchini, 1974).

Summary

In summary, it is my opinion that self-disclosure on the part of the child or adolescent represents a greater threat to the developing ego than it does to the adult. Both children and adolescents must focus their ego resources on mastering the developmental tasks with which they are faced. Premature uncovering of unconscious conflict may represent a serious threat to the ego's ability to maintain psychic equilibrium. As a result, the therapist who works with this population must constantly monitor the impact of the patient's self-disclosures on the therapeutic alliance, while helping him gain greater ego mastery of the intrapsychic conflicts with which he is faced.

The therapist who works with this population is more likely to be self-disclosing than the therapist who works with adults. I have argued that the interpersonal-object relationship between patient and therapist provides a crucial foundation for the psychotherapeutic process. The nature of this relationship is different with children and adolescents than with adults, since it occurs while the object relationship with the parents is ongoing. As a result, the child and adolescent therapist is more of a real figure in the life of her patients. This does not minimize the importance of work in the transference. Instead, it makes the therapeutic work more complex. Selective self-disclosures on the part of the child and adolescent therapist facilitate the therapeutic interpersonal-object relationship, and contribute to the child and adolescent's opportunity to identify with aspects of the therapist's personality.

References

Adatto, C.P. (1966). On the metamorphosis from adolescence into adulthood. *Journal of the American Psychoanalytic Association, 14,* 485–509.

Anthony, E.J. (1969). The reactions of adults to adolescents and their behavior. In Gerald Caplan & Serge Lebovici (Eds.), *Adolescence, psychological perspectives,* New York: Basic Books.

Arieti, S. (1974). *Interpretation of schizophrenia.* New York: Basic Books.

Blos, P. (1962). *On adolescence: A psychoanalytic interpretation*. New York: International Universities Press.
Blos, P. (1979). *The adolescent passage*. New York: International Universities Press.
Bornstein, B. (1951). On latency. *Psychoanalytic Study of the Child*, 6:279–285.
Bowlby, J. (1969). *Attachment*. New York: Basic Books.
Chelune, G.J. (1975). Self-disclosure: An elaboration of its basic dimensions. *Psychological Reports, 36*, 79–85.
Colm, H. (1964). A field-theory approach to transference and its particular approach to children. In Mary R. Haworth (Ed.), *Child psychotherapy: Practice and theory*. New York: Basic Books.
Cozby, P. (1973). Self-disclosure: a literature review. *Psychological Bulletin, 79*, 73–91.
Danish, S.J., DiAugelli, A.R., & Brock, G.W. (1976). *Helping skills verbal response rating tape*. Unpublished transcript, Pennsylvania State University.
Doster, J.A., & Nesbitt, J.G. (1979). Psychotherapy and self-disclosure. In G.J. Chelune (Ed.), *Self-disclosure: Origins, patterns, and implications of openness in interpersonal relationships*. San Francisco: Jossey Bass.
Fairbairn, W.R.D. (1952). *Psychoanalytic studies of the personality*. London: Routledge & Kegan Paul.
Flavell, J.H. (1963). *The developmental psychology of Jean Piaget*. New York: D. Van Nostrand.
Freidman, L. (1969). The therapeutic alliance. *International Journal of Psychoanalysis, 50* (2), 139–153.
Freud, A. (1976). The role of transference in the analysis of children. In Charles Schafer (Ed.), *The therapeutic use of child's play*. New York: Jason Aronson.
Freud, S. (1912). Recommendations to physicians practising psycho-analysis. *Volume XII: The standard edition*. London: Hogarth Press.
Freud, S. (1914). Observations on transference-love. *Volume XII: The standard edition*. London: Hogarth Press.
Giovacchini, P.L. (1974). The difficult patient: Countertransference problems. *Adolescent Psychiatry, 3*, 271–288.
Ginott, H.G. (1964). Problems in the playroom. In Mary R. Haworth (Ed.), *Child psychotherapy: Practice and theory*. New York: Basic Books.
Greenson, R.R., & Wexler, M. (1969). The non-transference relationship in the psychoanalytic situation. *International Journal of Psychoanalysis, 50*, 27–39.
Guntrip, H. (1971). *Psychoanalytic theory, therapy, and the self*. New York: Basic Books.
Holmes, D.J. (1964). *The adolescent in psychotherapy*. Boston: Little, Brown.
Jourard, S. (1964). *The transparent self (ed.1)*. Princeton: D. Van Nostrand.
Jourard, S.M. (1968). *Disclosing man to himself*. Princeton: D. Van Nostrand.
Jourard, S.M. (1971). *The transparent self (2nd ed.)*. Princeton, N.J.: D. Van Nostrand.
Jourard, S.M. (1971). *Self-disclosure: An experimental analysis of the transparent self*. New York: Wiley-Interscience.
Johnson, D.W., & Noonan, M.P. (1972). Effects of acceptance and reciprocation of self-disclosures on the development of trust. *Journal of Counseling Psychology, 19*, 411–416.
Kessler, E. (1979). Individual psychotherapy with adolescents. In J.R. Novello (Ed.), *Short course in adolescent psychiatry*. New York: Brunner Mazel, 1979.
Langs, R. (1978). *The listening process*. New York: Jason Aronson.
Marshall, R.J., & Marshall, S.V. (1988). *The transference-countertransference matrix: The emotional-cognitive dialogue in psychotherapy, psychoanalysis and supervision*. New York: Columbia University Press.
McCarthy, P.R., & Betz, N.E. (1978). Differential effects of self-disclosing versus self-involving counselor statements. *Journal of Counseling Psychology, 25*, 251–256.
Meeks, J.E. (1986). *The fragile alliance*. Malabar, Fla: Robert E. Krieger.
Meissner, W.W. (1986). *Psychotherapy and the paranoid process*. Northvale, N.J.: Jason Aronson.

Nilsson, D.E., Strassberg, D.S., & Bannon, J. (1979). Perception of counselor self-disclosure: An analogue study. *Journal of Counseling Psychology, 26*(5):399–404.
Papouchis, N. (1982). Intimacy and the psychotherapy of adolescents. In Martin Fisher & George Stricker (Eds.), *Intimacy*. New York: Plenum.
Pine, F. (1985). *Developmental theory and clinical theory*. New Haven: Yale University Press.
Renik, O. (1986). Countertransference in theory and practice. *Journal of the American Psychoanalytic Association, 34*(3):699–708.
Ross, A.O. (1964). Techniques of therapy. In Mary R. Haworth, Ed., *Child psychotherapy: Practice and theory*. New York: Basic Books.
Schafer, R. (1983). *The analytic attitude*. New York: Basic Books.
Springmann, R.R. (1986). Countertransference: Clarifications in supervision. *Contemporary Psychoanalysis, 22*, 256–277.
Stone, L. (1961). *The psychoanalytic situation*. New York: International Universities Press.
Sullivan, H.S. (1953). *The interpersonal theory of psychiatry*. New York: W.W. Norton.
Truax, C.B., Carkhuff, R.R. (1965). Client and therapist transparency in the psychotherapeutic encounter. *Journal of Counseling Psychology, 12*, 3–8.
Weiner, I. (1970). *Psychological disturbance in adolescence*. New York: Wiley-Interscience.
Winnicott, D.W. (1965). *The maturational processes and the facilitating environment*. New York: International Universities Press.

12

Self-Disclosure in Psychotherapy

WORKING WITH OLDER ADULTS

Lisa R. Greenberg

Introduction

A factory worker in her mid-60s recently came to me for treatment. She showed many symptoms of agitated depression and described herself as "always" having been extremely "nervous." She told me that it had always been her strategy to try to "erase" her feelings. Ten minutes into her first session, she hesitated in response to a question I had asked about her daughter, and then said, "Well, there was an incident...maybe subconsciously...no, let's go on." When I encouraged her to tell me what she was thinking, she reported an event that had occurred 20 years earlier, during which she had failed to protect her daughter as she thought proper. She was able to begin to see that her attempts to push aside her guilt had not worked for her, and to consider various ways in which her feelings about the incident had affected both her relationship with her daughter and her own sense of herself. She left the session somewhat teary but greatly relieved and committed to continuing therapy.

Like many other distressed older people, she had paid such a high price for so long for trying to minimize her own experience that the merest taste of a relationship in which her feelings were valued was enough to lead her to reveal highly personal material in a helpful, positive way. Is this woman unusual? Do older people as a group self-disclose easily and effectively, or hesitantly and with no clear results?

Lisa R. Greenberg • 428 Franklin Avenue, Nutley, New Jersey 07110.

Can those who do not disclose easily be helped to learn to do so? In a volume on the role of self-disclosure in psychotherapy, need the elderly even be considered as a separate group, or are the risks and benefits of self-disclosure, and even the content of what is disclosed, exactly the same as for others?

Role of Self-Disclosure for Older People

In considering the role of self-disclosure in the psychotherapeutic treatment of older adults, defining the concept of "self-disclosure" is an important first step. For the purposes of this chapter, I will use the term to refer to the process of verbally revealing to another information about oneself that is at least somewhat personal in nature.

Hatfield (1982) writes, "epidemiologists have accumulated an abundance of evidence that intimacy and self-disclosure help people maintain their mental and physical health," while also identifying the risks of too much disclosure. Do these conclusions, derived from various studies with the general population, apply to the elderly?

The answer appears to be yes, but this conclusion is more tentative and more ambiguous than might be imagined.

In examining the work of those who argue for the importance of intimate, self-disclosing relationships for the elderly, Lowenthal and Haven's (1968) well-known study of San Francisco residents over age 60 is a good starting point. As part of a much larger work, they asked the question, "Is there anyone in particular you confide in or talk to about yourself or your problems?" Their hypothesis, that having at least one close personal relationship might serve as a buffer against such age-linked social losses as role loss, reduction of social interaction, widowhood, and retirement, was confirmed. They found, for example, that a person who has been widowed within seven years and had a confidant had even higher morale than a married person without a confidant. The only crisis in which having a confidant did not protect a subject's morale was physical illness: the elderly subjects who were or had recently been ill were found to be seriously depressed, regardless of whether they had a confidant. The authors summarize:

> The maintenance of a stable intimate relationship is more closely associated with good mental health and higher morale than is high social interaction or role status, or stability in interaction and role. Similarly, the loss of a confidant has a more deleterious effect on morale, though not on mental health status, than does a reduction in either of the other two social measures. (p. 400)

Lowenthal and Haven also looked at both the characteristics of those who had confidants and the identity of the confidants themselves. They identified women as more likely than men to have confidants, and married people as more likely than widowed, who were in turn more likely than single people to have confidants. Among those who did have confidants, the confidant was equally likely to be spouse, child, or friend, with men much more likely to identify their spouse as confidant than women. The likelihood of having a confidant was greater for those above the mean socioeconomically, and for those with a more complex social life.

Murphy's (1982) work generated similar conclusions. She compared depressed and normal elderly people in the general population using several measures, including a version of the Bedford College Life Events and Difficulties Interview modified for the elderly, which allowed a rating of depth of intimacy. She found the lack of a confiding relationship to be a factor increasing one's vulnerability to depression. Like Lowenthal and Haven, Murphy found most elderly subjects to be "remarkably cheerful," even in the face of considerable difficulties, with the exception only of those who lacked a confidant. She notes that it is not those who are lifelong social isolates by choice who have difficulty, but those who have tried and failed to establish good relationships. It is also interesting that those whose confidants were seen as little as every two to three weeks were as protected against depression as those who shared a household with a confidant. This suggested to Murphy that the crucial factor protecting against depression in the elderly is the capacity for intimacy, which she felt to be a lifelong personality trait. Unlike Lowenthal and Haven, she did not believe that intimacy was related to social class.

In a later study (1985), Murphy compared the ratings of intimacy of interpersonal relationships for elderly subjects who did and did not recover from depressive episodes for a year. She found that those who had recovered were significantly more likely to report a positive change in the quality of their intimate relationships than were those who had either remained continuously depressed or who had recovered and relapsed. While cause and effect are obviously unclear here, a statement about the value of confiding relationships for at least some elderly seems to be implied.

Some work of my own is also relevant here (Greenberg, 1982). As part of a study designed primarily to explore life satisfaction among elderly female homemakers and retirees, a structured interview and the Osgood Semantic Differential were administered to 60 women ranging in age from 70 to 79. Of particular interest in this context is that, while many of these women spoke with pleasure of a sense of freedom, a joy in the feeling that "I do what I feel like doing" after a lifetime of caring for others, many others expressed the flip side of this and spoke eloquently of feelings of loneliness and isolation. Many widows spoke with sadness of not having a spouse, or any relationship with a man, while others specifically mentioned the pain of not feeling close to anybody. Several felt that developing new friendships was harder in their old age than it had been at other points in their lives. All these concerns seemed to be expressions of deeply felt desires for intimate, confiding relationships. While the lack of these relationships had not led any of these women to become depressed or in any other way symptomatic, the frequency and eloquence with which this issue was mentioned by women who were otherwise reluctant to acknowledge painful feelings is indeed a strong statement, spoken by older people themselves, of the felt need for confiding relationships in older peoples' lives.

Indications of the importance of relationships in which self-disclosure plays an important part come from other sources as well, including studies on the importance of reminiscence for the elderly. Reminiscing, defined by McMahon and Rhudick (1961) as the "act or habit of thinking about or relating past experiences, especially those considered most personally significant" (p. 292), can be either an internal or an interpersonal process, but, when interpersonal, seems likely to be an act of self-disclosure. McMahon and Rhudick's finding, that reminiscing serves many positive functions for the elderly, including maintaining self-esteem, bolstering a sense of identity, and working through loss, again argues for the value of self-disclosure for the elderly.

Lewis and Butler (1974) formalized the process of reminiscing in the elderly with their "life-review therapy." They believe that, particularly for people in their 60s, a process of "life-review" occurs, in which the older person looks back over his or her life, reviews and resolves conflicts and comes to terms with both past and present. They believe that life review can take many forms, but noted that it is greatly enhanced by the presence of listeners, in which case it becomes a process of self-disclosure, which the authors clearly believe has value.

As suggested, however, the notion that confiding relationships are of value for the elderly is not universally held. Jerrome's (1981) study of friendship and aging among middle-class British women is an example. Her research was anthropological in nature, and consisted of depth interviews and participant observation. Her 66 subjects ranged in age from their late 50s to mid-80s. Most relevant to this work is her conclusion that the main need in friendships among the elderly women she studied seemed to be for companionship in a pleasurable activity. She stated specifically that neither the exchange of help nor the exchange of confidences seemed important in these friendships. The relationships she described appeared to be close and sustaining ones for the people involved, and included much time spent together in a wide range of mutually enjoyable activities, including shopping, gardening, card playing, and, in particular, eating and drinking. Self-disclosure, however, simply did not appear to be an important component, at least as observed and reported by Jerrome.

Andersson's (1985) work provides some support for Jerrome's conclusions. Working in Stockholm, he designed and studied an intervention program for a group of elderly women who described themselves as lonely. The intervention consisted of neighborhood groups with between three and five members who met four times, the first and last time with a home-help assistant present. Each group meeting was a discussion of a particular topic. Interviews held six months after the meetings showed that participating subjects had less feelings of loneliness and meaninglessness, more social contacts, higher self-esteem, greater ability to trust, and lower blood pressure than before the program. There was, however, no change regarding the availability of a close friend or confidant.

In considering his results, Andersson cited Jerrome's breakdown of friendship into three levels of intimacy, the first being shared activity, the second, reciprocal help, and the third, an exchange of confidences. Referring to the work of Jerrome and others, he hypothesized that under the normal circumstances of daily life, the optimal level of intimacy appears to be the exchange of reciprocal help. The next level of intimacy, the exchange of confidences, or self-disclosure, he proposed as promoting adaptation only in times of social loss. Andersson, however, did not consider that such losses do come along particularly frequently in the lives of elderly people, and therefore, the presence of a confiding relationship could be viewed as protective for all older people. It should also be noted that the findings of both Jerrome and Andersson seem to be in some contrast with my own; the women who described to me feelings of loneliness seemed clearly to be seeking, not companions with whom to share particular activities or exchange help, but true friends with whom to share themselves.

Emery and Lesher's (1982) paper on the treatment of depression in the elderly is also germane. This work was identified as part of a series of depression-treatment outcome studies at the University of Southern California's Andrus Gerontology Centers, but appears to be anecdotal in nature. This work supports the idea that self-disclosure is not universally of value to the elderly, but may be helpful under certain conditions. These authors came at the problem from another angle, claiming that the value of self-disclosure for a particular individual depends not on that person's circumstances at a given time, but on personality. Specifically, they felt that the elderly can be divided into two personality modes, dependent and autonomous, and that these modes influence the causes, symptomatology, and appropriate treatment for a particular individual's depression. They saw the dependent elderly as introspective and eager to discuss feelings. For this group, despite a tendency to overdisclose, self-disclosure in psychotherapy was generally helpful, in part because it contributed to the formation of a closer bond with the therapist. On the other hand, according to these authors, encouraging self-disclosure in the treatment of typically underdisclosing, autonomous elderly depressed patients can cause problems. Their concern seems to be that self-disclosing will lead these fiercely independent people to conclude that it is only the therapist who is capable of solving their problems and that they themselves are helpless.

In summary, there is considerable evidence that relationships in which self-disclosure plays a role are as beneficial for the elderly as for the rest of us. Except for a small subgroup identified by Emery and Lesher, no one has found any negative effects of self-disclosure, despite the wide range in age, mental health status, and nationalities of the elderly populations studied, as well as the widely differing research methodologies used. Even those least enthusiastic about the value of self-disclosure generally agree that while it may not be of interest or value to a particular subgroup of the older population, such as Jerrome's healthy, community-based female British sample, it probably has value to other groups. When self-disclosure has been found to be of value, the value has often been considerable. For instance, Lowenthal and Haven argue for the importance of a confidant in protecting against social losses, and Murphy's data show that a confiding relationship helps to protect an elderly person from depression.

Psychotherapy and the Elderly

Before returning to consider the specific issue of the role of self-disclosure in psychotherapy of the elderly, it seems relevant to examine briefly some aspects of the literature. Many authors (e.g., Pfeiffer, 1976; Blum & Tallmer, 1977) have pointed to the small amount of psychotherapeutic treatment available to older people, despite their large numbers in the population. Pfeiffer notes that the elderly tend to receive either no psychiatric services at all, or total care in institutions. The missing aspect is outpatient psychological services, which are much more used by other segments of the population.

The absence of large numbers of older people in psychotherapy is often seen at least in part as a legacy from Freud (cited in Blum and Tallmer), who is well known to have been highly pessimistic about the usefulness of therapy for anyone over age 45. Other factors, both psychological and societal, are clearly involved as well. Tallmer (1982) cited the glorification of independence in this age group, and the corresponding notion of help-seeking as immature. Today's elderly are also not part of a birth cohort in which seeing a therapist is easily understood by peers or family. Pfeiffer (1976) also pointed to the importance of the misconception that, in the elderly, a degree of depression, emotional upset, and forgetfulness are to be expected, and therefore do not warrant treatment. These assumptions would clearly not be made if the same symptoms were found in a younger person. I can recall a psychiatrist arguing that a hospitalized man was suffering, not from a major depression critically in need of treatment, but from what he labeled "a masked old-age thing," for which treatment of any type would be useless.

Societal images of the elderly as entrenched in their ways and unable or unwilling to change also contribute to decreasing the likelihood that an older person will be referred for therapy. Once a referral is made and treatment is begun, societal pressures also seem to affect the length and nature of the treatment offered, with a bias toward briefer and less insight-oriented therapy for older patients. Lakin, Oppenheimer, and Bremer (1982), for example, speaking specifically of group treatment, advocated "an acceptant, encouraging, supportive and nonconfrontational mode" (p. 452), including the "mild amplification of feelings," and strong encouragement of sharing and comparing feelings and experiences. They believe that most elderly people prefer to discuss concrete issues, and they specifically discourage group leaders from focusing on intra-individual or interpersonal struggles within the group. It is noteworthy that, while the desire to focus on concrete issues would be viewed as a resistance by most therapists working with younger people, when seen in work with the elderly, it is accepted as a virtually immutable quality.

Other writers, including some who view themselves as advocates of psychotherapy for the elderly, also promote supportive rather than insight-oriented treatment strategies. Pfeiffer (1976), for example, discussed the need for "significant modifications in technique" in working with older people. Among other changes, he endorses increased activity in the treatment by the therapist, including "symbolic giving," and "specific or limited goals" for the work. He views old age as associated with loss, and saw the therapeutic relationship with an older patient as a symbolic replacement for these losses. He believes in the value of a long-term commitment to the patient but emphasized that this does not require frequent or prolonged contacts between patient and clinician, assumed by Pfeiffer to be a physician. He mentioned, for example, patients whom he felt were "symbolically connected" to him, though he saw them only twice a year. Of particular interest in terms of the issue of self-disclosure are Pfeiffer's comments that during his visits with these patients he showed them pictures of his family, and that he and the patient "share in each other's growth and accomplishments" (p. 197).

Goodstein's (1982) thoughts on psychotherapy with older people were similar, though, in contrast to Pfeiffer, he did state that some older people need primarily insight-oriented work. Others, identified by him as those with a history of coping well, benefit most from treatment that is supportive and cognitively oriented. Like Pfeiffer, Goodstein seemed to emphasize more supportive treatments, and he too encourages the therapist to make certain changes in technique. He suggested, for example, that therapists serve as "total health care coordinators" for their elderly patients, and he encourages the setting of specific, limited goals and tasks for the therapy. He also encouraged the use of self-disclosure by the therapist much as Pfeiffer does, i.e., to build the therapist into the patient's life as a replacement for losses suffered by the patient. He identified talking of common interests and feelings as potentially valuable in providing a "symbolic but safe implication of intimacy" (p. 414), and suggested that therapists play cards or checkers or even share an occasional brandy with their patients.

It is important to note that Goodstein was not suggesting these techniques be used to forge an empathic connection between patient and therapist, which would then be the basis for exploring troubling issues in the patient's life. Likewise, they were not to provide a direct look at the patient's ways of interacting and viewing the world. Social activities between patient and therapist were instead to be viewed as an end in themselves: in Goodstein's words, the therapist is to serve as "a permanent source of need fulfillment." In other words, the patient is to accept a substitute for true intimacy; he or she has been determined by the therapist to be no longer capable of forming true intimate relationships and so is being given a substitute instead.

Certainly, not all authors considering psychotherapy with the elderly share a bias toward supportive treatments. Tallmer (1982), for example, wrote of analytic treatment with elderly patients. She did feel that some changes in technique may be necessary, but her suggestions, such as modifying seating arrangements or lighting to accommodate hearing- or vision-impaired patients, are to be implemented when appropriate to allow a traditional treatment to occur, rather than to change the nature of the therapy itself, as suggested by Pfeiffer and Goodstein.

Cohen's (1981) thoughts on psychotherapy with the elderly also point to the value of insight-oriented treatment for older people. In his view, it is problematic to conceptualize the issues of old age primarily in terms of loss. Instead, he cites those who view old age as a time of transformation, which involves additions as well as losses, and his view of therapy includes a belief in the value of helping an older patient to explore and make use of what has been added. Cohen also cautioned that, in focusing on the specifics of psychotherapy with the elderly, there is a risk of neglecting much of what is known about psychotherapy in general, and is equally applicable to work with all patients, regardless of age. Related to this is Wylie and Wylie's (1987) contention, in one of the few case studies to be found of an analysis of an older patient, that the reluctance of an analyst to begin an analysis with an old patient is a countertransference resistance.

Self-Disclosure by Therapist

Having briefly summarized the writings of therapists who advocate supportive treatment for the elderly, and then those whose orientation is more analytic, it is interesting to observe that the issue of the therapist's self-disclosure arose only in the work of those, i.e., Pfeiffer and Goodstein, who advocate more supportive treatments. Furthermore, as alluded to earlier, both Pfeiffer and Goodstein seem to use self-disclosure to foster and maintain an empathic connection between patient and therapist, but not to deepen the therapeutic process and promote insight. The therapist's role is not to assist the patient in developing attitudes and skills necessary to build a better life, but simply to satisfy symbolically the patient's needs. This approach seems patronizing and is based on certain highly questionable assumptions.

Perhaps the primary assumption here is that "the elderly" can usefully be viewed as a homogeneous population. It is no doubt true that there are many elderly patients who, because of some combination of physical disability, psychiatric disturbance, and cognitive impairment, are truly unlikely to be able to form new relationships and to find many sources of gratification in their lives. For these people, assuming the therapist can determine who they are, using Pfeiffer's model of the therapist as a permanent symbolic substitute for lost relationships is probably valuable. Some support for this treatment strategy can be found in Murphy's finding, earlier cited, that even relatively infrequent contacts with a confidant protects against depression.

The danger, however, lies in believing that this treatment approach is appropriate for all older patients. For most old people, the role of therapist should be, as it is for patients of all ages, to foster growth and development, and to help the patient to be able eventually to gratify his or her needs outside the therapeutic relationship. Support for these goals as realistic can be found from several sources. Murphy (1985), for example, found her elderly subjects who ranged in age from 65 to 89, to have a "remarkable capacity" to form new close relationships after their depressive episodes had passed. Jerrome, too, found that most of her older subjects were able to increase their circle of friends to the degree they desired. If, in fact, most older people are able to form new positive, intimate relationships, at least when they are not depressed, this argues that the role of a therapist should be to aid older people in the resolution of their difficulties, and not to supply them directly with intimate relationships. Perhaps it is most significant that clinical researchers have not found a relationship between patient's age and therapy outcome (Blum & Tallmer, 1977), indicating that major therapeutic modifications may not be necessary for successful psychotherapy with the elderly.

This leads us to the question of whether self-disclosure by the therapist has a role in insight-oriented treatment with the elderly. It seems to me that, as with patients of other ages, self-disclosure by a therapist working with an elderly patient may or may not be helpful, may or may not be countertransferential, and may or may not advance the process. The factor that determines whether a particular self-disclosure by the therapist is helpful seems to me to be largely independent of the patient's age.

Several incidents come to mind. One was of unintended by unavoidable self-disclosure, which had positive consequences. Some years ago, I broke my foot and arrived at work in an inpatient psychogeriatric setting with a cast up to my knee. To my surprise, a very depressed and withdrawn man, after laughing (somewhat sadistically, it seemed to me) at my feeble attempts to walk, was able to consider my ability to continue to work and apparent good spirits. Previously, I had been seen as young, healthy, and problem-free, and therefore, as unable to comprehend his pain and inability to function. My cast, however, impelled him to ask some version of the question, "If you have that and are still OK, why aren't I managing despite my problems?" He began to shift from accepting his paralyzing depressions as inevitable to questioning his own investment in not functioning.

Similarly, when I became engaged to marry, one of my patients in both group and individual therapy was a psychotic woman in her early 70s, who had always been single. When I told her of my plans to marry, she reacted with a bizarre tirade comprising attacks both on me for my presumed abandonment of her and, even more vehemently, on herself for having failed ever to marry. With the help of me and my coleader and, perhaps most particularly of her elderly fellow group members, however, she was able to work through some of these feelings. She came away with at least a limited sense that there were many possible ways of living, and that it was by no means essential to have been married to feel that one's life has been of value.

This anecdote also points to a relation between the value of self-disclosure by the therapist and the age of the patient. Self-disclosure by a young therapist, often of something important in his or her present life, can at times serve to promote the patient's process of life review, as described by Lewis and Butler and previously discussed. Any mention at all of such events as marriage or pregnancy, for example, often triggers a flood of memories of the patient's own experiences of these major life events, and thereby provide an opportunity to work on any unresolved issues.

There is, however, also a caveat regarding a young therapist's self-disclosures to an older patient. Therapists at times attempt to use self-disclosure to communicate to patients that they understand and can empathize with the patient's experience, when, in fact, their own life may have been so different that their capacity for understanding and empathy is not as great as they would like. Today's elderly have had life experiences that differ dramatically from those of their therapists, particularly if their therapists are much younger. Often, therapy is occurring between one person who has directly experienced immigration, the Great Depression, and one, if not two, world wars. Setting aside issues that are purely personal, these differences alone are important. Rather than forcing an unreal connection by expressing too much empathy too quickly, or sharing a life experience that is only mildly similar to that of the patient, it is often more helpful for a young therapist to listen with attention and respect, and to be open to being educated. My sense is that comments that are intended by the therapist to build a connection with the patient by pointing to similarities between them are often instead felt as disappointing intrusions by the patients in that they remind the patient that there is, after all, a wide gap between them.

This leaves open the question of what self-disclosing statements by the therapist do and do not tend to be helpful. Perhaps most helpful are those remarks that the therapist freely makes about his or her own life, with no expectation of any particular response, while those that almost urge the patient to experience a connection that may or may not be real can be instead distancing and hurtful.

Self-Disclosure by Older Patients

Having discussed the issue of self-disclosure by the therapist in the treatment of elderly patients, the obvious remaining subject is self-disclosure by patients themselves. Lakin *et al.* (1982) report a relevant study designed to compare group behaviors of older (age 65+) and younger (college students) subjects in unstructured helping groups led by the authors. Self-disclosure was found to be significantly higher for all the older adult groups than for the younger groups, and also to differ in quality between the age groups. Older people talked easily about major problems, including loneliness and fear of abandonment, but the authors report an "almost stereotypic quality" in both the disclosures and the empathic responses they elicited. The authors contrast this to the behavior of the younger subjects, who, while generally more defensive and less disclosing, spoke with more affect when they did disclose. Discussions among the old were reported to be "less jagged"; the authors surmise that this is because these subjects have a firmer sense of their own identity and a related sense of confidence that others will feel as they do. The young, on the other hand, tend to feel alone in their feelings, making self-disclosure feel much riskier to them.

In some ways, my own experience has been consistent with the findings of Lakin et al. In conducting interviews for the research discussed above (Greenberg, 1982), for example, I too observed a willingness to self-disclose. In fact, subjects often seemed to welcome having an opportunity to talk about many aspects of their lives with an interested younger person. There was, however, in almost all cases, a clear reluctance to disclose any painful affect and, in particular, to acknowledge situations that caused feelings of shame or guilt.

This pattern of talking freely and easily in response to direct questions about one's life, but becoming reserved in discussing painful feelings, seems to occur frequently in clinical settings as well, and seems to me to have several bases.

One issue that comes into play concerns the ways in which today's generation of older people were socialized. For most people, fulfilling one's obligations to others was valued far above one's own feelings. As a woman in her 70s said to me regarding her view of being a housewife while in her 20s, "You didn't know from anything, how could you be unhappy? Like a caveman, he was happy in his cave, everybody believed the same." Clearly, she had been taught to minimize the importance of her own needs and feelings. This value system is in marked contrast with that of psychotherapy, in which the focus is on one's self and one's feelings. This contrast in values can be confusing and alarming for an older person encountering a therapist for the first time. My impression is that the elderly patient is often mystified by the therapist's inquiries, and is left wondering, "What does this person *want* from me?"

Many older people also walk into a therapist's office expecting an experience similar to that of seeing a medical doctor, and this too can present a barrier to self-disclosure. Instead of understanding therapy to be a collaborative process, the therapist is perceived as a "doctor" who administers a cure with little input from the patient. (My own grandmother refused for years to answer questions put to her by any clinician, claiming that if they were supposed to know so much, why did she have to tell them?)

Another factor leading many older people to refrain from speaking freely about themselves seems to be a fear of damaging the status quo. It is as if they are afraid of undertaking Lewis and Butler's (1974) life review, as if they might be unable to come to terms with their own choices, and therefore prefer to leave well enough alone. Here, what appears to be a reluctance to speak freely to another is actually a desire to avoid acknowledging certain realities to one's self. As a woman, filling out a form requiring her to choose between "painful" and "pleasurable" to describe herself, said to me, "Well, it would be a shame to say 'painful,' so I'll say 'pleasurable'." It seemed clear that she was afraid to look too closely.

A related barrier to self-disclosure among old people is their fear of being judged negatively for any feelings or behavior that violate their idealized image of themselves, which is often society's image as well. That is, they are to be nonaggressive, nonsexual, noncompetitive and, at least for women, nurturing of others. Acknowledging that this is not always the case may be particularly difficult when the therapist is much younger than the patient, and is transferentially experienced as the patient's child, in whose eyes one must be a mature adult. Countertransferentially, as well, there may be difficulty in accepting that a parental figure may not live up to the therapist's infantile expectations.

Having identified all these factors that at times contribute to making self-disclosure in therapy difficult for old patients, I must also say that these factors are in no way to be viewed as contraindications for psychotherapy for older patients, or as reasons to promote particularly directive forms of treatment. Rather, they can be seen as resistances to be worked on in therapy.

In addition, I also believe that there is a subgroup of older patients who, while they may experience some of these conflicts, put them aside extremely quickly and self-disclose easily, effectively, and with impressive results. The woman whose case introduced this chapter is among those for whom self-disclosure has always been actively discouraged, and yet who are so desperate to share their experiences that an opportunity to do so is eagerly seized. Patients like this are less resistant than the norm, and often benefit tremendously from short-term dynamic treatment.

Summary

This chapter has considered the issue of self-disclosure and the elderly from several perspectives. Most of the literature on the value of self-disclosing relationships for the elderly concludes that for the elderly, as for people of other ages, confiding relationships are of value, particularly in maintaining morale during periods of loss. This is a powerful argument in favor of psychotherapy, a particularly intense and valuable self-disclosing relationship, for older people. It is thus particularly unfortunate that old people tend to be underrepresented as therapy patients, and that the therapy that is done with this population tends often to be more directive and supportive than is the case with younger patients. While most investigators only consider the role of the therapist's self-disclosure in therapy with the elderly in discussions of supportive treatments, self-disclosure by the therapist can facilitate an insight-oriented treatment as well. For example, the therapist's self-disclosure can provide an opportunity for the patients to rework significant events in their own lives.

Barriers to self-disclosure by elderly patients are often observed. These include issues arising from the ways in which these patients were socialized, and others based on transference–countertransference dynamics. These barriers are minimal for many patients but, even for those for whom they are considerable, they are not obstacles that make therapy impossible, but therapeutic challenges that must be worked through as part of the valuable and gratifying work of treating older people in psychotherapy.

References

Andersson, L. (1985). Intervention against loneliness in a group of elderly women: An impact evaluation. *Social Science and Medicine, 20* (4), 355–364.

Blum, J., & Tallmer, M. (1977). The therapist vis-à-vis the older patient. *Psychotherapy: Theory, Research and Practice, 14* (4), 361–367.

Cohen, G.D. (1981). Perspectives on psychotherapy with the elderly. *American Journal of Psychiatry, 138* (3), 347–350.

Emery, G., & Lesher, E. (1982). Treatment of depression in older adults: Personality considerations. *Psychotherapy: Theory, Research and Practice, 19* (4), 500–505.

Goodstein, R.K. (1982). Individual psychotherapy and the elderly. *Psychotherapy: Theory, Research and Practice, 19* (4), 412–418.

Greenberg, L.R. (1982). Subjective experiences of elderly women as a function of employment history and experience of the past. Doctoral dissertation, Adelphi University. *Dissertation Abstracts International, 43* (03-B), 870–1054. (University Microfilms No. AAD82-19001).

Hatfield, E. (1982). Passionate love, compassionate love, and intimacy. In M. Fisher and G. Stricker (Eds.), *Intimacy*. New York: Plenum.

Jerrome, D. (1981). The significance of friendship for women in later life. *Aging Society, 1,* 175–197.
Lakin, M., Oppenheimer, B., & Bremer, J. (1982). A note on old and young in helping groups. *Psychotherapy: Theory, Research and Practice, 19* (4), 444–452.
Lewis, M.I., & Butler, R.N. (1974). Life-review therapy. *Geriatrics, 29,* 165–173.
Lowenthal, M.F., & Haven, C. (1968). Interaction and adaptation: Intimacy as a critical variable. In B. Neugarten (Ed.), *Middle age and aging.* Chicago: University of Chicago Press.
McMahon, A.W., & Rhudick, P.J. (1964). Reminiscing: Adaptational significance in the aged. *Archives of General Psychiatry, 10,* 292–298.
Murphy E. (1982). Social origins of depression in old age. *British Journal of Psychiatry, 141,* 135–142.
Murphy, E. (1985). The impact of depression in old age on close social relationships. *American Journal of Psychiatry, 142* (3), 323–327.
Pfeiffer, E. (1976). Psychotherapy with elderly patients. In L. Bellak & T. Karasu (Eds.), *Geriatric Psychiatry.* New York: Grune & Stratton.
Tallmer, M. (1982). Intimacy issues and the older patient. In M. Fisher & G. Stricker (Eds.), *Intimacy.* New York: Plenum.
Wylie, H.W., & Wylie, M.L. (1987). The older analysand: Countertransference issues in psychoanalysis. *International Journal of Psychoanalysis, 68* (3), 343–352.

13

Self-Disclosure in Group Psychotherapy

Sophia Vinogradov and Irvin D. Yalom

John, usually a silent member, opened a group meeting with a carefully planned statement about an episode of sexual abuse he had experienced as a child. He told the story in a deliberate manner with a flat expression. When he finished, there were a couple of minutes of silence, whereupon John said, half-jokingly, that he didn't give a damn if the group responded to him or not. Soon the disclosure evoked many reactions in the rest of the group. Another member, Steven, began to weep, recalling a past experience of sexual molestation and its subsequent influence on his sexual identity. Two other members offered him some words of support, which fell on deaf ears; this permitted the leaders to point out how hard it is for Steven to accept comfort from others. One member commented that she felt confused by the discrepancy between how much John revealed and his flat, rehearsed manner of revelation. Another member, Mary, had an entirely different set of responses to John: she felt that his overwhelming self-disclosure put pressure on other group members to respond in kind. She resented this pressure and felt manipulated by John. A lively and engaging session ensued, with many complex variations on the theme of self-disclosure.

Every group psychotherapist knows that, if a therapy group is to function optimally, members must disclose a great deal of personal material to one another. And yet, self-disclosure is important in individual psychotherapy as well. What distinguishes the two? What is unique about self-disclosure in the context of a group?

Sophia Vinogradov • Department of Psychiatry, Pacific Presbyterian Medical Center, San Francisco, California 94115. **Irvin D. Yalom** • Department of Psychiatry and Behavioral Sciences, Stanford University School of Medicine, Stanford, California 94305.

There are several answers to these questions. First of all, we may dichotomize disclosure into two forms: *vertical self-disclosure,* where one reveals material about one's past, or about one's outside life, and *horizontal self-disclosure,* where one examines the interpersonal effects and implications of revealing oneself. In the example above, John engaged in vertical self-disclosure and was joined in this by Steven, who shared early memories that had been evoked by John's disclosure. In this clinical situation, the leader deliberately refrained from reinforcing the vertical disclosure either by exploring it or by encouraging more vertical disclosure from John, Steven, or the other members. Instead, the leader encouraged the process of horizontal disclosure—by encouraging John to examine how he felt about sharing this material, by asking whose opinion was particularly important to him and how he felt about the support offered him (both the explicit support of other members and the implicit support of Steven, who, by revealing similar painful material, had given John a gift). The leader also encouraged a discussion of Mary's observations about John's style of delivery, and her feelings of having been coerced and manipulated. The examination of these aspects of horizontal disclosure was enlivening to the group and far more productive for them than the other clinical option of delving more deeply into the content of John's early sexual abuse.

Second, in group therapy, patient self-disclosure is greatly influenced by the attitude and role of the group leader, who is generally more self-disclosing than the individual therapist. The leader who judiciously uses his or her own person to relate authentically to others in the group creates an atmosphere in which sharing, mutual respect, and interpersonal honesty are modeled. Consider this vignette:

> In the tenth meeting of a sixteen session therapy group, one of the therapists, Irv, was called out of town because of his mother's death. Joan, his co-therapist, not wanting to intrude on Irv's privacy, explained his unexpected absence by vaguely referring only to a death in the family. When Irv returned to the group the following week, members acted curious, but were very uncomfortable when asking questions about his absence. At this point, Irv revealed to the group that he had been out of town because his mother had died, and he encouraged members to ask questions and to explore the rules of what they could and could not ask a therapist. Members had many strong and sympathetic reactions, and asked a series of appropriate questions: How was Irv doing? Would he like to use the group to work himself? How did he get help in times of distress? What was his relationship to his mother? Irv answered all questions openly and honestly, at times giving the members more information than they requested. The group seemed satisfied and turned to continue productive work on other issues.

In this example, the therapist's disclosure liberated the group; the members were persuaded that the therapist was coping well and that he had the energy available to work with them. Furthermore, the therapist's self-disclosure served as good modeling and encouraged the patients, in turn, to reveal more of themselves and to relate more honestly to others.

From the patient's point of view, self-disclosure occurring in the context of a group carries a higher risk than that occurring in a patient-therapist dyad. There is more chance of being misunderstood or rejected by a group of individuals who are, after all, fellow patients, and not paid to be supportive. In like manner, however, self-disclosure in group therapy has a higher return: Genuine acceptance by fellow group members carries a great deal of meaning and weight.

From the therapist's point of view, self-disclosure in group therapy plays a very different role than it does in individual work. Initially, it serves to increase group cohesiveness and it contributes to members' sense of sharing and belonging. It allows therapists to identify members who show deviant participation in the group, either those who reveal too little, or those who reveal too much too soon. And finally, self-disclosure, especially horizonal self-disclosure, is absolutely essential to the development of interpersonal learning in the group.

As our clinical vignettes illustrate, the process of self-disclosure and of developing closer, more genuine relationships within the context of the psychotherapy group is complex, and quite different from the process of self-disclosure in individual psychotherapy. Both patient and therapist play an important role in its development.

Patient Self-Disclosure in Group Psychotherapy

Self-disclosure, whether it takes place in group therapy or in individual therapy, takes many forms: Patients may reveal material involving past or current experiences, personal fears, fantasies or dreams, and hopes, aspirations, and concerns for the future. However, there is in group therapy an additional dimension of self-disclosure: Patients in a group setting may also reveal and explore their feelings towards the other members and interactions in the room, often referred to as *here-and-now disclosure*. This process plunges members into the "here-and-now" of the group's interactions and forms an integral step in the process of learning about one's interpersonal relationships (see Yalom, 1985). Here-and-now disclosure occurs in individual therapy as well, particularly when the patient expresses his or her feelings about the therapist as they arise during a session; however, it is more limited and unidirectional in nature, as the patient rarely receives similar feedback in return from the psychotherapist.

The Importance of Patient Self-Disclosure in Group Psychotherapy

If the timing and atmosphere are right, nothing commits individual members to a group more than to receive (or to reveal) some previously secret material. The entire group feels privileged when a member is able to disclose for the first time something that has been burdensome for years; the individual feels exhilarated as he or she is understood and fully accepted by the group. With gradually increasing levels of self-disclosure, the entire membership of a group strengthens its involvement, responsibility, and obligation to one another.

A large body of research evidence underscores the importance of self-disclosure in group therapy. First, high levels of disclosure in a group have been demonstrated to increase group cohesiveness (Bloch, 1981; Query, 1964; Johnson, 1974). People are apt to reveal more to those they like, and group members who reveal themselves are in turn more liked by others (Worthy, 1969). Patients who disclose early in the life of a group are often very popular, and the popularity of a patient in a therapy group correlates positively with therapy outcome (Yalom, 1967). As a general rule, patients who are ultimately successful in group therapy make more self-disclosing statements (Peres, 1947; Truax, 1965; Lieberman, 1973).

Some investigators consider self-disclosure to be so central to the healing or curative process of a group psychotherapy that they identify it as a therapeutic factor per se (Bloch, 1980). Certainly, interpersonal theorists such as Sullivan and Rogers have maintained that self-acceptance must be preceded by acceptance by others; in order to accept oneself, then, one must allow others to know and accept one as one really is.

Yalom has expanded this point by noting that—although self-disclosure is indeed intrinsically valuable—its real usefulness in group therapy occurs within the matrix of interpersonal learning (Yalom, 1985). Patients find self-disclosure to be an important act not only because of the sheer relief they feel from ventilating a secret, but because they can then go on to experience the interpersonal response from others to their disclosure. To reveal oneself, and then to be actively accepted and supported by others, is deeply validating. Patients often entertain some disastrous or shameful fantasy about revealing less-than-ideal parts of themselves; to allow others to see "the real me" and to have that fantasy disconfirmed is highly therapeutic.

Not only are patients rewarded by other group members for their disclosure, but they learn more about why it was difficult to reveal parts of themselves and about how this affects their relationships both in the group and in real life. Ultimately, this insight and this behavior change in the group—this interpersonal learning—is transferred into the patient's real life relationships.

The Process of Patient Self-Disclosure

Self-disclosure is a complex social and psychological act which is bound by one's role and one's situation. Time, place, and person all enter into the balance of what determines appropriate acts of self-disclosure. A challenging and helpful exchange between two senior members in an advanced interactionally oriented therapy group (e.g., "I finally feel able to tell you how arrogant I find you") may be threatening to neophytes in a less-advanced group, and may be downright destructive in an acute inpatient group of decompensated patients.

No matter what the timing or context, self-disclosure in the group must be guided as much by a sense of responsibility and empathy for others as by total openness and honesty. Hostile and destructive interactions can occur in groups under the guise of self-expression: "Okay, so I made a hurtful comment to Mark. But you told us that we should be perfectly honest about our real feelings!" The group therapist will find that, for some people, disclosure about overt angry or hostile feelings comes easily. The therapist will need to encourage such individuals to self-disclose at a deeper level, and to reveal the feelings that underlie and account for their anger or hostility—feelings that might include fear, envy, or sadistic pleasure.

The group therapist may also need to remind members that, if self-disclosure is to promote greater sharing and closeness, it must occur in a context of remaining constructive and responsible to others. Full self-disclosure is never possible; there will always be layers of reactions that we choose not to share with others: secret judgments about physical traits, impatience with intellectual mediocrity, stereotypes about social class, boredom, fleeting sadistic or sexual fantasies, and the like. We refrain from revealing these sorts of feelings because of more overriding concerns of empathy and responsibility. The therapist may, in fact, wish to emphasize that for many individuals high-risk disclosure consists not of making negative remarks to others, but of taking the chance to honestly and openly voice positive feelings in the group, feelings such as admiration, concern, attraction, and closeness.

Problems in Maladaptive Patient Self-Disclosure

Too little self-disclosure can prevail when the entire group is blocked and unable to share any personal material. There are many causes for this situation: distrust of the group leader, fear that the group may not be safe (usually because of the presence of a hostile or agitated member), concern about judgmentalism in the group (such as when some members seem extremely judgmental about marital fidelity). Occasionally there is concern about confidentiality; when members lack trust in the confidentiality of group material, they are reluctant to discuss personal issues. For example, a therapy group led on a university outpatient service was being videotaped for teaching purposes; because members felt threatened in their anonymity and privacy by the videotaping, the group remained very superficial and blocked in its interactions.

A therapy group as a whole can also fail to develop appropriate levels of self-disclosure when it lacks one or more members who are able spontaneously to reveal personal material and serve as pace-setters. This problem is generally amenable to appropriate modeling by the leader, who can demonstrate or encourage self-disclosing statements and foster a more revealing, more interactional kind of group.

Even in a group where most members are disclosing appropriate amounts of personal material, there may be individuals who are unable to reveal very much to others. Often a member will disclose little about him- or herself because of a sense of shame and fear of nonacceptance. And yet, without honest self-disclosure, the group is unable to relate to that member or to accept him or her in any kind of authentic way; without genuine acceptance by others, the individual has little hope of self-acceptance and little chance for experiencing a rise in self-esteem. As a general rule, too little self-disclosure by an individual member reduces his or her chances for forming meaningful relationships in the group.

Some individuals dread self-disclosure not because of shame or fear of nonacceptance, but because they are heavily conflicted in the area of control: to them, self-disclosure is dangerous because it makes them vulnerable to the control of others. When others in the group have made themselves exceedingly vulnerable through self-disclosure, then, and only then, is such a person willing to reciprocate.

Phillip, a member of a 20-session outpatient group, had gone through two unsuccessful marriages and was extremely distrustful of women. He kept prodding the women members in his group to lay their inner selves bare before he would reveal anything; this posture soon made the women members feel exploited and angry, creating a self-fulfilling prophecy in Phillip's relationships with women in the group.

In some group settings, particularly those involving professionals (such as a T-group for psychology interns, or a staff retreat for ICU nurses), honest self-disclosure is discouraged by a climate of competition or judgmentalism. In addition, if one reveals personal vulnerabilities or character flaws, one may be open to criticism about professional performance. In mental health fields in particular, one's professional competence is seen as overlapping heavily with one's emotional maturity—self-disclosure thus represents a double jeopardy, as it opens the individual to judgments about both personal health and professional competence.

In specialized groups oriented towards support (such as an eating disorders group), where members place a premium on being "nice" or "polite," self-disclosure often becomes equated with "taking up time for oneself" and not being supportive and concerned about others. In these cases, patients have made the mistaken assumption that self-disclosure consists solely of recitation, rather than a reciprocal, dynamically evolving process among all group members.

Some group members are so concerned about maintaining a socially attractive facade that they dwell on appearances: If they open up about their problems, will they appear to be friendless, lonely, pitiable? Others believe that they do not deserve the time and attention, that what they have to say about themselves is unimportant, and they therefore reveal things in an apologetic, hesitant, telegraphic manner. Other individuals, and these may be the majority of new group members, simply don't know how to self-disclose in an appropriate way.

Too much self-disclosure can be as maladaptive as too little. Some patients reason that if self-disclosure is desirable, then continuous and total self-disclosure must be even better. They fail to realize that it is not the amount of self-disclosure on an absolute scale, but its occurrence in the context of the relationship between discloser and receiver, that defines a healthy pattern of self-disclosure. Under normal circumstances, individuals disclose different types and amounts of material, depending on whether the receiver is a family member, a work associate, or a best friend (Jourard, 1950).

Some maladaptive disclosers disregard the nature of their relationships to the people they talk with, and indiscriminately "spill their guts" to any and all who fall within earshot. In group psychotherapy, the individual who reveals intimate material before knowing the group well, or who lets it be known that this same material has also been shared with mere acquaintances outside the group, perplexes the other members. First, a great deal of self-disclosure can frighten off unprepared recipients: What are the implications of this much sharing? What will the discloser want in return? Is this an implied demand that they must reciprocate in turn? Second, the group may feel devalued, even deceived, when it learns that supposedly intimate material confided by one of its members has in fact been related on numerous occasions to others outside the group.

Members who reveal early and promiscuously will generally drop out early in the course of group therapy (Yalom, 1966, 1985). Although patients should be encouraged to take risks in the group, to reveal themselves, and to obtain feedback and reinforcement for their behavior, they may—if they reveal too much too soon—exceed their own tolerance and that of the rest of the group. The member who has self-disclosed too early may feel so much shame in the group that the interpersonal rewards seem insignificant or unsatisfactory. Furthermore, such individuals may threaten other members who are willing to be accepting and supportive, but who are not yet prepared to reciprocate with an equivalent degree of self-disclosure. Consequently, they refuse to "join" with the discloser, who may be placed in such a vulnerable and isolated position that he or she often chooses to flee.

> Evelyn was a faithful but largely silent member of a newly formed support group for women engineering students. As the group began to become more interactive, other members started turning to Evelyn and attempting to draw her out. She steadfastly resisted these attempts, frustrating the group and perplexing the leaders.
>
> At the fourth meeting, during a rather general discussion on the subject of intimacy, Evelyn suddenly revealed that she was having an extramarital affair with her advisor, and that this was turning into an exploitative and abusive relationship. The other group members, although sympathetic, were stunned by this dramatic and unexpected revelation from a usually silent and resistant individual.
>
> During ensuing sessions, members found they were having a great deal of difficulty offering Evelyn helpful feedback. In addition, all further attempts at eliciting more material from her were useless; Evelyn "clammed up" again and refused to share anything more with the group. Three weeks later, she dropped out of the group without any forewarning.

Therapist Self-Disclosure in Group Psychotherapy

Group psychotherapists may—just like other members in the group—openly share their thoughts and feelings in a judicious and responsible manner, respond to others authentically, and acknowledge or refute motives and feelings attributed to them. In other words, therapists, too, can reveal their feelings, the reasons for some of their behavior, acknowledge the blind spots, and demonstrate respect for the feedback group members offer them.

This form of therapist self-disclosure, or *therapist transparency*, has two effects in the group: First, it counteracts the effect of transference, or irrational responses to the group leader. In the face of ever-increasing reality-based data revealed by the therapist, members find it more and more difficult to maintain their fictitious beliefs about the group leader. By gradually revealing more of him or herself, by reacting to the patient as a real person in the here and now, the therapist helps members to confirm (or disconfirm) attitudes and abilities attributed to him or her on the basis of unconscious fantasies. Second, the judicious use of therapist transparency models interpersonal sharing and honesty for the rest of the group. In this manner the therapist can reinforce norms of self-expression and self-exploration, while modeling responsibility and restraint.

Two Forms of Therapist Transparency

> A group leader noticed that, once again, Barbara, an unusually shy member, had not spoken at all during the session. She had sat quietly with a pained expression on her face, and now, towards the middle of the meeting, she was glancing frequently at her watch. "You know, Barbara," the leader said. "I've noticed you looking at your watch as if you're wondering when the meeting will be over. I sense some pain in you and I'd like to bring you into the group today—one of my roles is to help all members participate. Yet I feel caught in a dilemma; I feel paternal towards you, like I want to rescue you, but I often do too much of that and it feels like I'd just be infantilizing you. Also, there's a part of me that doesn't want the obligation of being your rescuer."

There are two aspects to therapist self-disclosure or transparency: personal, and professional. In personal self-disclosure, the therapist behaves and reacts in the real time of the group. He or she carefully chooses to reveal personal thoughts or feelings that are germane to ongoing interactions and that might facilitate the group process ("I don't want the obligation of being your rescuer," or "I feel paternal towards you"). This consists of providing (and accepting) honest, constructive feedback; of stimulating interpersonal learning by sharing reactions in the group; and of modeling nonjudgmental acceptance.

When therapists engage in professional transparency, they judiciously reveal the process guiding some of their therapeutic interventions and the results they feel they have obtained from those interventions. The professional transparent therapist allows patients to observe the manner in which the therapist's questions, thoughts, and conclusions are derived from the data at hand. This can occur when the leader makes comments during an actual session: "I feel caught in a dilemma, Barbara...If I call on you, I infantilize you. If I don't, I have concerns that you will get little from the therapy, or maybe that you will drop out of the group."

There are other useful techniques of professional transparency that are unique to group psychotherapy. Yalom (1985) suggests that the therapist write a brief synopsis after each session and mail it to group members, who can read the summary before the next session. Therapists can use this format not only to comment on events in the group, but to explain why they made the interventions they did, or how they reached certain conclusions.

Another technique allows group members to watch post-group sessions where the therapist, co-therapist, and any observers describe in detail their interpretations of the group and their reasons for arriving at those conclusions. Some rehash sessions even allow for a brief feedback period from group members (see Yalom, 1983).

Objections to Therapist Transparency

The primary sweeping objection to therapist transparency is based on the traditional analytic belief that the paramount therapeutic factor in psychotherapy is the resolution of patient–therapist transference. According to this model, the development of patient–therapist transference should be encouraged, and the group therapist should aid this by deliberately remaining opaque. In group therapy, however, other therapeutic factors are of equal or greater importance; some of these include altruism, vicarious learning, and cohesiveness. The therapist who judiciously uses his or her own person in the real time of the group greatly increases the therapeutic power of the group by encouraging the development of these other factors (see Yalom, 1985).

In modeling interpersonal transparency, the therapist can directly attend to here-and-now interactions occurring in the group, and can also help members examine some of the group process. In the clinical vignette where the therapist disclosed his mother's death to the group, this example of therapist transparency stimulated many important interactions and questions among members. Why had they found it so difficult to ask the leader about his absence? Now that he had told them about his mother, could they ask more about the nature of his relationship with her? Did they even have the right to ask the therapist if he would like to talk more about his mother? These issues in turn prodded several members into discussing their own relationships with their aging parents, while other members were led to examine some of their assumptions about what they can and cannot ask the group leader. By modeling, by showing respect for the process and for the group members, by demonstrating that he, too, believes it helps to talk, by letting members know that he was really all right and could work with them, the therapist was able to hasten the development of group cohesiveness and autonomy.

One objection therapists sometimes raise to self-disclosure is the fear of escalation, the fear that once they reveal themselves, the insatiable group will demand even more. But strong forces in the group oppose this trend; though members are enormously curious about their group leader, they also wish the therapist to remain unknown and all-powerful. When Joan, Irv's co-therapist, was asked why she had been so reluctant to give any details about his sudden absence, she revealed to the group that she had found herself in a dilemma; on the one hand, she had wanted to be completely open and honest with the group, while on the other hand, she had wanted to protect Irv's privacy. Rather than question her any further about her decision to protect Irv at the expense of the group, members were sensitive to the awkwardness she was describing and did not press her further. While group members will generally appreciate the responsible and growth-promoting use of interpersonal feedback from their leader, few will want therapists to discuss their own personal problems or professional insecurities (Cohen & Dies, 1976).

Guidelines to the Use of Therapist Transparency

There are many different approaches to therapist transparency, depending upon the therapist's personal style and goals in the group at a particular time. An important guideline can be obtained by asking oneself what the purpose of self-disclosure is at any given point in the group: "Am I trying to facilitate transference resolution? Am I model-setting in an effort to create therapeutic norms? Am I attempting to assist the interpersonal learning of members by working on their relationship with me? Am I attempting to support and demonstrate my acceptance of members by saying in effect: 'I value and respect you and demonstrate this by giving of myself'?" At all times, the therapist must consider whether transparency is consonant with other group therapy tasks.

Although therapist self-disclosure generally facilitates the group interaction, it is important to keep in mind that the group therapist's raison d'etre is not primarily to be honest or fully disclosing. If the group does not require any therapist transparency, the leader should not make special attempts to provide it—and certainly, no therapist should try to bootleg therapy for him- or herself from the group.

Furthermore, leader self-revelation must be guided by the different needs of the group members. Not all patients need the same thing from the therapist (or from the group). Some patients need to relax controls, need to learn how to express their emotions in an honest and responsible manner, whether they be emotions of anger, love, tenderness, envy, or frustration. They will learn the most from a leader who models spontaneous, sharing, affective interactions. Others need quite the opposite: They need to gain impulse control and learn to accept limits to the expression of their emotions; they may already be characterized by labile and immediately acted-upon affect. Such patients can learn from a therapist who shares his or her reactions to their impulsivity, and who shows them alternative ways of dealing with strong emotions. Finally, even the transparent and authentically self-disclosing therapist must provide some cognitive structuring, some intellectual integration to the group experience. Only in this manner can patients learn to generalize their group experiences to outside life.

Accepting Feedback as Part of Therapist Transparency

Therapist disclosures will be part of the here-and-now interactions of the group in that each disclosure reveals something of the inner world experienced by the therapist in the group setting. Feedback to the therapist about these disclosures will also be part of this cycle of interaction and reaction, and thus another form of self-disclosure occurs when the therapist receives and accepts accurate feedback from group members. There are several general principles that are useful to the therapist when he or she is receiving feedback from the group.

First, the therapist should take the feedback seriously by listening to it, considering it, and responding to it directly. The therapist should then obtain consensual validation: How do other members feel? Is the feedback primarily a transference reaction, or does it closely correspond to reality as confirmed by the majority of the group members? If it is reality-based, the therapist must confirm this in order to facilitate the patients' reality testing. When Barbara, the silent, pained patient accused her group leader of not making enough attempts to draw her into the group, the therapist responded: "Yes, there is some truth in what you say. I did know you wanted me to call on you today and I deliberately refrained from doing so. I've been drawing you into the group every week and it's beginning to feel burdensome to me. I feel I've got to resist my tendencies to take care of you so that you will begin to take more care of yourself."

Finally, the therapist should measure the feedback against his or her own internal experience: Does the feedback fit? Is there something important to learn from it? The leader who consistently finds herself being told by members that she comes across as distant and uncaring may find that this indeed reflects her inner state, and that, for the sake of her future professional development, she must understand these feelings and their impact on patients.

The leader's role will undergo a gradual metamorphosis during the life of any relatively stable interactional group. In the beginning, therapists will busy themselves with the many functions necessary to the creation of the group, with the development of a social system in which the many therapeutic factors may operate, and with the activation and illumination of the here-and-now. Gradually, however, the leader will begin to interact more personally with each of the members, and the early stereotypes the patients cast him or her into will become more difficult to maintain.

Concluding Remarks

Self-disclosure in group psychotherapy is an absolutely integral part of the therapeutic process, and carries risks and gains not associated with self-disclosure in individual therapy. It occurs when members reveal personal material about their outside lives and, even more importantly, when they explore their feelings and reactions to each other in the here and now of the group session. Appropriate and adaptive self-disclosure in the group is a complex function of timing, content, and reciprocity. Therapists play a more active and self-revealing role in this process than they do in individual psychotherapy, as they model responsible personal and professional transparency in the group.

References

Bloch, S., & Reibstein, J. (1980). Perceptions by patients and therapists of therapeutic factors in group psychotherapy. *British Journal of Psychiatry, 137*:274–278.

Bloch, S., Crouch, E., & Reibstein, J. (1981). Therapeutic factors in group psychotherapy. *Archives of General Psychiatry, 38*:519–526.

Cohen, M., & Dies, R. (1976). Content considerations in group therapist self-disclosure. *International Journal of Group Psychotherapy, 23*:71–88.

Johnson, D., & Ridener, L. (1974). Self-disclosure, participation, and perceived cohesiveness in small group interaction. *Psychological Reports, 35*:361–363.

Jourard, S.M., & Lasakow, P. (1950). Some factors in self-disclosure. *Journal of Abnormal Social Psychology, 56*:91–98.

Lieberman, M., Yalom, Y.D., & Miles, M. (1973). *Encounter groups: First facts*. New York: Basic Books.

Peres, H. (1947). An investigation of non-directive group therapy. *Journal of Consulting Psychology, 11*:159–172.

Query, W. (1964). Self-disclosure as a variable in group psychotherapy. *International Journal of Group Psychotherapy, 14*:107–115.

Truax, C., & Carkhuff, R. (1965). Client and therapist transparency in the psychotherapeutic encounter. *Journal of Consulting Psychology, 12*:3–9.

Worthy, M., Gary, A., & Kahn, G. (1969). Self-disclosure as an exchange process. *Journal of Personality Social Psychology, 13*:59–63.
Yalom, I.D. (1966). A study of group therapy dropouts. *Archives of General Psychiatry, 14*:393–414.
Yalom, I.D. (1967). Prediction of improvement in group therapy: An exploratory study. *Archives of General Psychiatry, 17*:159–168.
Yalom, I.D. (1985). *The theory and practice of group psychotherapy*. (3rd ed.). New York: Basic Books.

V

Extratherapeutic Manifestations

14

Criteria for Therapist Self-Disclosure

Judith C. Simon

Introduction

The psychotherapeutic relationship is unique to interpersonal relationships. The role definition includes agreement that one person, the patient, will openly discuss his or her personal life, while the therapist will function in a manner that will further the patient's psychotherapeutic gains. The hours spent together generate a special closeness and intensity, discussing primarily the patient's emotional life.

Inherent in any ongoing intimate relationship is each person's learning about the other. Implicit to the goal of a psychotherapeutic relationship, however, is a one-way intimacy in which the patient is the primary self-discloser. Discussion of the therapist's personal life is not necessarily part of the relationship. However, the therapist cannot avoid imparting some personal information; for example, the way the office is decorated, personal dress, the management of appointments, and nonverbal body language all give the patient clues about the therapist.

Since therapists' personal revelations are frequently a component of psychotherapy, questions arise regarding when, why, and what is disclosed.

When Freud first discussed transference and, later, countertransference, he acknowledged the impact of the therapist's personality and responses on the psychotherapeutic work (1959). Therapeutic neutrality was the goal. Therapist self-disclosure came to be viewed as the antithesis of the detached observer. It is important to distinguish between neutrality as a therapeutic stance and therapist self-disclosure as

Judith C. Simon • 329 South San Antonio Road, Los Altos, California 94022.

a therapeutic technique. They are not mutually exclusive. Freud spoke of being like a mirror but not "like an inanimate thing" (1959). The therapist was to function as a blank screen, mirroring the patient while adding nothing that did not originate in the patient. According to Freud, the components of neutrality included passivity, anonymity, and mirroring, and these were free of countertransference distortions. Annie Reich said (1951), "To be neutral in relationship to the patient... does not imply, of course, that the analyst has no relationship at all to the patient." She, among others, maintained that psychotherapy is a process within the context of an intimate and caring relationship that can be warm and supportive and can either include or exclude intentional therapist disclosures.

Therapists vary greatly in how they value, define, and maintain neutrality in their work. Currently, the trend is away from neutrality and toward increased activity, including intentional verbal self-disclosure by the therapist (1983). The societal trend towards a holistic approach to health care and more equal relationships between patients and their health-care providers have impacted psychotherapy relationships.

There is a paucity of material regarding this clinical issue. The general body of psychotherapy literature traces the evolving thinking within the following categories: neutrality, countertransference, the real relationship, therapist self-disclosure, and management of special circumstances in a therapist's personal life (Yalom, 1980; Alger, 1973; Rogers, 1961). Specific attention to therapist self-disclosure appears in the very recent literature (Greenson, 1971; Palombo, 1987; Rosie, 1980; Weiner, 1974). These writings cover a variety of research, including studies with simulated patient populations, explorations with patient populations, and anecdotal material. The literature reflects widely divergent viewpoints. Agreement does not exist regarding recommendations to disclose or not.

The Study

I explored criteria for intentional verbal self-disclosure by experienced therapists who practice long-term psychotherapy. "Intentional self-disclosure" was defined as verbal behavior through which therapists consciously and purposefully communicate ordinarily private information about themselves to their patients.

Eight experienced therapists were interviewed. "Experienced" was defined as having 10 or more years of private clinical work. These eight were selected by ranking 27 returned questionnaires on a scale from high to low disclosing and choosing those four who fell at each of these extremes. They represented the three psychotherapy disciplines of clinical social work, psychiatry, and psychology.

These two groups of four therapists comprised the subjects for the research and were labeled the high disclosers and low disclosers, respectively. The demographic differences between the two groups are worthy of note. The high disclosers were older and more experienced than the low disclosers. There was one woman and three men in each of the subject groups. Two psychiatrists and two psychologists comprised the high-disclosing group and one psychiatrist, one psychologist, and two clinical social workers formed the low-disclosing group.

Findings

Three themes, theoretical orientation, the psychotherapy relationship, and therapist self-awareness, emerged from the interviews and provide the context for the discussion of the criteria for therapist self-disclosure.

Theoretical Orientation

Therapists' theoretical orientation was the major determinant of therapist self-disclosure. The distinction between the two groups was reduced to whether one viewed the psychotherapy process as focused on working through patients' transference, or on the interconnection between therapist and patient.

The high disclosers labeled their orientations eclectic, humanistic, existential, and "here and now." Their mentors were Arthur Ellis, Carl Rogers, Fritz Perls, and Werner Erhard. They viewed the therapeutic factors in their work as truth, love, communication, understanding oneself, and the human bond. The stance of friendliness and personal connectedness was consistent with their theoretical conception of quality psychotherapy and therapist self-disclosure was regarded as enhancing these factors. Transference, insight, and interpretation were not useful concepts for them.

The low disclosers considered use of transference as the integral aspect of their work and were therefore generally opposed to therapist self-disclosure. Many of their therapy hours are spent exploring the patients' projections on them which they consider to be the primary curative component in the process. One subject discussed creating a context of deprivation:

> The deprivation is important in the treatment, especially with neurotic patients, because that mode encourages their projections, so I don't want to

answer their questions too quickly, it's more valuable to help them to explore. "Deprivation" is a bad word, but that's the one Freud used. It conveys harshness. I don't mean that.

These therapists wanted to share enough not to be artificial, but not reveal so much as to structure any more than necessary and risk getting in the way of the patient's projections. Self-disclosure may reinforce the social quality of the relationship and thereby burden the patient with information to process along with fantasy.

Their mentors were Freud, Karen Horney, Frieda Fromm-Reichman, and Ralph Greenson.

The Psychotherapy Relationship

Viewpoints about the psychotherapy are a reflection of theoretical orientation. Both the high and the low disclosers viewed the purpose of the psychotherapy relationship as the improved mental health of the patient. All agreed that the therapist is an agent of change, that therapists' personalities and styles are facets of the psychotherapeutic relationship and that respect, empathy, compassion, and realness are essential components of the psychotherapy relationship. They all reported that they consciously use themselves in their work and value being real with their patients. However, there were differences in the definition of "realness," in views on the therapist's role, and the psychotherapy relationship.

The intent of the high disclosers was to create a connection with the patient that would provide a context for growth. They saw their work as based on a real and human relationship. "Real" meant being genuine, honest, fully open,and personally involved and not creating illusions. These high disclosers spoke of the therapeutic relationship as a human exchange with mutual personal sharing. "This being together, openly sharing together, connecting, the relationship, that's what therapy is!" said one subject. Another commented, "What really heals in therapy is the truth." They talked about therapy as the offering of the therapist's total self to the healing process. The high disclosers were critical of the traditional psychoanalytic model for its hierarchical implications and its encouragement of patient projections as the context for the work. They valued equality in the relationship and disagreed with the traditional neutral stance. One referred to Freud's writings as having taught him to be respectful, caring, and equal, which he interpreted as encouraging free disclosure. "Freud was very helpful with his patients. He talked with them, walked with them. He was interested in their family problems and revealed some of his. He was real."

This group presented divergent opinions regarding boundaries in the therapeutic relationship ranging from "all boundaries are open when patient and therapist meet" to valuing the importance of respecting patients' cues regarding their psychological borders. None of the high disclosers felt that there was much difference between the psychotherapy relationship and a close friendship. They all were clear that while they would not socialize with current patients, social relationships with former patients were considered acceptable if desired by both parties. This was compatible with their view that the psychotherapy relationship ends when psychotherapy terminates.

Therapist satisfaction was a facet of the high disclosers' conceptualization of the psychotherapy relationship. The more they were able to be open and sharing participants in the relationship, the more growth potential for both parties.

All the low disclosers saw themselves as "real," but in a different sense. Their definition of real included being respectful, warm, attentive, empathic, and "not dishonest"; that is, honest but not fully open. These therapists were as clear as the high disclosers that these traits were essential therapist characteristics, but used themselves differently. Genuineness was discussed as conveying emotional sincerity, empathy, and responsiveness. For these therapists, nondisclosing is not dishonesty, but rather reflects their commitment to neutrality as the appropriate therapeutic stance. The low disclosers reported that they reveal as little as possible without being artificial or totally depriving. They viewed the psychotherapy relationship as separate from the real world, but not incognizant of it. Quoting a subject:

> There is an agreement that we will look at what happens in here as though it is real. It is real, but only within the confines of this arrangement. If you have to break the arrangement, it's sort of like the theater—the roof leaking in the theater. Then you refund people their money, or tell them the roof is leaking. But you don't say, "This is part of the play."

The issue of equality in the psychotherapy relationship elicited strong reactions from the low-disclosing therapists as well as the high disclosers. They were cognizant of the fact that their neutral stance evokes criticism and suggests that they present themselves as superior to their patients. These therapists insisted that equality-inequality is not the issue. When the patient is enabled to understand that the therapist is being supportive and empathic while encouraging transference, a sense of teamwork emerges, not hierarchy. While it is true that both patient and therapist are equal in terms of their human rights and the complexity of their psychological makeup, the therapist is more expert than the patient in the realm of emotional problems and their solutions. To deny this is to deny the validity of one's own training.

Consistent with their viewing the psychotherapy relationship and their roles in it as distinguished from other relationships, these therapists were opposed to socializing with current or former patients. They did not regard the professional relationship as ending when therapy is terminated. Patients were thought to carry an incorporation of their relationship with their therapists that would be tainted by another kind of contact. Additionally, these therapists assumed a professional duty to not contaminate the patient/therapist relationship in a manner which could preclude a patient's freedom to return to therapy.

Therapist Self-Awareness

The two subject groups held contrasting viewpoints about therapist self-awareness. Consistent with this, the high disclosers had considerably fewer hours of personal psychotherapy experience than the low disclosers.

The high disclosers, in regarding the psychotherapy relationship as mutually satisfying for therapist and patient, felt that it was less significant whose material was being discussed than that the patient and therapist were interacting in a deep and meaningful way. This connection provides the context for their own growth along with their patients'. Personal psychotherapy was indicated only when the therapist faced a crisis.

Therapists who utilize transference as the primary material believe that they have to be maximally self-aware to minimize distortions. One statement reflected the sentiment of the group: "I have to know what's mine and what's the patient's."

These therapists addressed their self-questioning before revealing themselves. They acknowledged an occasional pull to share special news with patients. One subject described his personal joy after the birth of a son and his wish to share that with any interested person. "But it wasn't my place to discuss that with patients, it was my wish, and I had to be able to contain it. I was sufficiently aware of my personal need and the conflict it caused in me... so I went back to my therapist."

The two groups clearly utilize different models, viewpoints, and paradigms in their psychotherapy practices. Internal consistency within each group was high as they discussed their concepts of the psychotherapy relationship, their theoretical orientations, and personal awareness. This consistency persists in the findings specific to the criteria for therapist self-disclosure.

Criteria

All eight subjects self-disclosed at times and utilized the same criteria for self-disclosure. The differences emerged in the therapists' individual determinations regarding when, what, and why to self-disclose. Frequency of self-disclosure varied widely and was a function of therapists' theoretical orientations. Decisions to self-disclose were based primarily on clinicians' conceptualizations of the curative components in psychotherapy, or what several stated as "the way I do therapy."

The high disclosers were quick to share themselves. Their orientation prescribed that the indications for self-disclosure were ever-present and they were not as contemplative of their reasons for disclosing or as concerned about supplying as firm a theoretical basis for their criteria of disclosing as were the low disclosers.

This same phenomenon was observed in the interviews. When asked why they might disclose something, the high disclosers frequently responded quickly by saying, "I just do," whereas the low disclosers paused, thought, and gave a response such as, "I do that because it furthers the patient's sense of reality." In contrast to the low disclosers, none of the high disclosers labeled therapist self-disclosure a psychotherapy technique.

Five categories of criteria emerged from the subjects: to model and educate, to foster the therapeutic alliance, to validate reality, to encourage the patient's autonomy, and, for the high disclosers only, therapist personal satisfaction. Clearly, there was overlap among the criteria utilized in this study: responses were categorized by their most prominent feature.

Modeling

Modeling emerges as the most common criteria for therapist self-disclosure. Therapists reported that they often served as models of adult behavior by demonstrating problem-solving approaches, coping skills, self-acceptance, and assertiveness. All of the subjects said that they used self-disclosure to model more frequently with adolescent patients than with adults because of the adolescent's need for help with the developmental task of becoming more autonomous. Identification with the therapist was viewed as helping patients face life and was encouraged by the therapist's appropriate self-disclosures.

Both the high and low disclosers felt that handling an error made with a patient presents therapists with an important opportunity to model the ability to err and the capacity to apologize.

The high disclosers felt modeling was an essential component of psychotherapy and that by showing their patients their own honesty and openness they were modeling relationships in general. One subject wanted to model someone who was transparent and who could demonstrate a way to live without fear or secrets, a stated psychotherapy goal of his. They believed that good therapists are models and in so being, communicate to their patients, "You can do these things, too."

These therapists freely disclosed personal information to illustrate behavior in specific situations in addition to modeling openness in general as essential to a functioning relationship.

Personal information was readily offered, especially to adolescent patients, and these therapists viewed this as re-parenting and/or education about the adult world. Personal experiences of their teen years which paralleled their patients' were freely disclosed. Adolescents' questions about the therapist's experiences in the adult world were also responded to fully. Examples cited were career evolution, earning capacity, and marital problems.

I explored use of therapist self-disclosure when there are stressful circumstances in the therapist's life. All high disclosers felt that it was very important to fully disclose information about these kinds of crises, primarily to model a way of coping. "Teach them how to deal with it, including what you did that helped and what you did that didn't help." In the same vein, two of these subjects recommended revelation of information about any personal crisis or significant occurrence. "I might even reveal that I fight with my wife. People don't often know that it's okay to get angry at someone close."

Fewer examples of modeling were presented by the low disclosers, although modeling was also their primary criteria for self-revelation. While they rarely self-disclose in order to model with neurotic adult patients, modeling with adolescent patients was an appropriate deviation from their usual nondisclosing stance. For example, "Some of these kids haven't had decent adults to look up to. If I can provide that, I'm not going to withhold because I'm a Freudian." They freely told stories about their own adolescence to offer themselves for identification.

One therapist said that he sometimes shared a personal experience that showed his bad judgment to model that "even the idealized therapist is not a perfect person."

All of these subjects have shared their own reactions to difficult personal situations in order to indicate that their patients' intense feelings were appropriate. Examples included their emotions in responding to the death of a parent and the frustrations and fatigue of early parenting.

Three felt that they would model with more disturbed patients to show them ways of coping with specific situations. The emphasis was on *specific*. These therapists were inclined to share emotions with this population to demonstrate that emotional responses were, indeed, sometimes appropriate. A common example was "That would make me angry too." They did not present themselves as overall objects of identification. Encouraging imitation in social situations, for example, dining out, and interactions with co-workers, were also uses of therapist self-disclosure with the purpose of modeling.

Two of these therapists felt that universalizing was a successful tool to reduce some insecurities, and that they included themselves as models in this respect. "Sometimes we're just at the mercy of the powers that be" was a common phrase.

Fostering the Therapeutic Alliance

Fostering the therapeutic alliance was the second most common criterion cited. All of the subjects reported that they were more inclined to disclose early in the psychotherapy process for this reason. Patients often ask for specific personal information during the first or second interview and this was universally viewed as expression of the patient's anxiety and need to assess the trust potential with the therapist. The manner in which the subjects responded to these kinds of questions varied according to their theoretical orientations.

The high disclosers willingly gave whatever information patients requested during any phase of treatment. In the early stages, their purpose was to reduce alienation, lessen patients' anxiety and establish the working alliance. The therapists saw this as critical for the building of trust and communicating to patients that they were genuine, human, and real. They expressed their strong commitment to being truthful and honest in every situation, and stated that the therapeutic alliance depends on this absolute honesty. Understanding and empathy were viewed as facets of the working alliance, and these therapists disclosed to convey their compassion.

Patients' curiosity was respected. This quote reflected the sentiment of the high-disclosing therapists: "Curiosity makes sense. I think people are particularly anxious when they come to a therapist... wanting to know who they are dealing with." Not answering questions would be offensive and increase rather than reduce anxiety. The subjects could not cite a reason not to reveal anything that was asked.

Self-disclosures were discussed as a tool to end impasses. Responding to a patient's perception of never being understood by sharing a similar experience or feeling can enable the work to progress. One therapist related listening to his patient talk about an early jail experience. This therapist had had a similar experience as a young adult and became aware that the patient's material elicited an intense reaction that he was unable to contain. He chose to share his experience to refocus his attention on the psychotherapy.

All high disclosers speculated that their way of handling having received a black eye in a fight would reflect their interest in fostering the therapeutic alliance. "I'd be embarrassed...but honesty is very important. It's a matter of them believing me or not, and they must believe me and my honesty. I'd tell the truth." When asked if they might equivocate about the details with any patient, they all hesitated, and concluded that they would have to be truthful.

The determination not to disclose was reported as sometimes being in the interest of maintaining and/or furthering the therapeutic alliance. They reported specifically withholding personal information for this reason. For example, two said that they wouldn't share their news of prospective grandparenthood with a woman who was experiencing fertility problems because that information was potentially painful. These high disclosers were clear that they would not reveal personal sexual information, considering such disclosures inappropriate to most social interactions. Allowing an invasion of their privacy would alter their objectivity with their patients and interfere with the therapist-patient connection. These subjects' deviations from their usual stance of absolute honesty reflects a conceptualization of their professional boundaries which was not otherwise apparent.

Self-disclosing interventions to further the therapeutic alliance were less frequent for the low disclosers, except for early sessions. In the interests of not adding to their patients' anxiety at the outset of therapy, these therapists stated that they would probably answer demographic questions during the first session. One subject said that he would answer personal questions out of courtesy, explaining that until the therapeutic alliance and agreements were set, the usual social manners were necessary. One presented this in terms of the patient's need to feel secure and comfortable. "I think of this more like a character analysis of the person, and then what type of information that person will need to feel secure."

They were clear that they would rather not answer these questions but acknowledged that they usually did. Several subjects reported that the way in which they refused to respond to early inquiries laid the groundwork for establishing the therapeutic agreements. "I might use a patient's question, straightaway, as an opportunity to show him that I won't readily reveal, and that nonrevealing on my part is an aspect of the process."

In general, patients' curiosity was seen as an opportunity for further exploration. They all felt that if the material was fully explored and still seemed very important for the patient, that they would briefly share it. This applied to inquiries about their personal data and to observations about their state of health. One expressed a common feeling: "I don't think there's any point in being mysterious for its own sake."

Furthering the therapeutic process when there is an impasse was reported as a criterion for self-disclosure by these low-disclosing therapists. In this regard, one said, "I share only if the patient's progress is being totally hampered by something related to my personal life." One said that he might share that he'd had good news, if the patient seemed sidetracked by his good mood. "It would probably get me back on track too. It would discharge it in the moment and get us both back to work."

Responding to the hypothetical vignette about the black eye, these therapists felt that this was exactly the kind of situation where their disclosure would close off a valuable opportunity for the patient's exploration.

This group saw their decisions not to disclose as protection of the therapeutic alliance. Because maintaining the therapist-patient boundary was an aspect of the alliance, they were careful not to blur it by introducing irrelevant personal material.

Establishing and maintaining the alliance with low functioning patients was discussed as an aspect of the determination to self-disclose. One subject discussed his work with disturbed patients who sometimes "needed" personal information "to maintain a state of homeostasis within the therapeutic hour." One of the low disclosers stated that his task was to help them with boundary issues and that he would "gently and minimally disclose and inquire why they needed to know, and what if they didn't know." In work with ego-impaired patients, strictness about self-disclosure was seen as potentially threatening to the working alliance.

Sometimes the patient's refusing to know anything about the therapist and not asking for a disclosure was viewed as significant to the alliance. Examples included a therapist's broken arm and patients who, over the years, never ask anything. These therapists regard these occurrences as appropriate times to explore why the patient didn't want to know. In these instances, the subjects said that they probably would reveal some information.

Validating Reality

One of the goals of psychotherapy, as reported by the therapists in the study, is the enhancement of the patient's ability to cope with and respond appropriately to reality factors. However differentiated the psychotherapy relationship may be from the outside world, the impact of reality factors on the psychotherapy process cannot be ignored. Both groups reported therapist self-disclosure as a technique to enhance patients' abilities to deal with real-life occurrences. Special reality circumstances may arise in the therapist's life during the course of psychotherapy that demand some response by the therapist.

The high disclosers, in their particular view of "truthfulness" in psychotherapy, felt that validation of the patient's reality remained an important aspect throughout the psychotherapy process. By being open and truthful they were always facilitating the patient's grasp of reality. One subject said that such disclosures help "patients to be able to validate their perceptions of what's going on with me. If they're wondering—the more feedback I can give them, the more accurate they can be about 'that's my stuff and the other stuff is her stuff'."

Subjects were asked how they would respond to a patient's comment, "You look ill. Are you okay?" All said that they would answer directly to confirm their patients' perceptions with enough detail to make it real for patients. Responses ranged from a simple, "I'm a little sleepy" to including details, for example, "My kid was up a lot last night and I didn't get much sleep." Two subjects said that they would then explore the meaning of the query for the patient. The other two felt that the question reflected the patient's sensing something awry and they would respect and confirm the patient's perception by saying something like "I guess I am sluggish today."

Circumstances do arise during the course of therapy that necessitate direction by the therapist. The subjects were asked how they would handle their illnesses, vacations, and special occasions in their lives. These high-disclosing therapists have shared and believe that therapists should disclose fully about their own illnesses and absences from work. Consistent with their orientations that the truth heals, and that experiencing reality with the therapist enhances the patient's ability to react to personal reality, these therapists freely disclose children's weddings, toothaches, marital problems, surgery details, and deaths of loved ones.

The low disclosers acknowledged that reality sometimes intrudes, even for psychoanalytic psychotherapists. These subjects felt that to pretend that their personal reality is a facet of the patients' projections is to confuse and betray the patient. As noted above, the kinds of realities that the therapists enumerated related to therapists' illness, losses, and joys. The low-disclosing therapists were in agreement that they had to validate their patients' reality when they made observations that were accurate. To ignore their observations undermines their ability to trust themselves in relationships. Therefore, they would share minimal information. In response to "You look ill. Are you okay?" these subjects all agreed that they would first explore the patient's motivation behind the question and then share truthfully and briefly, if indeed they were feeling less than well. They would not volunteer any details.

In managing their own illness, these subjects felt that the information patients requested related to their needs to know what was going to happen to their treatment. One said, "I'd recommend disclosure of enough to allow the patient to deal with it realistically. When you're sick you're going to have to violate the contract, the frame, involuntarily, and that's different from a patient wanting to have information." A patient failing to ask about an obvious injury to the therapist could be viewed as an avoidance of reality. These subjects felt that they would reveal some information in this situation to push the patient to confront reality.

Encouraging the Patient's Autonomy

Although not as frequently cited as the above criteria, therapists commonly use self-disclosure to increase a patient's sense of self.

Consistent with the high disclosers' commitment to openness, these therapists felt that self-disclosures communicated respect for their patients' autonomy as well as their own. An aspect of this was their belief in equality between therapist and patient and this was reported to be most successfully communicated through personal disclosures. They wanted to let patients know that they were regarded as peers. One therapist said, "When I tell a patient about my life, I am telling him 'I like you, I trust you, I respect you.' That's got to make him feel like a mensch!"

These high-disclosing therapists also mentioned withholding personal revelations to be respectful of their patients' autonomy. They were careful not to be intrusive with revelations that could be painful or overload a fragile patient.

The low disclosers reported that respect for patients was communicated by their demeanor, commitment, and attentiveness. Management of errors the therapist makes provides an opportunity to encourage patients' autonomy. These clinicians would acknowledge an error and apologize, thereby imparting to patients that they are entitled to respect. Equality is not a consideration. As noted above, these therapists do regard their patients as equal human beings who seek the therapist's expertise.

Diagnosis was a major factor in these therapists' determination to disclose with the purpose of enhancing patients' autonomy. All the examples given referred to patients labeled "low functioning" or "borderline," who needed to see their therapists as whole persons. Sharing information about location of vacations with borderline patients was generally regarded as an appropriate self-disclosure. They also addressed patients who need to merge as a part of the psychotherapy process. "Sometimes that's manifest in wanting to know a lot about you. And I would probably gently help them with those boundaries. I would give them information, briefly, and inquire why they felt they needed to know." One of the subjects commented that, with this purpose in disclosing, timing was more important than what was revealed.

Therapist Satisfaction

While all the subjects reported satisfaction from their work, the fulfillment derived from practicing psychotherapy was different for the therapists in the two groups.

The high disclosers were very clear about the gratification they obtained from their patients. They chose orientations that support therapist openness, and it is the mutuality of openness in the psychotherapeutic relationship that provides much of their professional satisfaction. They acknowledged their own enjoyment of their friendly relationships with patients and their belief that therapist and patient both grow in the relationship. Therefore, their conceptualization of criteria for therapist self-disclosure was casual and relatively unstructured.

Two of these therapists said that they would pursue discussions with patients about most topics of interest to the therapist. For example, they agreed that they would elicit information about a patient's vacation if the destination was of personal interest.

The low disclosers also reported satisfaction from the psychotherapy relationship. However, therapist satisfaction was not a criterion for self-disclosure. For them, it was the psychotherapy process and relationship, including intellectual stimulation, that provided fulfillment.

Discussion

The original research question, "What are the factors in therapist self-disclosure?" can be answered concisely. The main factor is therapist theoretical orientation. At the same time, it is clear that this concise answer, while accurate, is inadequate. Numerous other factors impact therapist disclosure. Theoretical orientation, the psychotherapeutic frame, the psychotherapeutic relationship, the therapist's personality, and therapist self-awareness are all themes associated with therapist self-disclosure.

The four high-disclosing therapists defined their orientations similarly: they agreed on loose boundaries between themselves and their patients; they opposed therapeutic neutrality; they espoused equality; and they were active participants in the interchange between themselves and their patients. The four low-disclosing therapists also defined their orientations consistently: they agreed about defined boundaries; they valued neutrality; and they believed in being fairly inactive in interactions with their patients to encourage transference.

Attitudes about transference both exemplified and were crucial to the differences between the two subject groups. Therapists who believe that transference work is the crux of the psychotherapy process self-disclose minimally. Therapists who reject transference work do not hesitate to self-disclose.

Viewpoints about the psychotherapy frame were consistent with the above distinction. That the high disclosers were more casual about boundaries was evident in their attitudes about time, money, personal artifacts in their offices, and telephone calls. The low disclosers, consistent with their neutral frame, maintained this stance with regard to time, money, office decor, and calls.

The low-disclosing therapists were more contemplative about their roles in the psychotherapy process. These clinicians were frequently silent for several moments during the interviews, obviously thinking about their responses. This behavior reflected their general stance of thoughtfulness and intentionality when self-disclosing. In contrast, the more spontaneous responses of the high disclosers were seen as being congruent with their stances and their less self-reflective styles.

The issue of the "real" relationship within the psychotherapeutic relationship was viewed very differently. A therapist who is real, as defined by the high disclosers, adheres to a code of truthfulness and genuineness. Such a therapist actively uses him or herself and freely discloses personal information. In contrast, the low-disclosing therapists' conceptualization of "real" in psychotherapy meant the actual person-to-person relationship, and "genuine" meant being direct, attentive, respectful, and responsive to patients. This "realness" can be manifest without self-disclosure.

Equality as an aspect of the psychotherapeutic relationship underlies the topic of therapist self-disclosure. Is the therapist suggesting his or her own superiority by being neutral?

High-disclosing therapists regard their use of self-disclosure as an important way to communicate their care, respect, and parity with their patients. According to their thinking, therapists who maintain neutrality and do not share themselves are withholding respect and care and are elevating their own status.

For low-disclosing therapists, maintenance of the neutral stance is consistent with their theoretical orientation, and not a technique to establish superiority. They are no less committed to communicating care and respect to their patients, but feel that this is accomplished by their undivided attention and adherence to a professional style that they regard as the most facilitative of patients' growth. As human beings they are equal to their patients; as professionals they contribute their expertise and, in that regard, they are not equal (Weiner, 1983).

When and why a therapist self-discloses is also an extension and/or reflection of the therapist's personal style. In this study, the four high disclosers were very interactive and congenial. They were unusual and colorful personalities who were "out front" with their likes and personal philosophies. The interviews were entertaining, lively, and lengthy. In contrast, the low disclosers' interviews were briefer and more focused. They were more formal and restrained (neutral?) in their manner. These interviews were less lively and more intellectually provocative.

Offices were decorated in a manner consistent with orientations. For example, one high discloser proudly displayed family photographs. Another had numerous art objects reflecting an ethnic interest. These therapists had more desire to share themselves and did so physically as well as verbally. The low disclosers' offices were austere by comparison. Colors were more muted and the displayed art less reflective of personal taste.

One can question which office style is more appropriate and/or supportive of psychotherapeutic work. Clinicians and patients must feel comfortable and supported in the therapist's office. The therapist's attention to the physical environment is important, whether it be a clear reflection of the therapist as a person or an aspect to support the therapist's professional stance. Sensitivity to one's patient population was considered. The therapists' personal dress also reflects the therapist as a person and, in this study, their attire was consistent with their orientation and office decor.

Therapist self-awareness was assessed by the questioning of personal psychotherapy experience. There appeared to be a relationship between valuing self-awareness and working with transference. When working within a neutral frame and encouraging patients' transference projections, knowing oneself is important. The high disclosures did not regard self-awareness as being related to their professional functioning.

The fact that all the subjects utilized similar criteria for therapist self-disclosure and that all the subjects did self-disclose leads to the conclusion that self-disclosure is a fact in most psychotherapy. The similarity in the purposes of therapist self-disclosure expressed by all the subjects blurs some of the striking differences between the two groups. The high disclosers did not think through their processes in making disclosures because they valued overall openness. They were not concerned about being too revealing since they considered self-revelation an integral component of the therapy process as well as their personal styles. For the low disclosers, intentional self-disclosure demanded thought. It was this discriminative thinking process in contrast to readiness to self-disclose that differentiated the two subject groups.

Several further issues emerged from this study. Diagnosis as a facet of therapist self-disclosure was explored. All the subjects gave less attention to it than to the other criteria, which leads to the tentative conclusion that diagnosis is a minor criterion.

Stage of therapy also emerged as a minor criterion. All subjects reported that they were more likely to disclose in the early phases of psychotherapy either to further the alliance, relieve the patient's tension, or to be courteous. The mention of courtesy suggests that there is a period of adjustment to the psychotherapy process to which therapists are sensitive.

The issue of physical touch between therapist and patient, although not part of this study, can be viewed as a facet of therapist self-disclosure. Several subjects did mention touch. Three of the low disclosers indicated they never have physical contact with their patients. The high disclosers volunteered that they often hug a patient on leaving and, consistent with their styles, if they feel like making physical contact, they do. (There was no suggestion that any of this physical contact went beyond casual touch.)

The managing of reality within the psychotherapy context presents a challenge, as was confirmed by the literature and the findings. Therapists' intense personal stress impinges upon professional functioning. The "appropriate" way to manage this is probably consistent with one's theoretical orientation, but our reality, as therapists, is that we, too, can be overwhelmed with our own personal stresses and not respond in the optimal manner with respect to our patients' well-being.

There is an absence of agreement regarding the management of personal circumstances in the therapist's life. Divergent recommendations and experiences are represented in the study and the literature (Abend, 1982; Dewald, 1982; Flaherty, 1984; Goldberg, 1984; Weiner, 1974). I have experienced fall out from another therapist's inability to be professional while he was coping with a terminal illness. This raises the issue, how to respond to a patient who had such an experience with a previous therapist? How much, if anything, should be disclosed about the former therapist's illness and his/her struggle to be professional while personally stricken? Can we expect ourselves to maintain a professional stance when we are in great physical and/or emotional pain? What is the impact on our patients of being real, i.e., self-disclosing, in these situations?

The issue of patients liking the therapist is a thread that was evident in this research and in the surveyed literature. It is possible that an aspect of the high disclosers' friendly style is wanting to be liked by their patients. Studies suggest that some patients like therapists who self-disclose, but that liking one's therapist does not correlate with successful psychotherapy outcomes (Simonson, 1974; Truax, 1971). This raises questions regarding patients' selection of therapists. How do and how should prospective patients go about selecting a therapist?

There is clinical value in therapists becoming more aware of the early process of assessing their patients. The distinction between counseling and psychotherapy suggests a very different use of therapist self-disclosure. The counseling process connotes briefer, less in-depth exploration with more emphasis on coping skills and environmental manipulation. Modeling, the most frequent criterion for self-disclosing, is a very successful technique in this kind of work. Psychotherapy, on the other hand, is usually more insight-oriented, and therefore self-disclosure to foster the alliance is the most relevant criterion. The lack of confidence in utilizing therapist self-disclosure might be addressed by a clearer conception of the kind of therapy being practiced. The low disclosers, with their basic anti-disclosure viewpoint, might be excluding a useful tool in their supportive or counseling work with some patients.

Further study might contrast experienced therapists with beginners. Less experienced therapists may not have clearly conceptualized their theoretical orientations and their frequency of disclosing may reflect their personal styles and/or anxieties. Therapists who are moderately experienced are probably, as a group, the least disclosing. They may be trying the hardest to adhere to classical teachings and maintain a professional stance.

Highly experienced therapists, as suggested by this study, make determinations regarding self-disclosures in a manner consistent with their professional conceptualizations as evolved from years of study, personal growth, and clinical practice.

References

Abend, S.M. (1982). Serious illness in the analyst: Countertransference considerations. *Journal of the American Psychoanalytic Association, 30* (2), 365–379.

Alger, I. (1973). Freedom in analytic therapy. *Current Psychiatric Therapy, 9*, 73–78.

Dewald, P.A. (1982). Serious illness in the analyst: Transference, countertransference, and reality responses. *Journal of the American Psychoanalytic Association, 30* (2), 347–363.

Flaherty, J.A. (1984). Self-disclosure in therapy: Marriage of the therapist. *International Journal of Group Psychotherapy, 34* (2), 442–452.

Freud, S. (1959). Recommendations to physicians practising psychoanalysis. In E. Jones (Ed.), *Collected papers*, Vol. II. New York: Basic Books.

Goldberg, F. (1984). Personal observations of a therapist with a life-threatening illness. *International Journal of Group Psychotherapy, 34* (2), 389–396.

Greenson, R.R. (1978). The real relationship between the therapist and the psychoanalyst. In R.R. Greenson (Ed.), *Explorations in Psychoanalysis*, New York: International Universities Press.

Palombo, J. (1987). Spontaneous self-disclosure in psychotherapy. *Clinical Social Work Journal, 15* (2), 107–120.

Reich, A. (1951). On countertransference. *International Journal of Psychoanalysis, 32*, 25–31.

Rogers, C.B. (1961). The concept of a fully functioning person. In C.B. Rogers (Ed.), *On becoming a person*. Boston: Houghton Mifflin.

Rosie, J.S. (1980). The therapist's self-disclosure in individual psychotherapy: Research and psychoanalytic theory. *Canadian Journal of Psychiatry, 25*, 469–472.

Simonson, N.R., & Bahr, S. (1974). Self-disclosure by the professional and paraprofessional therapist. *Journal of Consulting and Clinical Psychology, 42*, 359–363.
Truax, C.B., & Mitchell, K.M. (1971). Research in certain interpersonal skills in relation to process and outcome. In A.E. Bergin & S.L. Garfield (Eds.), *Handbook of psychotherapy and behavior change: An empirical analysis*. New York: John Wiley.
Weiner, M. (1972). Self-exposure by the therapist as a therapeutic technique. *American Journal of Psychotherapy, 31*, 42–51.
Weiner, M. (1974). Personal Openness with Patients: Help or hindrance. *Texas Medicine, 76*, 60–65.
Weiner, M. (1983). *Therapist disclosure*. Baltimore: University Park Press.
Yalom, I.D. (1980). *Existential psychotherapy*. New York: Basic Books.

15

Self-Disclosure in Holocaust Survivors

EFFECTS ON THE NEXT GENERATION

Arlene Cahn Gordon

Introduction

> The Holocaust was woven into the fabric of life.
>
> It was always there. The natural tapestry of my life. It was my first memory. There was never a time in my life where there wasn't an Auschwitz.
>
> It was very much a part of my life. Growing up I wondered what it was like not to be a child of a survivor.
>
> It was always a way of splitting time. Before the war and after the war.

No child is born in a vacuum. As a child grows, she becomes aware of the culture of which she is a part as she simultaneously distinguishes her own place within and her effect upon that culture. A child's entry into culture is facilitated by her parents. As is evident in the above quotations, children of Holocaust survivors enter a world that is colored by the Holocaust. An event they did not directly experience is felt to be a pervasive part of their own lives.

I suggest that the manner in which the Holocaust is negotiated between parent and child, the way it is "woven into the fabric of life," is related not only to the child's understanding of the world, but of herself. The study discussed in this chapter concerns the relationship between self-disclosure in survivor parents and their children. I will present evidence that suggests that the manner in which survivors disclose their Holocaust experience is related to their children's ability to disclose their

Arlene Cahn Gordon • 15 Dogwood Drive, West Orange, New Jersey 07052.

own experiences. It is this ability to disclose or acknowledge one's own experience that is considered of central importance in facilitating intimate relatedness with others and, in a different sense, with oneself.

Self-Disclosure in Stages of Survival

Those who survived the Holocaust endured a systematic attempt to strip them of every fiber of their humanity. They experienced constant fear and anxiety regarding their fate, uprooting, and loss of family, friends, and possessions. In the majority of cases they suffered physical and psychological brutality. After living through the horrendous traumas of the war, survivors were faced with rebuilding their lives and their sense of trust in a world gone mad before their eyes. For many, getting married and having children became a way to reenter the world of the living and compensate for the incomprehensible losses (Freyberg, 1980). Rushing into these "marriages of despair" (Danieli, 1982) often led to placing all hope on the children. When survivors became parents, they assumed the universal role of introducing and sharing their world with their children.

Let me start, as do children of survivors throughout their lives, with an attempt to understand the role of self-disclosure in survivors, at each of the stages described above. Self-disclosure is viewed here as an acknowledgment of experience to oneself and/or to others. It includes two processes: first, the symbolizing of experience, a process of maintaining verbal or nonverbal representations of experience within an individual; and second, the acknowledgment or naming of experience by linking internalized representations of all kinds to words. Those who survived one of the worst assaults on humanity had to rework these essential human tasks, those of self and other-directed disclosure, at each stage of their lives. Observing their monumental task highlights the inextricable link between self-disclosure and intimate relatedness within and across generations.

During the war individuals had to alter the way they interacted with and reacted to the world. Consider those who survived internment. Authors consistently describe a series of stages through which concentration camp prisoners passed (Bettelheim, 1960; Chodoff, 1963; Frankl, 1959; Krystal, 1968; Niederland, 1968). Essentially, they describe the breakdown, by external observation, of relatedness with oneself and one's world. Initially, prisoners experienced an acute fright reaction which resulted in a dazed state and depersonalization. This phase was followed by a period of apathy and emotional numbing. Krystal maintains that those who survived did so on the basis of automatization of functions, and restriction of cognitive and emotional life solely to the task of survival. The feelings ceased to be, on the surface, because one could not live with such feelings of disgust and terror. On some level, acknowledgment of one's experience, which is proposed as critical to a sense of relatedness, was so intolerable it actually interfered with adjustment.

Emotional numbing to external reality is thus viewed as one coping mechanism necessary for survival. What was it that helped survivors maintain the will to live, given the necessity of what Eitinger (1961) refers to as "psychic anesthesia"? A key variable in survival may have been survivors' ability to rely on internalized experience. Eagle (1984) suggests that the cognitive-affective links provided by both interpersonal relations and by interests and values contributes to psychological integrity in extreme conditions. When normal interpersonal relations are disrupted, values and interests which have been internalized become even more crucial in survival.

Rapaport (1958) talks about the "stimulus nutriment" needed by the ego in order to function. The ego maintains autonomy from the id by "stimulus nutriment" from the environment, and the ego maintains autonomy from the environment by "stimulus nutriment" or affective signals from the id. Those experiencing sensory deprivation, for example, fare better if they are capable of engaging in fantasy and reverie. Inmates of concentration camps who were able to sustain a rich inner life were better off than those who, without "stimulus nutriment" from their inner life, were more dependent on the environment, which in their case was intolerable. In explaining the usefulness of escaping from the environment by dependency on an inner life, Eagle (1984) states that "because the very inner life into which one escapes, by its very nature, is characterized by (internalized) cognitive and affective links to others, one's retreat is personal and yet not autistically personal" (p. 193).

Eagle's discussion helps resolve an apparent contradiction between types of behavior necessary for survival. On the one hand, there was tendency to become numb, to remain apathetic, and to deny the horrible thoughts and feelings about one's experience. One the other hand, individuals survived by maintaining an investment in ideals, in fantasy—in an inner life. Survivors cut off their cognitive-affective links to current reality, but retained the links to internalized objects.

The capacity to maintain internal representations of once-present objects in their absence, first achieved when a child develops object constancy, is dependent on symbol formation. Those who survived maintained their capacity to symbolize experience. These symbolizing processes were the crucial factor that allowed them to remain related, by reliance on internalized objects.

What happened after liberation? Making the transition from excessive reliance on fantasy and internalized objects to the reality of their current world and the possibility, indeed necessity, of establishing new relationships, led to severe emotional turmoil for many. Included in that turmoil was the difficulty of acknowledging what had happened to their lives, to themselves, and to others. While I will highlight some of the hurdles to appropriate acknowledgment of experience, it is important to emphasize the great variation with which survivors met and overcame them. The numerous books, studies, and first-person accounts by survivors, for example, attest to the ability, commitment, and strength of many to disclose their experiences.

One extremely difficult area of acknowledgment was mourning for those who died. Survivors were generally unable to mourn during the war. Their very survival was at stake, and they were unable to acknowledge their losses while saving themselves. After the war, the magnitude of their losses, the necessity to rebuilt their lives, and the overwhelming, unmanageable nature of their feelings often prevented adequate mourning. Klein (1971) states that most survivors experienced despair, suicidal thoughts, and fantasies of bringing lost relatives back to life and obtaining revenge. Denial of the death of loved ones ensued.

Freud (1917), discusses depression resulting from loss in terms of a failure to form symbols. In his paper "Mourning and Melancholia," he states that "the melancholic displays something else besides which is lacking in mourning—an extraordinary diminution in his self-regard...In mourning it is the world which has become poor and empty; in melancholia it is the ego itself" (p. 246). Freud suggests that the various self-accusations of the melancholic are really reproaches against a loved object, which have been shifted from the abandoned objects onto the melancholic's own ego. There is an identification of the ego with the abandoned object. By self-punishment, melancholics succeed in "taking revenge on the original object and in tormenting their loved one through their illness, having resorted to it in order to avoid the need to express their hostility to him openly" (p. 251).

Freud's conceptualization of melancholia stresses turning against the internalized object, which I relate to turning against the symbol. The importance of maintaining internalized objects, discussed by Eagle (1984), is here threatened. The survivor may not let the internalized, symbolized object survive, but turns against his/her own ego by identification with the lost object. From this perspective, a survivor who cannot acknowledge his/her losses has lost a sense of relatedness or intimate connection with not only significant others from his/her life, but with a part of him/herself.

Following the war, survivors also faced a kind of "turning against the symbol" from external sources. Danieli (1982) states that survivors encountered negative reactions and attitudes that led to a "conspiracy of silence" about the Holocaust. The survivors' experiences were too horrifying for most people to listen to. Even those who consciously wanted to listen, avoided asking questions, which they rationalized by a belief that they didn't want to add to the survivors' pain. Danieli discusses the consequences of this conspiracy of silence for survivor families. Feeling betrayed by the inability of their relatives to share their sense of loss, grief, and rage, survivors felt even more isolated. Some survivors had sustained the horrors of the war in order to bear witness: the imposed silence was particularly painful for them. The importance of self-disclosure, of intimate sharing and acknowledgment of the past, was evident in many survivors' reactions to this barrier. Some families sought out and clung to fellow survivors, establishing groups, organizations, or communities based on common experiences or residence before the war. Some survivors withdrew into their current families and used their children as their constant, captive audiences.

Many authors have suggested that survivors' experiences interfered with their ability for "good enough" parenting (Barocas & Barocas, 1980). Survivors have been described as emotionally unavailable, overprotective, and using their children for their own conscious and unconscious needs (Barocas & Barocas, 1973; Freyberg, 1980; Phillips, 1978; Sigal & Rakoff, 1971). Rakoff, Sigal, and Epstein (1967) discuss how children are expected to give meaning to their parents' lives and to restore the lost objects, goals, and ideals of their parents. The children are expected to become extensions of their parents, as well as symbols of all that their parents lacked in their own lives. Many of the problems described in children of survivors have been related to their parents' inability to allow their children to assume individual identities.

Impairment of symbolizing processes in survivors may be related to their parenting difficulties. Freyberg (1980) states that mothers were frequently bewildered with their role, having lost access to their introjected prototype of a good mother. Sonnenberg (1972) comments that the ego functions necessary for parenting are lost to some extent in every survivor. I suggest that these parenting difficulties are related to impairments in parents' overall ability to symbolize. Those survivors who did not maintain internalized good objects, i.e., whose capacity to symbolize was impaired, most likely had more difficulty as parents themselves.

The purpose of this brief outline of the role of the self-disclosure at subsequent stages of survival is twofold. First, it is to suggest the critical role of acknowledgment of experience in maintaining a sense of relatedness with oneself and one's world. Second, and directly following from the first, focusing on the difficulties of self-disclosure in the extraordinary experiences of Holocaust survivors begs the question of how one's acknowledgment of traumatic life events affects subsequent generations.

Self-Disclosure: A Developmental Framework

The importance of examining the relationships between acknowledgment of experience and relatedness within and between generations is also based on several theoretical assumptions. Developmentally, symbolizing and acknowledging one's experience is the process by which a child is introduced to his/her world, initially in the interaction with parents: Eventually, it is the process by which one becomes an active participant in society. Through the process of naming experience, a human being identifies and attributes meaning to thoughts, thereby establishing a sense of identity. Symbolizing of experience is the means by which one comes to understand not only oneself, but one's social world and culture.

Consider the relationship between language, thought, and culture within the family system. The family is the initial "culture" to which a child is exposed. It is the world of symbols produced by the family that introduce that family and the larger world to a child. It is also those symbols with which the child learns to think and to communicate. Kaye (1982) states that mind and language would not develop without the fit between infant and adult behavior. Parents help children make their intentions clear and make their expressions fit the conditions and requirements of the "speech community" or culture. Bruner (1983) discusses the interdependence of mother and child in the development of language. Even before a child asks a single word, language formation begins. "Mother and infant create a predictable format of interaction that can serve as a microcosm for communicating and for constituting a shared reality" (p. 18). Vygotsky (1962) refines the role of social relations as the root of mental development. Communication, he says, is the origin of the mind.

This theoretical framework suggests the tremendous influence of the parent's communication with the child on the child's symbol formation development. Not only words themselves, but formats of interaction between parent and child serve as the basis for the child's development of language, thought, and communication. I suggest that variations in the nature of parent communication contribute to the individual differences in symbolic processes and communicative ability in children.

Referential Activity: A Measure of Self-Disclosure

Having outlined some of the hurdles to appropriate symbolization of experience for survivors, and the importance of such symbols in the parent-child relationship, I became interested in finding a way to empirically investigate the effects of survivors' ability to acknowledge experience on their children. I theorized that the success with which those hurdles were overcome varied, and that that variation significantly impacted upon survivors' relationship with their children as well as their children's own symbolic processes. In other words, I proposed that survivors' ability to disclose their own experiences would affect not only their relationship with their children and what their children know about them, but their children's relationship with others and knowledge of themselves.

In order to investigate the above proposition empirically, a measure of acknowledgment of experience was needed. I have drawn extensively from the work of Bucci (1982, 1984) and Bucci and Freedman (1978, 1981), who have investigated the process by which individuals name their experience. They propose a dual-code model of representing experience. One represents or codes experience verbally, in words and definitions. One also represents or codes nonverbal experience, in sensory, affective, motoric, and temporal representations. These authors introduce the term referential activity to describe the process of making symbolic links between words and inner experience. This process is the basis of both understanding speech and speech production. In comprehending another person, one enters memory with a word and retrieves a referent which is either an image or another word. In producing speech one retrieves representations from memory and generates words. In other words, we store our experiences in many ways, through our senses, emotions, bodily sensations, and words. Referential activity is the process of accessing and translating that inner experience, those stored nonverbal, experiential representations, into words. It may be considered as the active cognitive function involved in self-disclosure. I am also suggesting that it is a way to measure a person's access to or knowledge of him/herself.

These authors suggest that individuals vary to a large extent in their ability to name their experience or find the right words. This variation is reportedly not correlated with measures of intelligence (Bucci & Freedman, 1978). Two studies of referential activity helped crystallize my investigation. First of all, the ability to acknowledge experience, referential activity level, was related to depression (Bucci & Freedman, 1981; Bucci, 1982). Clinically depressed patients had lower referential activity at the beginning of their hospitalization than immediately before discharge. The more depressed an individual, the less able to link experience to word. Secondly, Jaffe (1985) related mothers' referential activity to their speech interaction with their children, which was related to the children's separation tolerance. These studies are significant because they relate the ability to acknowledge experience, referential competence, to two of the major difficulties discussed in relation to both survivors and children of survivors, namely depression and separation individuation problems.

Given the results of the referential activity studies described above, consider the following: (1) Depression evident in survivors is related to their difficulties communicating their war experiences. (2) In children of survivors, depression may be related to their inability to "name" their own experience and that of their parents. (3) The prevalence of difficulties with separation in children of survivors may also be associated with difficulties in their capacity to form symbols. While depression and separation have been studied extensively with this population, the mediating variable, symbol formation, has not been addressed.

The Study of Self-Disclosure in Survivors and Their Children

The current study proposes that the ability to acknowledge one's experience, to contain it in language, is the mediating variable between the actual experience, in this case the Holocaust, and one's level of adjustment. An individual's sense of relatedness to others and to oneself is the aspect of adjustment I focus on. Furthermore, on the basis of Jaffe's findings, I suggest that a mother and a child's ability to acknowledge experience will be related, and this might help us to understand possible intergenerational effects of the Holocaust. We would then expect to find a positive correlation between a survivor's ability to acknowledge Holocaust experiences and her child's ability to acknowledge her own experiences—acknowledgment that is considered fundamental to the experience of self-relatedness or self-intimacy. Furthermore, we would expect this relationship for other intense events: In this respect this relationship in Holocaust survivors would represent a catastrophic extreme intensification of a human pattern that is universally shown. The present study was formulated to examine the relationship between mother and daughter's acknowledgment of experience in all participants, a children of survivor and a control group, as well as to compare the groups to determine if there was any special effect of the Holocaust on this relationship.

Forty adult women whose mothers were Holocaust survivors and 40

Jewish women of American-born mothers participated in this study. The study was restricted to mothers and daughters for statistical reasons, given the sample size. The other three basic nuclear family relationships need to be considered in the future. The criteria for participation, for children of survivors, included having a mother who was either interned by Nazis in forced labor camps or concentration camps, or who was in hiding from the Nazis and/or participated in the underground resistance. Children of survivors were recruited through second-generation organizations and from referrals of professionals, researchers, and clinicians in the field. Participants ranged from 18 to 45 years of age. Half the children of survivors in the sample were participants in such organizations and were recruited from this membership while half had not participated in any such groups. Control women were recruited by asking children of survivors to refer female Jewish friends who, to their knowledge, were not children of survivors.

All participants were initially contacted by phone and asked if they would be willing to take part in a study about daughters' knowledge and communication with their mothers about their mothers' life experiences. Meetings took place at the convenience of the participants, usually in their own homes, for approximately 1½ hours. Participants completed a structured interview and two taped 5-minute monologues.

Let me stress that I was not interviewing mothers directly: I was determining mothers' ability to acknowledge experience based on the administration of a structured interview to their daughters. The structured interview was designed to assess the nature of mothers' communication in two ways. Participants were asked specific facts about their mothers' experiences, and were also asked to describe the quantity of their mothers' communication. The first measure, number of specific facts known about mothers' experiences, is interpreted as an indirect, objective indicator of mothers' communication. This is based on the assumption that a survivor mother's prewar and war experiences could only be known by the daughter if the mother acknowledged them to someone at some point in her life. It was not possible, or necessary, to determine whether the information daughters knew was told to them directly by their mothers or by other relatives, friends, or from overhearing conversations. What was important, what was being measured, was the amount of information acknowledged by the mother in some way. The second measure, of participants' perceptions of the quantity of their mothers' communication, is a more direct but subjective assessment of mothers' ability to acknowledge their experiences.

These measures of mothers' acknowledgment of experience were correlated with measures of daughters' acknowledgment of their own experience, specifically their level of referential activity. Women with more active and direct referential connections in their verbal style, in other words, with high referential activity levels, are seen as better able to link verbal and nonverbal aspects of experience to words. In this study, two monologues were used and scored for referential activity. Participants' verbal style was measured by a monologue during which they were asked to speak for 5 minutes about any interesting personal life experience. This monologue was rated as to level of specificity, concreteness, clarity, and overall imagery level, to obtain an overall measure of referential activity. The second monologue was used to assess participants' ability to translate their own representations of their mothers' experiences into words. Children of survivors were asked to speak for 5 minutes about their mothers' experiences during the war, and controls were asked to speak about the most difficult experience of their mothers, before they were born. This monologue was also rated along the four dimensions of specificity, concreteness, clarity, and overall imagery level.

As noted, individuals vary in referential competence. All participants in this study were asked to speak about an interesting personal life experience. Some women, for example, chose the birth of a child as such an experience. A comparison of two excerpts on this topic shows the wide range of expressive features related to referential activity which are apparent in different discussions of similar events. The first excerpt is from a woman who scored above average in referential competence:

> And uh, I'll never forget the night we went into labor, cause that day my husband had gotten up at 5 AM to go to work, and I had gotten up with him and never gone back to sleep. But I was reading and sewing and doing all these last-minute things. And that morning I was on the phone with my girlfriend, flipping through the calendar and deciding I'm not having this baby for another 10 days. And uh, we went out to dinner, came home very tired. . . and then my water started to break, but it trickled out so you, I was sure I was incontinent at the age of 27. It was the most horrible, horrible feeling. And here I'd been up since 5 AM and I'm exhausted. . .

In this excerpt the language is clear and rich in descriptive detail. Concrete examples of specific actions and feelings bring the event to life. In contrast is a sample from a low-referential activity monologue:

> Um, let's see. Giving birth. (Chuckles.) That was a real exciting thing. That was a traumatic experience. Um, never expecting to go natural I went natural. That really is like number one in life experiences. Um, you know I had a wonderful doctor and my husband was very supportive. Um, everything really went smoothly even though I wanted to get uh, epidural needle and everything, um I was able to do it without anything. And it's been great, you know.

This example of low referential activity narrative is vague and full of generalities. There are few descriptive details. It is difficult, as a listener, to conjure up an image of this actual event. Both excerpts describe an event of major significance in these women's lives, but the ability to access specific, detailed, sensory, and imagistic language to describe these events differs dramatically.

The first major finding in the study is that, as expected, there was no significant difference between children of survivors and controls on measures of standard referential activity level. In other words, participants' ability to acknowledge their own experiences did not differ in the two groups. This finding upholds previous studies which stress that children of survivors are not less "competent" or less well-functioning than other people (Kestenberg, 1972; Klein, 1971; Phillips, 1978; Pilcz, 1979). As with the variety of symptoms discussed in the literature, referential activity level varied in children of survivors as in other individuals.

Given this anticipated null finding, we then looked at the relationship between referential activity and the measures of participants' mothers' communication. For children of survivors only, there was a significant relationship between a mother's ability to acknowledge her Holocaust experiences and the child's ability to acknowledge her own experiences. Specifically, the more facts children of survivors knew about their mothers' lives before and during the war, and the more frequent they perceived discussions about the war to be, the higher the children of survivors' referential activity level on the five-minute monologue, in which they talked about their own personal experience. This relationship was not significant in the control group.

There was a significant relationship in all participants, however, between their mothers' ability to acknowledge her difficult experiences, assessed by how many facts participants knew, and daughters' referential activity in the second monologue, in which they spoke about those difficult experiences. I will discuss the significance of this finding further on.

Unique and Universal Implications

The central finding of this study is that survivors who are able to acknowledge and communicate their traumatic Holocaust experiences have children who are better able to symbolize their own experiences; survivors who cannot talk about the Holocaust have children with more impaired capacities to discuss experiences in their own lives. How is it that a woman's knowledge of her mother's war experiences 40 years ago is related to her own discussion of giving birth, traveling to a foreign country, or dealing with her boss (some of the topics discussed in children of survivors' monologues)? I will address the significance of this relationship in terms of the unique nature of the Holocaust and its importance for the lives of children and survivors. I will also address what I consider the more universal implications of this relationship between symbolic processes in parents and children.

What was immediately apparent in conducting this study was that *all* children of survivors know that their parents went through the Holocaust. Whether or not specific experiences were discussed, this knowledge was "always there" for most. Thus the existence of the Holocaust as a representation in the minds of survivors and their children remains, regardless of the degree of clarity, specificity, concreteness, or imagery level.

Equally apparent as a central issue in this study, is that children of survivors want and need to know about their parents' Holocaust experiences. One woman said, "I was a real snoop. I hid in closets to overhear her talk to her cousins. Them she talked to." Prince (1985) states that the "drive to know" about the Holocaust is a common characteristic shared by all children of survivors. I conceptualize this "drive" as a manifestation of a general psychological tenet, that there is a tendency towards health in all individuals. Maslow conceives of self-fulfillment as the main theme in human life. Self-actualization is the desire to become all that one is capable of becoming (Hjelle & Ziegler, 1976). Children's desire to know their parents' Holocaust experiences can be understood in this light. Children of survivors seek knowledge of their parents' experiences not only for their own health, but in order to realize their full potential.

A series of common themes emerged in children of survivors who had difficulty acknowledging their own experiences, which were distinct from those who were better able to do so. Children of survivors with low referential activity ratings described their mothers' discussions about the Holocaust as infrequent or limited in some way. Some mothers could not speak about their experiences at all. Some spoke only of positive events; negative events or feelings were denied or not fully symbolized. Some mothers were ambivalent; they would talk, but made it clear that discussions inflicted pain.

Consider the following quotes from children of survivors with low referential activity ratings:

> Sometimes I'd ask. She'd always change the subject. I knew not to discuss it. I got a bad response. I let bygones be bygones.

> I think the most important aspect of my life is that my parents are survivors. She doesn't really talk about the war. When she speaks, she speaks about before the war or after the war.

> My mother was able to talk freely about life after the war, but she did not want what happened to her during the war to intrude. She never verbalized it. It was too painful. She still denies her background has had an effect on her. It's become pivotal to me. Not that I went seeking it. It started to intrude in my consciousness.

We can see in these comments how important their mothers' Holocaust experiences were even to those children of survivors who didn't hear about them, and in spite of their mothers' attempts to keep the experiences from their children. Children of survivors wanted and needed to hear their mothers' experiences.

Children of survivors with high referential activity ratings, in general heard a great deal. Painful feelings were not denied. The children sought information even though it was difficult. They also appeared to know how to regulate their questioning and listening so they did not become overwhelmed, even though they may not have felt that they could regulate their participation. Consider the following quote from a woman with high referential activity scores:

> I just remember them sitting at the kitchen table. My room was directly across from the kitchen. I could look from my bed, into the room, and see the light. The only time I think my mother would really let herself go, to all her feelings about the war, was to my aunt. My mother and my aunt, they'd go into great detail. I tune, I usually tune it out because it's too much for me. I wanted to know all the details, but not all at once. And sometimes they just talk and talk I don't know how many hours into the night. Before the war, during the war, after...

This woman knew how to regulate what she heard even though she felt it was too much at times. The important factor is that the information was accessible, if she wanted it.

In the following quote, the central thesis of this study is clearly articulated by a child of survivors herself:

> She doesn't understand why the war affects me. She was in the camps. I said 'Mom, I've heard about the war since I was a baby.' She thinks it's separate. She doesn't understand how much little words accumulate and are your life experience.

Children of survivors' mothers' words *are* their own experience. Without these words, part of children of survivors' own experiences are missing.

Why? This study suggests that parents' war experiences are an important and pervasive part of children of survivors' own experience and as such, the clearer, the more contained, and the more differentiated Holocaust representations are, the clearer children of survivors' other experiences are as well. As mentioned above, the majority of children of survivors in this study described the pervasiveness of the Holocaust in their lives. Consider these examples of how the Holocaust representations intruded on everyday events in their own lives:

> Anything would trigger a discussion. A sound, a reminder. When someone was barbecuing, my mother said that's what it smelled like in the camps.

> My mother would never wear yellow. She wouldn't let me. Then she'd tell me about the yellow armband.

> My mother would go shopping early in the morning or late at night. She couldn't stand to wait on line for food.

These examples portray specific instances of everyday life that, through survivor mothers' communication, became colored by the Holocaust. It is the accumulation of these instances that forms the backdrop of experience, resulting in many children of survivors characterizing the Holocaust as a central factor in their own lives.

The pervasiveness of the Holocaust in children of survivors can be further accounted for by returning to the initial culture of the child, the facilitating environment provided by the mother. Kestenberg (1972) states that, although the task of acknowledging one's parents' experiences is important for anyone growing up, it is different for children of survivors because it includes "a reality which defies trust in human nature." The Holocaust shook the most basic foundation of personality—trust. A child with a basic sense of trust sees the social world as a place of safety and stability, and views people as nurturant and reliable (Hjelle & Ziegler, 1976). For survivors of the Holocaust, their view of the social world and of humanity was shattered by reality. In order to continue functioning in current reality, they must maintain a degree of trust in everyday events, while living with the memory that every aspect of that reality, in the past, was unsafe. In most personal tragedies, while specific elements of the world become dangerous, one's basic foundation remains at least manifestly stable and trustworthy, to a reasonable degree.

The constant struggle to differentiate what is trustworthy from what is a threat, the earliest fundamental stage in psychosocial development, according to Erikson (1963), is viewed as a key factor accounting for the pervasiveness of the Holocaust in the lives of survivors and their children. In order to establish basic trust, every aspect of current life must be differentiated from its past associations and assigned new meaning in the shared world of the survivor and her child.

For example, when a survivor verbalizes her reaction to the color yellow, the child learns it is the yellow armband of the Holocaust that symbolizes evil, and not everything yellow; the significance of "yellow" becomes contained. In contrast, when the survivor is threatened by "yellowness," by uniforms, by a sound or a smell, and cannot make the connections to her past, her child in some sense "inherits" such diffuse fears. Thus, while connections to the past pervade all current reality, the ability to label these connections determines the extent to which the past is contained or perpetuated.

While this process of discrimination and labeling is necessary in every parent–child unit, I suggest that survivors have an additional symbolic step to perform. They must in a sense relearn what is safe in the external world and symbolize the distinction effectively, in order to communicate to their child a sense of the world as safe. Other individuals do this, to a large extent, once only as they are growing up. While particular events may be emotionally loaded and signify aspects of their own past that were not considered safe, for survivors it was their entire universe.

A possible implication of this finding is that the more able an individual is to acknowledge her experience, the less likely it is to be acted out or to cause adjustment difficulties such as depression or separation-individuation problems. The testing out of this inference would be a logical next step for research.

What are the more universal implications of the relationships found in this study? I'd like to return to the significant relationship found in all participants between referential activity based on the second monologue and number of facts known about mothers' difficult experiences. It may not be surprising that the more specific facts participants knew about their mothers' terrible experiences the more specific and clear they could describe the event. This finding might be explained simply as a function of memory; the more facts children heard, the more facts they can tell. The relationship between knowledge of facts and the expressiveness and evocativeness of their description is more difficult to explain in such direct terms. Based on what is known about referential activity, what appears to be measured in this case is what these women have internalized and symbolized of their mothers' experiences in verbal and nonverbal representations of their own.

Consider the following excerpt from a child of survivors' monologue about her mothers' experiences symbolized in a dream which her mother had told her:

> One day, one night I should say, she had a dream. And she dreamt that she was back in Tarnigov, which was a very happy place for her. You know, she loved that town. And she dreamt that, um, she walked into the center of the town, and she saw her father. And she ran to him and she said, "Papa, Papa, aren't you happy to see me?" And he said, "Yes, yes an—but I wanna tell you that the, you know, the linens are here and the silver is there, and this, these valuables I put here for you." And then he started walking away. And she said, "Where are you going? Aren't you—I just got home. Aren't you happy to see me?" And he said, "Yes, but you must listen very carefully." And he

> just went on and on and on. And then he went into a house and started walking up the stairs. And she said, "Where are you going?" And she ran, tried to go up the stairs behind him. And he said, "No, no, no, you can't come with me now." And he went up the stairs and disappeared. And she said that she woke up screaming. That she was so frightened by this dream that she couldn't even tell anybody about it...

This woman with high referential activity describes her mother's dream with a sense of immediacy because, in a sense, the experience is "alive" within her. It may not even be an accurate summary of what she was told. It is now her memory of her mother's experiences in multilayered symbolic form.

Of importance for this discussion is that referential-activity scores from these monologues about parent experiences were correlated with specific facts known in all participants. While the correlation was greater for children of survivors, the important finding with this monologue was that there was a significant relationship between referential activity and mothers' communication factors in both groups. By this relationship, the study recognizes a more general phenomenon, that is so clear in the survivor population—and that is that parental acknowledgment of one's own experience is related to one's children's symbolic ability.

Confirmation of the generalizability of this study will come through further research. This study has implications for children of survivors of other large-scale, man-made disasters as well as more general human interaction. Lifton (1968) has compared personality traits in children of Hiroshima survivors to children of Holocaust survivors. The transmission of symbolic impairment may also be evident in such devastating disasters. In addition, this research may have implications for children whose parents have experienced physical or psychological trauma, illness, or loss of various types. The development of groups of children of alcoholics and children of the chronically ill, like children of survivor groups, suggest the general importance, for one's own health, of labeling parental trauma. Eventually, with more sensitive instruments, it may be possible to identify the symbolic transmission processes of more universal life-crisis issues on children's symbolic activity. This study did not tap the process of acknowledgment of specific traumas and the consequences of a failure to do so. While I suggest that this process is in many ways unique in children of Holocaust survivors, there is also overlap with other personal traumas and cultural disasters, and this needs to be studied.

Therapeutic Implications

What are the implications of these findings for the treatment of Holocaust survivors and their children? Children of survivors need to acknowledge their parents' Holocaust experiences in order to develop the capacity to acknowledge their own. Yet for many, their needs have been frustrated by their parents' limitations. In order to prevent a kind of intergenerational transmission of the failure to acknowledge painful experiences, therapists must provide the environment in which the Holocaust experience can be brought out, and not contribute to the referential activity failure by their own countertransference reactions and resistances.

Even where survivors are unable to label their experiences, children of survivors nevertheless maintain nonverbal internalized representations of the Holocaust as this study has shown. Thus, they can be helped to link their own images and words, even if they do not have access to their parents' words. The therapeutic process can repair, for children of survivors, the paradoxical not knowing that which they have always known. This is a central function of the therapeutic process in general; this is its power. For a child of Holocaust survivors, this process must include symbolizing one's parents' Holocaust experiences in the process of acknowledging one's own history as well as one's current reality.

Conclusion

Self-disclosure occurs in a social context; it is fundamental to the experience of relatedness with others and ultimately with oneself. This study began with a theoretically based assumption, that one's ability to acknowledge experience is acquired in a relationship with one's parents. It concludes, based on empirical data, that a child's ability to acknowledge experience is affected by the parents' ability to do so. I am thus suggesting a powerful intergenerational connection between self-disclosure and relatedness. This connection may account for a continuous ripple effect of traumatic experiences on subsequent generations. It is also the connection that allows for the eventual containment of the effects of traumatic events. Self-disclosure within a relationship, be it with parent, child, friend, or therapist, allows one to extend and enhance the fabric of life woven by previous generations.

References

Barocas, H., & Barocas, C. (1973). Manifestations of concentration camp effects on the second generation. *American Journal of Psychiatry, 130*, 820–821.

Barocas, H., & Barocas, C. (1980). Separation-individuation conflicts in children of Holocaust survivors. *Journal of Contemporary Psychotherapy, 11*(1), 6–14.

Bettelheim, B. (1960). *The informed heart*. New York: Avon Books.

Bruner, J. (1983). *Child's talk: Learning to use language*. New York: W.W. Norton.
Bucci, W. (1982). The vocalization of painful affect. *Journal of Communication Disorders, 15*, 415–440.
Bucci, W. (1984). Linking words and things: Basic process and individual variation. *Cognition, 17*, 137–153.
Bucci, W., & Freedman, N. (1978). Language and hand: The dimension of referential competence. *Journal of Personality, 46*, 594–622.
Bucci, W., & Freedman, N. (1981). The language of depression. *Bulletin of the Menninger Clinic, 45*(4), 334–358.
Cahn, A. (1987). *The capacity to acknowledge experience in Holocaust survivors and their children*. Unpublished doctoral dissertation, Adelphi University.
Chodoff, P. (1963). Late effects on the concentration camp syndrome. *Archives of General Psychiatry, 8*, 323–333.
Danieli, Y. (1982). Families of survivors of the Nazi Holocaust: Some short- and long-term effects. *Stress and Anxiety, 8*, 405–421.
Eagle, M.N. (1984). Object-seeking and object relations. In *Recent developments in psychoanalysis*. New York: McGraw-Hill.
Eitinger, L. (1961). Pathology of the concentration camp syndrome. *Archives of General Psychiatry, 5*, 371–379.
Erikson, E. (1963). *Childhood and society*. New York: Norton.
Frankl, V.E. (1959). *Man's search for meaning*. Boston: Beacon Press.
Freud, S. (1951). Mourning and Melancholia. In J. Strachey (Ed. and tran.), *The standard edition of the complete psychological works of Sigmund Freud*. London: Hogarth Press. (Originally published, 1917.)
Freyberg, J. (1980). Difficulties in separation-individuation as experienced by offspring of Nazi Holocaust survivors. *American Journal of Orthopsychiatry, 50*(1).
Hjelle, L., & Ziegler, D. (1976). *Personality theories: Basic assumptions, research and applications*. New York: McGraw-Hill.
Jaffe, L.E. (1985). *Maternal symbolic and psycholinguistic behaviors and the child's evolving capacity to tolerate separation*. Unpublished doctoral dissertation, Adelphi University.
Kaye, K. (1982). *The mental and social life of babies: How parents create persons*. Chicago: University of Chicago Press.
Kestenberg, J. (1972). Psychoanalytic contributions to the problem of children of survivors from Nazi persecutions. *The Israel Annals of Psychiatric and Related Disciplines, 10*, 311–325.
Klein, H. (1971). Families of Holocaust survivors in the kibbutz. *Psychological Studies*, 67–92.
Krystal, H. (1968). *Massive psychic trauma*. New York: International Universities Press.
Lifton, R.J. (1968). Observations on Hiroshima survivors. In H. Krystal (Ed.), *Massive psychic trauma*. New York: International Universities Press.
Niederland, W.G. (1968). An interpretation of the psychological stresses and defenses in concentration camp life and the late after-effects. In H. Krystal (Ed.), *Massive psychic trauma*. New York: International Universities Press.
Phillips, R.E. (1978). Impact of Nazi Holocaust on children of survivors. *American Journal of Psychotherapy, 32*(3), 370–378.
Pilcz, M. (1979). Understanding the survivor family. In L. Steinitz & D. Szonyi, *Living after the Holocaust: Reflections by children of survivors in America*. New York: Bloch Publishing Company.
Prince, R. (1985). Knowing the holocaust. *Psychoanalytic Inquiry, 5*(1), 51–61.
Rakoff, V., Sigal, J., Epstein, N. (1967). Children and families of concentration camp survivors. *Canada's Mental Health, 14*, 24–26.
Rapaport, D. (1958). The theory of ego autonomy: A generalization. *Bulletin of the Menninger Clinic, 22*, 13–35.

Sigal, J., & Rakoff, V. (1971). Concentration camp survival: A pilot study of effects on the second generation. *Canadian Psychiatric Association Journal, 16*, 393–397.
Sonnenberg, S. (1972). Workshop report: Children of survivors. *Journal of the American Psychoanalytic Association, 22*, 200–203.
Vygotsky, L.S. (1962). *Thought and language*. Cambridge: M.I.T. Press.

16

From Secrecy to Self-Disclosure

HEALING THE SCARS OF INCEST

Mary Gail Frawley

Sexual abuse of children is a phenomenon that has only recently emerged from society's skeleton closet as a topic to be discussed and researched. Incidence figures generated by two large random sample epidemiological studies indicate, however, that approximately 38.0% of all women have been sexually abused before the age of 18, with about 4.5% having been sexually victimized by a biological, adoptive, step-, or foster father (Russell, 1986; Wyatt, 1985). The sexual violation of her physical and emotional integrity by a father figure thus appears to be an experience common to over 3.3 million American women. It is an experience grounded in secrecy; secrecy imposed by the perpetrator with promises and threats ranging from the gently insidious to the brutally forceful. It is an experience out of which arises a plethora of negative psychological sequelae, including an impaired capacity for emotional and sexual intimacy. Finally, it is an experience the healing of which often begins with the survivor's self-disclosure.

A review of book titles on childhood sexual abuse reflects the central role secrecy plays in this experience: *Conspiracy of Silence: The Trauma of Incest* (Butler, 1978), *I Never Told Anyone* (Bass & Thornton, 1983), *The Common Secret* (Kempe & Kempe, 1984), *The Family Secret* (Hill, 1985), *The Best-Kept Secret* (Rush, 1980), *The Secret Trauma* (Russell, 1986), *No More Secrets* (Adams & Fay, 1981). Secrecy is the cornerstone of incest and is

Mary Gail Frawley • Pomona Clinic, Robert L. Yeager Health Complex, Pomona, New York 10970. The author thanks Michelle Collins, Michael O'Toole, and Ann Kuehner for their review of this manuscript and for their valuable editorial suggestions.

imposed by the abusing father with a variety of intimidations, some of which are poignantly captured by Charles Summit in his 1983 article, *The Child Abuse Accommodation Syndrome*:

> This is our secret; nobody else will understand...Don't tell your mother—she will hate you; she will hate me; she will kill you; she will kill me; it will kill her; she will send you away; she will send me away; it will break up the family and you'll end up in an orphanage...If you tell anyone, I won't love you anymore; no one will love you; I'll spank you; I'll kill your dog; I'll kill you. (p. 181)

The imposition of secrecy is usually effected with such success that the incestuously abused child often reaches adulthood with the incest secret intact. At the more extreme levels of preservation, the incest may remain repressed within the unconscious of the survivor, thus constituting a secret even from the victim herself or, in multiple personality, may be contained within a separately functioning personality who has only marginal interaction with the birth personality. If, on the other hand, the child does disclose while the incest is occurring, she may be disbelieved, vilified, or ignored, rather than validated and supported.

The pervasiveness of secrecy was evident in the author's study of 82 survivors of father-daughter incest (Frawley, 1988). Results indicated that 56.0% of the women did not disclose their incest until adulthood; the mean age of adult disclosure was over 29 years. Of the 36 women who did disclose while the incest was happening, 78.0% failed to receive any support from the disclosure target. For the majority of father-daughter incest victims, then, their victimizations become actual and internalized core developmental experiences that are relegated to the shadows of secrecy; key aspects of their lives that are rendered unknowable by and unshareable with others or sometimes even themselves. The intense affects attached to the incest memories, and the isolation in which both become enshrouded, alienate the child/women from an entire realm of her development, resulting in deficits in her sense of relatedness to self and others.

The long-term negative sequelae of father–daughter incest are numerous and may seriously interfere with the survivor's adult functioning. Table 1 illustrates negative effects perceived by 82 father–daughter incest survivors to be connected to their childhood abuse (Frawley, 1988). Other symptoms frequently mentioned in the incest literature include promiscuity, prostitution, somatic complaints, chronic anxiety, impulsivity, eating disorders, and increased risk of incestuous abuse of the survivor's own children. Most of these symptoms can be conceptualized as reflective of impairments in the woman's ability to relate intimately and empathically to herself and others. These relational capacities are diminished by domination of internalized bad objects

Table 1. Incest Survivors: Perceived Negative Effects of Incest, N = 82

Variable name	Percentage
Low self-esteem	95.1
Difficulty trusting men	86.6
Chronic guilt	82.9
Major depression	81.7
Sexual dysfunction	76.8
Difficulty trusting women	58.5
At least one suicide attempt	53.7
Drug or alcohol abuse	47.6
Parenting difficulties	45.1
Sexual abuse by person other than father figure	42.7
Adolescent running away	31.7
Adult rape	26.8
Adult physical abuse	26.8
Adolescent pregnancy	20.7

(Fairbairn, 1943) and by representations of interactions with others that have been generalized (Stern, 1985) to form templates of relational expectations regarding self, others, and self-in-relation-with-others.

It is perhaps in the area of sexual functioning that the incest survivor's impaired capacity for interpersonal intimacy is most clearly evidenced. David Scharff (1982) postulates that sex is a physical interaction in the real world which links each person with his/her internal objects and is thus influenced by the quality of the child's object relationships from birth onward (p. 9). Scharff thus implies that sexual functioning reflects a capacity for emotional intimacy with self and other that is founded on early relationships with both parents. Similarly, Fairbairn (1941) asserts that mature genitality emerges from a libidinal attitude toward self and other that is based on early object relationships. In healthy development, these childhood relationships engender a capacity to merge temporarily with another while retaining a sense of personal separateness, a capacity reminiscent of Erickson's (1980) stage of Intimacy and Distantiation versus Self-Absorption.

The incestuous family clearly mitigates against development of the relational capacity necessary for functional and pleasurable sexual intimacy. Instead, as indicated by Scharff, the father's assault on his daughter's bodily integrity, his betrayal of the parental bond, and the mother's failure to protect the child are parenting deficits which result in the adult survivors' inability to "let down their own massive bodily shield to allow appropriate penetration physically or emotionally. . ." (p. 82). It is more encompassing to view that shield as both bodily and psychic.

The author's dissertation research was designed to study sexual functioning among adult survivors of father-daughter incest (Frawley, 1988). Sexual functioning was conceptualized as emanating from a capacity for emotional intimacy reflective of childhood relationships with both parents. Eighty-two incest survivors participated in the research and comprised the largest sample of former incest victims to have been studied at that time. They were compared on a number of measures of sexual functioning with 76 control women who had no history of childhood sexual or physical abuse. Results indicated that the incest survivors experienced physiologically manifested sexual dysfunctions to a significantly greater degree or significantly more frequently than control women. The survivors were also significantly more likely to experience guilt regarding sexual matters and activities, and reported significantly less satisfaction with the quality of their current sex lives. While all women in the study experienced greater sexual dysfunction in more emotionally laden relationships—with husbands or with lovers for whom there were deep emotional feelings—than in casual relationships, the incest survivors were incrementally more dysfunctional than controls in the emotionally closer dyadic contexts. Significance for these results was achieved at least at the $p<.01$ level. These results generally support other empirical investigations of sexual dysfunction among incest survivors (Becker & Skinner, 1983; Becker, Skinner, Abel, & Treacy, 1982; Finkelhor, 1984; Fromuth, 1986; Gold, 1986; Jehu, Gazan, & Klassen, 1985; Landis *et al.*, 1970; Meiselman, 1980; Van Buskirk & Cole, 1983).

Personal accounts by adult incest survivors (Allen, 1980; Armstrong, 1978; Bass & Thornton, 1983; Ward, 1985) and reports from clinicians working with former incest victims (Banmen, 1982; Cohen, 1983; Forward & Buck, 1978; Gelinas, 1983; Gordy, 1983; Kaufman, Peck, & Tagiuri, 1954; Kempe & Kempe, 1984; McGuire & Wagner, 1978; O'Hare & Taylor, 1983; Renvoize, 1982; Rosenfeld, Nadelson, Krieger, & Backman, 1979; Ward, 1985; Westerlund, 1983) also support a connection between childhood incestuous abuse and adult sexual dysfunction. Charlotte Vale Allen (1980), an incest survivor, describes her experience of sex as follows: "It was a matter of accommodating a tremendous, invading weight while my head traveled through stage after stage of recoil and shock and I tried to convince myself that I was a grown woman doing what grown women do" (p. 225). Another survivor, a participant in the author's study, wrote: "I feel that the worst result of incest for me was sexual dysfunction—it was what brought me to psychotherapy...I simply could not continue pretending to enjoy it one more minute after so many years of trying, trying, trying" (Frawley, 1988). To reframe the struggle, these women were engaged in a losing battle to construct a mutually safe, empowering relationship that combined emotional and sexual intimacy.

If secrecy is the mainstay of father–daughter incest, and if an impaired capacity for emotional and sexual intimacy is one of the tragic long-term consequences of childhood incestuous abuse, it can be postulated that disclosure of the incest secret to a validating, believing other may begin a process of healing that can reopen channels of intimate relatedness to self and other. Before discussing the effects of disclosure, however, it is important to remark on the ways in which disclosure can be elicited by clinicians.

Many women with incest in their pasts have "completed" one or more psychotherapies without ever having mentioned their sexual abuse (Courtois, 1980; Faria & Belohavek, 1984). In some cases, these women may have been desperately hoping just to be asked so that they might begin to speak (Herman, 1981; James, 1977, in Swanson & Biaggio, 1985). It is crucial, therefore, that clinicians ask about sexual abuse during every intake. In one study conducted by Briere and Zaidi (1988), 100 intake reports on nonpsychotic women presenting to an urban psychiatric emergency room were reviewed in two phases. In the first review, 50 charts were randomly selected and the intake report was checked for a history of sexual abuse; 6.0% of the charts reflected such data. Clinicians were then instructed to question intake patients for previous sexual victimizations. Another 50 postinstruction intake reports were randomly reviewed and, this time, researchers found that 70.0% of the women interviewed reported having been sexually abused at some point in their lives. Not surprisingly, an incest survivor who has carried her secret into adulthood may not be able to disclose unless she feels certain that the therapist believes that childhood sexual abuse occurs and that he/she can tolerate hearing the woman's story. The clinician who asks about past sexual victimizations during intake conveys to the patient that she/he does know and believes that children are sexually abused, that those victimizations are important clinical material, and that he/she is prepared to join with the former victim in working through the memories and affects linked with any childhood abuse.

Many other women may enter treatment with their sexually abusive experiences repressed. In these cases, the therapist's knowledge of and attention to the signs and symptoms of sexual abuse may allow her/him to help the patient unlock repressed memories, thus facilitating working through and recovery. Courtois (1988), Ellenson (1986), and Gelinas (1983) fully discuss presenting and historic characteristics that alert the therapist to possible childhood sexual abuse.

Once psychotherapy begins with an incest survivor, the work may evoke strong affective responses in the clinician. The material regarding specifics of the abuse may, for instance, engender powerful feelings of anger—at the perpetrator, the nonabusing parent, and toward the victim, revulsion, fear, eroticism, a wish to rescue, a wish to avoid. Additionally, for the therapist/survivor, this work may evoke particularly potent memories and feelings related to her own abuse. It is thus important, as Courtois (1988) and Herman (1981) indicate, that therapists treating incestuously abused women carefully work through their attitudes and affects towards childhood sexual victimization in general, and any abuse in their own pasts in particular, to ensure that they can provide service to the incest survivor that encourages continued disclosure and discussion.

Finally, these patients often present with characterological disorganization and defenses likely to evoke strong positive and negative countertransferential reactions not necessarily directly linked to the incest material. As Fairbairn (1943) and Scharff (1982) discuss, the betrayal of trust inherent in incest and the confusion bestowed on the child by having to adapt to the invasion of her physical and psychic boundaries by a loved and needed parent often results in severe splitting of the ego. This once-adaptive survival mechanism can lead to the discontinuous self and other representations and to the defensive constellation consistent with borderline personality structure as described by Kernberg (1984). The clinician's own ability to sustain an openness toward intimate relatedness within appropriate therapeutic boundaries throughout the Sturm und Drang of treatment with an incest survivor organized at the borderline level of ego structure will certainly be associated with the patient's progress in increasing her own capacity for intimate relatedness. Implied support for this view is contained in articles by Epstein (1979), Gorney (1979), and Racker (1972) in which they discuss transference/countertransference and the interpersonal context of psychoanalytic work.

Before discussing the considerable positive effects of disclosure on an incest survivor's overall functioning and capacity for intimate relatedness, it is important to note that disclosure of the incest secret may initially engender increased disorganization and symptom exacerbation (Courtois, 1988; Gelinas, 1983; Herman, 1981). Gelinas indicates that revealing an incest history may release a flood of painful memories and affects connected to the original trauma. She points out that women may, during this initial stage of treatment, experience disorganizing flashbacks and/or reenact some portion of their abuse. Similarly, Courtois asserts that self-punitive behavior may be evoked by the betrayal of and disloyalty to the family represented by the very act of disclosure. These after-effects of disclosure can be postulated to reflect the return of repressed bad objects (Fairbairn, 1943) to whom the incest survivor remains unconsciously and tenaciously attached. A group at greater risk for suicide than women without histories of sexual victimization (Bagley & Ramsey, 1985; Briere & Runtz, 1986), incest survivors may attempt or complete suicide when disclosure evokes very painful and/or very rageful previously repressed feelings about their abuse (Courtois, 1988). Attempted or successful suicides can, in these cases, be viewed as vicious attacks on and by the woman's parental introjects.

Simone, an attractive 36-year-old incest survivor, had disclosed her incest for the first time when she came to therapy around problems in her seven-year, childless marriage. At intake, Simone stated that she had unresolved feelings about her childhood incestuous abuse and about her father, who had suicided 15 years earlier. In addition to the sexual abuse, Simone had been terribly neglected as an infant by both parents—left alone in a crib for hours while they drank at a neighbor's house—and was verbally denigrated by her mother into adulthood.

It became clear early in Simone's therapy that she was truly "possessed" by punitive introjects (Fairbairn, 1943) who deemed her useless and a totally unworthy being. Gradually, the therapy itself became an instrument of self-torture as Simone ruminated virtually nonstop about her sessions, her memories of her traumatic childhood, and her feelings about those memories. Rage was one emotion Simone expressed during the last weeks of her therapy; rage towards her mother for not protecting her and towards herself for "letting" the abuse happen, as well as for not working "hard enough" in her therapy. She also expressed anger and disappointment toward the author for the latter's inability to read Simone's mind; for not simply intuiting all that Simone had difficulty disclosing herself. While suicidal and homicidal ideation were expressed, intent and a concrete plan were denied. Despite her disclaimers, Simone suicided four months after beginning treatment, overdosing with Seconal, as her father had done. Later, it became evident that while Simone had been open about her incestuous abuse, there was much about her that remained secret. In particular, Simone hid her intention to die. She never mentioned that she kept a large supply of Seconal in her bedside night table, or that she was quietly saying good-bye to family and friends for a month prior to her death.

Simone's suicide can certainly be conceptualized as a rageful act against and by her parental introjects. It may have also been a desperate act of loyal attachment to her internalized father or, conversely, an enactment of a threatened punishment for disclosure. It was simultaneously an expression of rageful hatefulness and despairing hopelessness toward family, friends, and therapist. Ultimately, however, Simone remained unknowable and unreachable, isolated with her horrific internalized object world, unable to use treatment to reopen pathways to ameliorative intimate relatedness with another.

Despite the turbulence, and even tragedy, that may follow a survivor's initial disclosure of her incest, the opportunity to reveal the secret and to discuss her abusive experiences with another more usually signals the beginning of recovery from the incest trauma for many former victims (Brunngraber, 1986; Courtois, 1988; Herman, 1981; Westerlund, 1983).

Since, by definition, women who have not disclosed their incest secret are unavailable to researchers, it is difficult empirically to validate the importance of disclosure. In the author's study (Frawley, 1988), however, a significant correlation was found between the age at which a woman first disclosed her incest and several measures of adult sexual functioning, with disclosure later in life related to more frequent or more severe sexual dysfunction. Significance was achieved at least at the $p < .05$ level. These results are consistent with Brunngraber's (1986) findings, generated in a study of 21 adult incest survivors, that disclosing their incest experiences to others was considered by the women to be positively related to overall adjustment to their past victimization. Similarly, Courtois (1980) found that all 30 adult survivors of childhood sexual abuse that she interviewed deemed participation in her research helpful. They specifically cited the importance of the catharsis involved in discussing their experiences with a nonjudgmental other. These findings indeed suggest that an incest survivor's self-disclosure is crucial to reopening intra- and interpersonal channels to intimate relatedness. Beyond findings like these, it is in clinical work with incest survivors that the central role of disclosure in revitalizing a capacity for intimacy is most evident.

Various books and articles discuss individual and group treatment strategies for work with incest survivors (Blake-White & Kline, 1985; Courtois, 1988; Faria & Belohavek, 1984; Forward & Buck, 1978; Gordy, 1983; Herman, 1981; McGuire & Wagner, 1978). While, to the author's knowledge, there have been no systematically conducted outcome studies on the retrospective treatment of father–daughter incest, a number of writers concur that many of the long-term negative sequelae of incest are amenable to treatment through psychotherapy.

In the author's own clinical experience, several incest survivors have demonstrated marked improvement in their capacity for intimate relatedness subsequent to disclosing their incest histories. Angelina, for instance, is a 40-year-old woman who had not disclosed her incest secret until beginning psychotherapy for anxiety and depression following the end of her 16-year marriage. During that marriage, Angelina experienced chronic vaginismus—involuntary contraction of the vaginal muscles that prevents penetration. It was also clear that the lack of sexual intimacy between Angelina and her husband paralleled an emotional distance in which they shared few aspects of their internal worlds, relating primarily around the concrete events in their mostly separately organized lives. Although she clearly recalled her father's incestuous abuse, this woman did not connect her sexual dysfunction nor her emotional distance from her husband with her childhood experiences. After a year and a half of psychoanalytic psychotherapy in which her incest and her relationship with both parents have been primary foci, Angelina has established a more mutually enriching relationship with a man in which emotional and sexual intimacy are both possible and enjoyable. Although sexual intercourse can sometimes be unsettling for Angelina, she has had no recurrence of vaginismus since revealing her incest history in treatment.

A dramatic instance of the ameliorative impact of disclosure is represented by the author's work with Betsey, a 38-year-old mother of three. Betsey presented for outpatient therapy subsequent to a brief psychiatric hospitalization precipitated by a drunken rampage in her boyfriend's apartment that was perpetrated while she was there alone. Three months prior to the hospitalization, she had impulsively left her husband of 15 years and their three children to live with a new man. The rampage was connected to overwhelming feelings of confusion and guilt over this behavior which stood in sharp contrast to her historical presentation as a "good girl." At intake, Betsey reported a two-year history of bulimia nervosa then in remission, a six-month habit of episodic, solitary alcohol abuse, and even more recent episodic self-mutilation during which Betsey would cut her forearms with a razor. Childhood sexual abuse was denied at intake.

Over the first six months of treatment, Betsey cut her arms, or at least wanted very much to cut herself, as often as once a week. It became clear that the cutting often followed a session during which the author failed sufficiently to validate Betsey's "badness." While this woman seriously distorted the extent and depth of her badness, her behavior toward her family had, in fact, been destructive. As the author learned verbally to validate that destructiveness, Betsey could begin also to examine the pain and hopelessness that led to the behavior she so hated. Acknowledging the truth of her malevolence thus created a holding environment for Betsey in which she was freed to begin to integrate more worthy parts of herself. At this point, the cutting diminished but did not abate entirely.

During this time, Betsey also frequently dissociated in session, without exception after she had been discussing her father in some context. The part of her "floating on the ceiling" would report that the part of her sitting in the chair was numb from the waist down and that "someone" was pushing down on her head and shoulders. The dissociative episodes, combined with other aspects of her history and symptoms, strongly suggested that this woman was a father–daughter incest survivor who had repressed the memories of her abuse.

After about six months of therapy during which the author would occasionally question Betsey about possible childhood sexual experiences, Betsey had a dissociative experience at home with her boyfriend during which she reenacted her father's pushing her to her knees to perform oral sex on him. During this episode, she revealed to her boyfriend that her father had threatened to cut her arms off if she ever told about the abuse. The self-mutilation was clearly an enactment of the threatened punishment and was evoked as her memories of the abuse neared consciousness through the therapy.

Since Betsey reenacted her abuse, she has gradually recovered more memories and can now tolerate remembering without dissociating. There has been no self-mutilation since that time, and Betsey now says, "I wouldn't even want to cut myself. It never hurt before but I know it would hurt me to do it now." While she still has much work to do in therapy, Betsey has begun to develop a more compassionate attitude toward herself and she is beginning to repair the relationships with her children. Within the therapy, Betsey's eye contact has markedly increased and there is an emerging interest in the therapist as a person rather than as someone who is simply fulfilling a professional role. Betsey was once unable to walk down the hall with the author to her office because it made her "too nervous" to be that close to and somewhat out of role with the therapist. Recently, however, she loped down the hall alongside the author chatting animatedly about a newspaper article she had read that day. It is quite apparent that, in Betsey's case, regaining the memories of her childhood incest and discussing them with another human being has improved this woman's capacity for intimately knowing and relating to herself and others.

Many clinicians who treat incest survivors recommend group therapy as a primary or important ancillary treatment modality (Courtois, 1988; Gordy, 1983; Herman, 1981; Westerlund, 1983). Group therapy affords the former incest victim the opportunity to expand her disclosure network; to reality-test negative self-concepts with women who share similar traumatic histories; and to develop within the holding environment of the group more intimate relatedness with self, other, and self-in-relation-with-other.

A survivor group run by the author confirms the recommendation of others in the field; the group experience seems to stimulate increased trust in self and other, in part through expanded self-disclosure in an environment of safety and common ground. In this group of women ranging in age from 20 to 50, it has been particularly poignant to observe the "re-mothering" and "re-daughtering" taking place within the group. Most of the mothers in the group regret what they perceive as an inability on their part to relate empathically to their own children when the latter were young; relationships with girl children with whom the survivors identified were often especially distant and strained. The women in the group who are not parents have hungered for freely given maternal nurturance all their lives and have raged in silence against their own mothers who were not able to provide that kind of relationship. The "mothers'" need to give without damaging and the "daughters'" need both to rage and to receive have been voiced within the group. This experience is reparative for the "mothers" who can now re-mother themselves while responding to the "daughters" with nurturance and acceptance of their rage. At the same time, the "daughters" have an opportunity to repair their relationships with their internalized mothers by introjecting new maternal experiences. For all these women, the group provides expanded channels for intimate relatedness.

Father–daughter incest is a damaging, core developmental experience which, although it occurs in childhood or adolescence, continues to haunt the survivor's adulthood, precluding intimate relatedness with self and other. It is an experience often secretly stored in the skeleton closet of the adult survivor's psyche. Disclosure of that secret to an accepting, believing other may signify initiation of a healing process. Often long and painful, the healing begun with disclosure can ultimately result in a revitalized capacity for intimacy, for knowing and being known by self and other.

References

Adams, C., & Fay, J. *No more secrets*. San Luis Obispo: Impact Publishers.

Allen, C.V. (1980). *Daddy's girl*. New York: Berkley Books.

Armstrong, L. (1978). *Kiss daddy goodnight*. New York: Pocket Books.

Bagley, C., & Ramsey, R. (1986). Sexual abuse in childhood: psychosocial outcomes and implications for social work practice. *Social Work Practice in Sexual Problems*, 33–47.

Banmen, J. (1982). The incidence, treatment and counseling of incest. *International Journal for the Advancement of Counseling*, *5*, 201–206.

Bass, E., & Thornton, L. (1983). *I never told anyone*. New York: Harper & Row.

Becker, J., & Skinner, L. (1983). Assessment and treatment of rape-related sexual dysfunctions. *The Clinical Psychologist*, *36*, 102–105.

Becker, J., Skinner, L., Abel, G., & Treacy, E. (1982). Incidence and type of sexual dysfunction in rape and incest victims. *Journal of Sex and Marital Therapy*, *8*, 65–74.

Blake-White, J., & Kline, C. (1985). Treating the dissociative process in adult victims of childhood incest. *Social Casework*, *66*, 394–402.

Briere, J., & Runtz, M. (1986). Suicidal thoughts and behaviors in former sexual abuse victims. *Canadian Journal of Behavioural Science*, *18*, 413–423.

Briere, J., & Zaidi, L. (1988). *Sexual abuse histories and sequelae in psychiatric emergency room patients*. Paper presented at the annual meeting of the American Psychological Society, Atlanta, GA, Aug.

Brunngraber, L.S. (1986). Father-daughter incest: Immediate and long-term effects of sexual abuse. *Advances in Nursing Science, 8*, 15–35.

Butler, S. (1978). *Conspiracy of silence: The trauma of incest*. New York: Bantam Books.

Cohen, T. (1983). The incestuous family revisited. *Social Casework*, 154–161.

Courtois, C.A. (1980). Studying and counseling women with past incest experience. *Victimology, 5*, 322–334.

Courtois, C.A. (1988). *Healing the incest wound*. New York: W.W. Norton.

Ellenson, G.S. (1986). Disturbances of perception in adult female incest survivors. *Social Casework, 67*, 149–159.

Epstein, L. (1979). The therapeutic use of countertransference data with borderline patients. *Contemporary Psychoanalysis, 13*, 248–275.

Erikson, E.H. (1980). *Identity and the life cycle*. New York: W.W. Norton.

Fairbairn, W.R.D. (1941). A revised psychopathology of the psychoses and psychoneuroses. *Psychoanalytic studies in the personality*. London: Routledge & Kegan Paul.

Fairbairn, W.R.D. (1943). The repression and the return of bad objects. *Psychoanalytic studies of the personality*. London: Routledge & Kegan Paul, 1984.

Faria, G., & Belohavek, N. (1984). Treating female adult survivors of childhood incest. *Social Casework, 65*, 465–471.

Finkelhor, D. (1984). *Child sexual abuse*. New York: The Free Press.

Forward, S., & Buck, C. (1978). *Betrayal of innocence*. New York: Plenum Press.

Frawley, M.G. (1988). The sexual lives of adult survivors of father-daughter incest. *Dissertation Abstracts International, 49*. (University Microfilms No. 88-06, 457.)

Fromuth, M.E. (1986). The relationship of childhood sexual abuse with later psychological and sexual adjustment in a sample of college women. *Child Abuse and Neglect, 10*, 5–15.

Gelinas, D.J. (1983). The persisting negative effects of incest. *Psychiatry, 46*, 312–332.

Gold, E. (1986). Long-term effects of sexual victimization in childhood: an attributional approach. *Journal of Consulting and Clinical Psychology, 54*, 471–475.

Gordy, P.L. (1983). Group work that support adult victims of childhood incest. *Social Casework*, 300–307.

Gorney, J.F. (1979). The negative therapeutic interaction. *Contemporary Psychoanalysis, 15*, 288–337.

Herman, J. (1981). *Father-daughter incest*. Cambridge, MA: Harvard University Press.

Hill, E. (1985). *The family secret*. New York: Dell.

Jehu, D., Gazan, M., & Klassen, C. (1985). Common therapeutic targets among women who were sexually abused in childhood. *Social Work and Human Sexuality, 3*, 25–45.

Kaufman, I., Peck, A., & Tagiuri, C. (1954). The family constellation and overt incestuous relations between father and daughter. *American Journal of Orthopsychiatry, 24*, 266–277.

Kempe, R.S., & Kempe, H. (1984). *The common secret*. New York: W.H. Freeman.

Kernberg, O. (1984). *Severe personality disorders*. New Haven: Yale University Press.

Landis, C., Landis, A.T., Bolles, M.M., Metzger, H., Pitts, M.W., D'Esopo, D.A., Moloy, H.C., Kleegman, S.J., & Dickinson, R.L. (1970). *Sex in development*. College Park, MD: McGrath Publishing Company.

McGuire, L.S., & Wagner, N.N. (1978). Sexual dysfunction in women who were molested as children: One response pattern and suggestions for treatment. *Journal of Sex and Marital Therapy, 4*, 11–15.

Meiselman, K.C. (1980). Personality characteristics of incest history psychotherapy patients: a research note. *Archives of Sexual Behavior, 9*, 195–197.

O'Hare, J., & Taylor, K. (1983). The reality of incest. *Women changing therapy*. Englewood Cliffs, NJ: Haworth Press.

Racker, H. (1972). The meanings and uses of countertransference. *Psychoanalytic Quarterly, 41*, 487–506.
Renvoize, J. (1982). *Incest*. London: Routledge & Kegan Paul.
Rosenfeld, A., Nadelson, C.C., Krieger, M., & Backman, J.H. (1979). Incest and sexual abuse of children. *American Academy of Child Psychiatry, 18*, 342–353.
Rush, F. (1980). *The best kept secret*. New York: McGraw-Hill.
Russell, D.E.H. (1986). *The secret trauma*. New York: Basic Books.
Scharff, D.E. (1982). *The sexual relationship*. Boston: Routledge & Kegan Paul.
Stern, D.N. (1985). *The interpersonal world of the infant*. New York: Basic Books.
Summit, R.C. (1983). The child abuse accommodation syndrome. *Child Abuse and Neglect, 7*, 177–193.
Swanson, L., & Biaggio, M.K. (1985). Therapeutic perspectives of father-daughter incest. *Child Abuse and Neglect, 7*, 177–193.
Van Buskirk, S.S., & Cole, C.F. (1983). Characteristics of eight women seeking therapy for the effects of incest. *Psychotherapy: Theory, Research and Practice, 20*, 503–514.
Ward, E. (1985). *Father-daughter rape*. New York: Grove Press.
Westerlund, E. (1983). Counseling women with histories of incest. *Women and Therapy, 2*, 17–31.
Wyatt, G. (1985). The sexual abuse of Afro-American and white women in childhood. *Child Abuse and Neglect, 9*, 507–519.

17

Issues in the Disclosure of Perinatal Death

Douglas J. Peddicord

In late 1978 a son was born to my wife and me. Thirteen weeks premature and weighing just under two pounds, he died, after struggling courageously for 11 days, on Christmas Eve. The events of his birth, life, and death changed things—my sense of myself, my understanding of the world, my feelings about life—to an extent that is difficult to convey even now. And at the time very few people seemed willing to see, to acknowledge, to understand that.

For me, part of the process of working-through involved the dictum that one becomes expert in what one must. Nearly two and a half years of research then, which included in-depth interviews with 35 parents (20 mothers, 15 fathers) who had suffered a stillbirth or infant death within the preceding 4–10 weeks, produced a dissertation (Peddicord, 1982) and a clinical familiarity with an experience that forces individuals to make contact with what Stricker and Fisher in their Preface call "the dark, fearful, and often untouched areas within. . . ."

The Problem of Perinatal Death

In modern society there is a common belief that the successful birth of a child is a most "natural" and uncomplicated process, and that the loss of an infant—to miscarriage or stillbirth or neonatal death—is an

Douglas J. Peddicord • 9402 Sunfall Court, Columbia, Maryland 21046.

uncommon experience. Despite the fact that more deaths occur in the first few days of life than in any subsequent period of childhood, such an event seems nearly unthinkable, an affront to the spectacular advances of medical technology and treatment in this century. But, in reality, depending upon the definition of perinatal mortality utilized, (ranging from a generally accepted time frame between the 20th week of gestation and the 28th day of life to much broader limits, such as from conception to one year after birth), these "rare" tragedies actually occur from 70,000 to 250,000 times each year in the United States alone.

Though a great many mothers and fathers are forced to confront one of the truly nightmarish anxieties of parenthood, until quite recently researchers and clinicians largely shied away from the topic of perinatal death. Thus, as late as 1970, Kennell, Slyter, and Klaus, while noting detailed descriptions of mourning responses of adults to the loss of a spouse, parent, friend, or terminally ill child, could state that theirs was the first report in English on the reactions of parents to the loss of a newborn. The taboo nature of the subject and dearth of research allowed for caregiver assumptions marked by avoidance and denial:

> Not too many years ago it was common practice for the physician of a mother who just had a stillbirth to deny her physical contact with the dead baby's body, prescribe tranquilizers to minimize her grief, and recommend forgetting about the sad event as soon as possible, perhaps by quickly attempting another pregnancy. (Leon, 1987, p. 186)

Rando (1986) asserts that the loss of a child is unlike any other, that parental grief is especially severe, often complicated and long lasting, and marked by major symptom fluctuations over time. Lippman and Carlson (1977) state: "Throughout the literature is the pervasive theme of loss, of feeling devastated, and of the need to find the means to meet and overcome these traumatic experiences" (p. 171). Investigators agree that mothers (and fathers, in general) mourn and that this is usually manifested in an acute grief reaction, as delineated initially by Lindemann (1944). On occasion, marked pathological reactions such as severe depression, reactive psychosis, and significant somatic difficulties have been noted (Cullberg, 1971). Feelings of guilt and lowered self-esteem in the mothers of deceased infants have been cited frequently (Benfield, Leib, & Reuter, 1976; Peppers & Knapp, 1980; Miles & Demi, 1986).

Unique Characteristics of Perinatal Death

A number of authors have commented that the loss of an infant is as much a loss of potential as a loss of a real object; instead of the fulfillment of a happy expectation there is a substitution of death. And this is a "special kind" of death. As one father put it:

> What upsets me most is the unfulfilled potential of that child...like that it wasn't a real person. It's almost like if we could not have children and always wanted one—it's that same sort of unfulfilled potential that is the saddest thing to me, provokes the most in me. And at the same time the little being that was and now isn't, isn't and it's...there is nothing to remember really. Like with a funeral people can get together and talk about the good times they had (with the person) but for us there really weren't any good times to be talked about. (Peddicord, 1982, p. 89)

It is a unique situation to have in some way intimately known the person one has lost (a feeling especially true for mothers), while in another way not to have known him or her at all. Parents often feel isolated by the "emptiness" of the relationship with the dead infant, cut off from communicating with others because their "memories" are largely unfulfilled fantasies and hopes—and, as we shall see, there is little encouragement to share the reality of what one mother called "the overwhelming sadness of leaving the hospital no longer pregnant but without a baby" (Peddicord, 1982, p. 88).

Mazor (1970) points out that the wish to have children contains mixed motivations: a desire to share and experience love in a new way, to create a family, to attain an identity as generator and nurturer, on the one hand; and attempts at narcissistic gain such as the fantasy of being reborn, creating an extension of or better version of oneself, insuring against loneliness, on the other. Because parents experience not only the loss of a child or potential child but also secondary losses of hoped-for changes in their own identities, special difficulties in mourning occur. (In brief, the processes of mourning, as explicated in the psychoanalytic literature, include: withdrawal of libidinal energy from the object; loosening of cathexes or ties to the object; benign identification with and introjection of the object; and freeing of the ego and a resumption of normal functioning.) According to Furman (1976):

> In mourning an infant a parent faces a particularly difficult task because (1) he can only utilize the painful long process of detachment, since identification would not prove adaptive (how can a parent become part child again?) and (2) he deals not only with the loss of a loved one but also with a loss of a part of himself (parental attachment consists of a mixture of object love and self-love)...The child has not yet become a person to be loved in his own right, and his death represents primarily a loss of self and of self-esteem to the parent. The inner adaptation to such a loss differs from mourning the death of one who has been known and loved as a unique individual. (p. 234)

If parents who suffer a perinatal death must deal with the unusual loss of a potential rather than an established relationship and the difficulties of mourning both the lost child and their own narcissistic injuries, they do so in a social context that Rando (1986) characterizes as "uniquely strange and callous" (p. 38). She says:

> Other parents are clearly made anxious by bereaved parents as they recog-

> nize that this unnatural event could happen to them and their own children. Bereaved parents represent the worst fears of these other parents and they become the victims of social ostracism and unrealistic expectations as other parents attempt to ward off the terror generated within them...It is common for bereaved parents to experience feelings of abandonment, helplessness, and frustration as reactions to their experiences with other parents. They often complain that they feel like "social lepers." (p. 38)

Peppers and Knapp (1980) explain:

> The unusual character of the grief response in relation to infant loss is also determined by...the way infant death is defined and perceived in our culture. The community—friends, neighbors, and even relatives—neither perceives, nor responds to, infant death in the same way as it does to the deaths of older, loved persons. The community tends to disregard the infant as a real, living person, and thus to disassociate "normal grief" in response to the loss of an older person from "pseudogrief" in response to infant loss. The death of an infant is defined not so much as a "tragic" occurrence for the family as simply an "unfortunate" one. Consequently, the community expects the mother's reaction to this "unfortunate" event to be short-lived and temporary. (p. 28)

A central characteristic of parents' experience is that their loss is not validated, and this becomes a primary impediment for mothers and fathers to disclose genuinely to others the fierce anguish they suffer.

The Impact on Parents

In the author's formal research, in addition to clinical interviews, two paper-and-pencil measures have been utilized to assess the experience of parents. The first is a questionnaire, similar to that employed by other investigators, (Benfield *et al.*, 1976; Benfield, Leib, & Vollman, 1978) containing 10 common symptoms (sadness; crying; difficulties eating; sleep disturbance; feelings of weakness or exhaustion; irritability; social withdrawal; feelings of guilt or responsibility; preoccupation thinking or dreaming about the baby; anger) which, taken together, could be considered a measure of grief or mourning. The second, the Tennessee Self-Concept Scale, is a multidimensional instrument that has allowed some understanding of the effects of perinatal death on self-esteem.

Mothers

Simply put, mothers mourn more than do fathers in reaction to a perinatal death; they report more sadness, more crying, more sleep difficulties, more preoccupation, more anger, more guilt. Such findings seem unsurprising in light of the truly intimate (literally symbiotic) relationship a mother has with her unborn child, an experience the father cannot share. While the fetus "becomes real" for the mother with its movement during the course of the pregnancy, until birth it is not in reality a separate person—it is a part of the mother, and utterly dependent upon her. This factor of complete responsibility for the development and nurturing of a potential person appears to offer the most straightforward explanation for the greater grieving of mothers. It is also consistent with the suggestion of Parkes (1965) that the intensity of mourning after a loss is proportionate to the closeness of the relationship prior to death.

Unlike fathers, almost all mothers manifest moderate to severe guilt in reaction to a perinatal death. These mothers have "failed" in the tasks of developing and nurturing, and their statements (which contain indications of magical thinking, such as fantasies of being punished by God or beliefs of having directly harmed the fetus with thoughts or feelings) indicate that it is this failure—to themselves, to their husbands, and (fatally) to their infants—that evokes the characteristic response of guilt.

Although in the tenets of psychoanalytic theory it is the hostile components of ambivalence, including death wishes, that produce guilt at the death of a significant person, I would suggest that guilt is in fact a "realistic" response to the uniquely responsible position of mothers; how could one not feel guilty, for example, for failing to save from death even an unknown person one "could" or "should" have saved? In this situation, as Gardner (1969) points out, guilt may be essentially a defense against a truly existential anxiety—the magical thinking stemming from a wish to somehow control the uncontrollable, even at the expense of taking the blame for it. But this defensive guilt can create a profound isolation: The mother is afraid to disclose the "secret" (of her culpability) to others; and, if she does, others (including—often especially—her husband) cannot tolerate the pain of her guilt, deny her the primal responsibility she feels, and thus resist sharing her experience and foreclose the potential for genuine intimacy.

Mothers incur not only guilt in relation to their "incompetence," but also a loss of self-esteem; again by comparison to the statements of fathers, they are more self-derogatory, feel more diminished, and experience themselves as more fragmented, less integrated. Freud (1917) states that when the object-choice has been effected on a narcissistic basis with death "the shadow of the object (falls) upon the ego" (p. 249). The mother, a piece of herself gone, often feels that her purpose, her function, has been lost; "I feel empty. . . I should be taking care of a newborn—I don't feel like a woman who just had a baby." She may speak of losing in an implicit competition with other women her age to have children, and of failing to produce a gift, a grandchild, for her own mother. Her experience is shameful, and frightening:

> The newly bereaved mother may be reluctant to reveal typical reactions such as transient hallucinatory experiences of a baby crying or the powerful urge to steal another mother's infant for fear that she would be considered insane. She may consciously suppress her tendency to cry in response to any reminders of babies fearing that if she is not able to control her grief, it will overwhelm her and never end. (Leon, 1987, p. 187)

It can feel that there is no longer an acceptable, an adequate self to disclose, to share, and she is further demeaned by comments such as "It was God's will" or "It's for the best" or "You're young, you'll have another."

Fathers

To say that fathers display less mourning than do mothers is not to say that they do not grieve. However, their relationship to the infant is less intimate, and they mourn both less intensely and more quickly. By comparison to mothers, fathers seem almost one step removed from things and the focus of their attention is more diffuse. The most commonly felt concern is of the need to be in *control*—"I was blocking out my feelings because I wanted to have my head clear to make decisions"; "I couldn't really show much feeling, I needed to support my father and her father, I was paying attention to everyone—only when I was alone did I break down" (Peddicord, 1982, p. 93). Fathers talk of practical issues, such as the need to make decisions regarding burial or the difficulties of being the one who had the task of informing family and friends of the infant's death or the conflicts felt in regard to competing responsibilities, i.e., to wife, work, surviving children, etc. Some do feel shortchanged by their role—"Everyone was telling me to be strong for her and was asking about how she was doing, but I was hurting too!"—but, on the whole, fathers seal over the experience as quickly as possible: "I think I did all my crying at one time"; "I fight very hard for what I can have, when I can't have it I drop it like a hot potato. . . when the (twins) were dead they were gone and I put it back behind me very fast" (Peddicord, 1982, p. 93).

While mothers are internally focused in the aftermath of a perinatal death, wondering "Why me?" or "What did I do?," fathers, when not attending to the myriad tasks others seem to leave to them, tend to be intellectualized, focused on abstract questions such as "What does it mean?" Though they are unlikely to identify a diminishment of personal identity, some do report feeling fundamentally changed by their loss. They talk of feeling less in control of life, more at the mercy of "fate." Some become more religious or more concerned with the ultimate meaning of life. New perspectives are realized; for example, that having dealt with genuine life and death, it can be hard to continue treating work or career as the most important thing in one's life or, simply, that "half of the details that keep you so busy are really incidental" (Peddicord, 1982, p. 90). They question their values, their purpose. And some fathers (especially those without other surviving children) feel disoriented—having rearranged their lives, even changed jobs, in preparation for parenthood, only to be faced with needing to reorder priorities, goals, etc., yet again.

Their behavior limited by a cultural role that discourages expression of feelings, and reluctant to confront (as mothers do) the vulnerability and powerlessness inherent to their experience, fathers not infrequently couple avoidance with acting-out. The diversion offered by working too much or drinking too much or having an affair takes away the sting of a shameful knowledge—that he too has "failed" in the attempt to create a new life, has failed at the primary paternal function of protecting his child.

Barriers to Disclosure

Parents confronted with a perinatal death live out a dreaded fear come true, are denied a happy expectation the rest of the world takes for granted. Yet at a time when they most need support, most need "narcissistic supplies," mothers and fathers find their grief discounted, their pain minimized.

In the death of an infant a primal separation anxiety is enacted—fear of loss/abandonment becomes loss/abandonment. Fisher (1982) points out that resistance (whether to therapy per se or to the sharing of experience or to intimacy) can be understood as "humanity's constant effort to avoid the pain of feeling, thinking, or reexperiencing nonbeing" (p. 117). The literal nonbeing of the infant is nightmarish, and the resistance—of parents to the acceptance of the event forced by the reality principle, and of others to the possibility of establishing an identification, of genuinely sharing the parents' experience—is the central barrier to self-disclosure and authentic relatedness.

In the Couple

Schiff (1977) makes the point that, despite common assumptions that at least this tragedy can be faced by the couple together, grief is in fact a highly individual experience and often places enormous stresses on the marital relationship. Fish (1986) puts it straightforwardly:

> For parents who have lost infants, expect high levels of disagreement and misunderstanding. . . much higher levels of grief in mothers than in fathers, greater eagerness in the father to return to normal (especially in sexual relations), and consequent high stress on the marriage and consideration of divorce, especially by mothers. (p. 426)

What factors could account for such significant communication difficulties within the couple, the one relationship in which empathy and acceptance might be presumed? First is that husbands and wives go through the experience of an infant's death separately and differently. Symbiotically connected to the fetus/child, mothers frequently feel dependent upon and at the mercy of the medical professionals treating them; fathers, meanwhile, may become agents of those same professionals, e.g., sometimes the father is informed of the baby's death first and the task of telling the mother then falls to him. And, as previously mentioned, fathers are usually the ones who make the practical decisions on issues ranging from medical treatment of the infant to burial arrangements. In ways, then, husbands and wives are not equal participants in the event—in general, they are treated and they behave independently. An equally important factor is that mothers and fathers mourn incongruently; simply, fathers get through the process more quickly and want to talk about their feelings, their "failings," much less.

In the author's research (Peddicord, 1982) support for the notion that the quality of a couple's relatedness has a significant impact on their experience of a perinatal death was found. For instance, those rated positively on *ability to talk to spouse* reported more crying, but showed higher self-esteem, more satisfaction with his/her body (body image), and a better sense of personal worth; while those rated negatively evidenced more guilt and greater inadequacy, and were less likely to express a desire for further pregnancies. In brief, those who could disclose themselves within their relationship were less diminished by their loss and more confident about facing the future than those who could not.

Family and Friends

While parents themselves often feel confused about their reactions to the death of an infant, other people seem to be even more disoriented by confrontation with an event that is somehow taboo, (in part because "in 20th century America people simply don't lose babies"). Although many parents speak of feeling supported by family and/or friends, almost all recognize as well a profound discomfort on the part of others and frequently the mother or father feels responsible for this, and then endures "failing" an attempt to "make things better" (the way they should be) yet again.

It is not uncommon for the birth of a child to promise a great deal—perhaps a potential for a change in the relationships of the parents to their own parents is involved or perhaps a maintaining of the family line, the very survival of a given family. The disappointment of expectations across generations is felt keenly by mothers. At times they feel called upon to console their own mother on the loss of "her" child (grandchild), and experience their own pain as seemingly secondary. Several mothers interviewed by the author felt demeaned by their mothers or mothers-in-law who, after the infant died, recommended against further pregnancies. This "protection" was perceived as a lack of confidence, an indicator of the mother's inadequacy; e.g., "My husband's mother had a lot of kids and can't really understand why someone could have trouble being pregnant" (Peddicord, 1982, p. 97).

If they have "disappointed" family, parents—especially mothers—often feel that they have "lost" in relation to friends. Commonly, bereaved mothers feel painfully envious of pregnant friends, are unable to accept the sympathy of female friends who have children, feel incredibly angry at women who smoke or drink or otherwise do not "do it right" (as they did) only to deliver healthy babies. Sad, angry, and tainted by failure, mothers (and, in tandem, fathers) often find themselves shunned by friends if premorbid levels of activity and mood are not returned to quickly. In our society the young cherish a belief in the ability to control life, to plan it, to make it perfect—and parents who have lost an infant are viewed, consciously or unconsciously, not as victims of a random or fateful or uncontrollable tragedy, but as the architects of their own failure and, as such, unacceptable.

Given the preceding commentary, it is not surprising that mothers and fathers most often feel that genuine disclosure of their experience is precluded. As one father, seen on follow-up some months later, commented, "I've never known such aloneness as that funeral only my wife and I went to...that tiny white casket sitting on the ground...the feeling of that I don't think anyone could really understand."

Caregivers

Although the explosion of malpractice insurance rates has made the specialty more difficult to pursue, obstetrics is still a generally happy field of medicine and the tenor of the times is that there is nothing more natural, nothing more free of risk, nothing less in need of interference by the medical establishment than the birth of a child. While that may be true 92%–96% of the time, for pregnancies that progress past the first trimester, it appears that physicians, as well as parents, feel distressed by the 4%–8% of cases that do not end happily, the cases that constitute their "failures." Most often men, and trained to be in control always, like fathers they have difficulty tolerating, let alone expressing, feelings of vulnerability and powerlessness in the face of tragedy, and like fathers they tend to use avoidance and rationalization. Nearly half the mothers interviewed by the author said that their doctors responded inadequately at the point in time when the pregnancy went from normal and uneventful to potentially catastrophic, for example, with premature labor—they felt placated, not taken seriously, treated as hysterical. Mothers often felt "dumped" or "abandoned" then when transfer to the care of attending physicians at a high-risk, regional neonatal center was initiated—and frequently the doctor who had been following the pregnancy did not make further contact with his patient.

In trying to "protect" parents from the reality of their experience, caregivers at times make stunningly incorrect assumptions. For instance, a nurse commented to an unmarried, teenage mother that her loss, a stillbirth, must have been in some way a relief (presumably because her circumstances for raising a child would have been so difficult); the young woman experienced the interaction as denigrating and cruel, because she was counting on the child to give her "purpose...I was finally going to *do* something...I had something to put my life into" (Peddicord, 1982, p. 107). Another assumption is that a stillbirth is somehow less real, less painful, than the loss of a live-born infant, but the mother (and, to a lesser extent, father) has in fact lived with the fetus for a number of months and what she (he) deals with is not simple removal of a "benign tumor." One mother said, "After so much attention in the delivery room the night before, no one came in to talk or help me clean up or anything...but I *had had* a baby!" (Peddicord, 1982, p. 100).

Sometimes caregivers assume a model of grieving that proceeds by neat "stages." Not uncommonly parents are characterized then as mourning incorrectly; not talking, not sharing their feelings enough, for example, or remaining "stuck" in anger and guilt (emotions that caregivers find especially uncomfortable, unreasonable). But the experience of parents cannot be grasped so easily; a willingness to understand the meaning of this death/loss to this particular person, to appreciate this individual's character structure and defenses, to allow and feel a pain that threatens to annihilate the self, is required. Grief is not so much a problem to be solved as a process in which caregivers can be genuine participants. Self-disclosure and intimacy are two-way streets and for most caregivers the resistance is too great—they neither disclose (to the other or to themselves) their own internal contents nor do they truly apprehend the experience of the mothers and fathers with whom they come in contact.

Self-Disclosure and Its Effects

Although researchers have expressed concern about intruding upon parental grief, participation rates reported in studies of perinatal death have been unusually high. Mothers and fathers feel deep needs to understand and to be understood, and consistently are grateful for opportunities to tell their stories. Many intuitively believe that only another bereaved parent can fully appreciate (and tolerate) the tragedy and in self-help groups such as The Compassionate Friends and AMEND the act of sharing one's experience, of self-disclosure, becomes a part of the parent's search for meaning, imparts some purpose to the child's life and the parent's loss. Hopeful of helping others, parents recognize that revelation by one who has also lost a part of himself/herself not only validates the grief but suggests that it can be survived.

In my research, and in several psychotherapy treatment situations since, I have made parents aware that I suffered the loss of a newborn son in the past. With many parents I have found that some degree of sharing and/or straightforward education—offering information gathered from the literature or supportive comments regarding the normalcy of a parent's reactions or some personal experience—has served to reduce the individual's anxiety to a manageable level and elicited a freer responsiveness. Disclosure and openness offer the parent permission to see, to feel, to touch his/her wounds and thus to mourn. This stance suggests that the author, having lived it, will not be overwhelmed by the anxiety provoked by a perinatal death, so even "crazy" thoughts, feelings, wishes, impulses, etc., can be expressed.

Though analytically oriented and most comfortable with being a reasonably neutral object onto which patients project, in the situation of my research and several therapies since, for me it would have felt inauthentic not to disclose. Acknowledgment of personal experience seemed not an intrusion or countertransference manifestation, but a bridge to genuine relatedness. From the point of view of the patient, who is already intensely preoccupied with a sense of narcissistic inadequacy, the intact, undamaged (idealized) therapist may evoke rage and the belief that he/she can never empathize with the patient, can never know what it is to have failed so horrendously. Leon (1987) comments about one case, the mother's "transference was marked by both admiration and envy of her female therapist. She has the powerful conviction that everything desirable and valuable was in her therapist's domain" (p. 188). While transference distortions can be analyzed and worked through if the patient remains in treatment, an intense initial negative transference can be overcome (and the opportunity for treatment preserved) by the therapist's disclosure of shared experience, which establishes both a present identification and a hope for the future, i.e., "if the therapist could be repaired perhaps I can be also." A genuine person, the self-disclosing therapist can (as in all therapies) be hated too, but the patient is less likely to worry that her/his own disclosures will induce abandonment.

With the common unwillingness of friends, family, and even caregivers to tolerate the primitive anxiety engendered by the death of an infant, to acknowledge the parents' loss in a genuine way, or even to allow mourning to occur, often the greatest pain of a perinatal death is in the aloneness it creates; internal devastation and emptiness are matched by external isolation. It is that barrier to intimacy which self-disclosure by a caregiver or therapist can breech, which self-disclosure by a parent can overcome.

References

Benfield, D.G., Leib, S.A., & Reuter, J. (1976). Grief response of parents after referral of the critically ill newborn to a regional center. *New England Journal of Medicine, 294*, 975–978.

Benfield, D.G., Leib, S.A., & Vollman, J.H. (1978). Grief response of parents to neonatal death and parent participation in deciding care. *Pediatrics, 62*, 171–177.

Cullberg, J. (1971). Mental reactions of women to perinatal death. In N. Moriss (Ed.), *Psychosomatic Medicine in Obstetrics and Gynecology, Third International Congress*. London: Karger-Basel.

Fish, W.C. (1986). Differences of grief intensity in bereaved parents. In T.A. Rando (Ed.), *Parental loss of a child*. Champaign: Research Press.

Fisher, M.N. (1982). The shared experience: A theory of psychoanalytic psychotherapy. In M.N. Fisher & G. Stricker (Eds.), *Intimacy*. New York: Plenum.

Freud, S. (1917/1958). Mourning and melancholia. *Standard Edition of the Complete Psychological Works of Sigmund Freud* (Vol. 14). London: Hogarth Press.

Furman, E. (1976). Caring for the parents of an infant who dies: Comment. In M.H. Klaus & J.H. Kennell (Eds.), *Maternal-infant bonding*. St. Louis: C.V. Mosby.

Gardner, R.A. (1969). The guilt reaction of parents of children with severe physical disease. *American Journal of Psychiatry, 26*, 636–644.

Kennell, J.H. Slyter, H., & Klaus, M.H. (1970). The mourning response of parents to the death of a newborn infant. *New England Journal of Medicine, 283*, 344–349.

Leon, I.G. (1987). Short-term psychotherapy for perinatal loss. *Psychotherapy, 24*, 186–195.

Lindemann, E. (1944). Symptomatology and management of acute grief. *American Journal of Psychiatry, 101*, 141–148.

Lippman, C.A., & Carlson, K. (1977). A model liaison program for the obstetrics staff. In C.E. Hollingsworth & R.O. Pasnau (Eds.), *The family in mourning: A guide for health professionals*. New York: Grune & Stratton.

Mazor, M.D. (1979). Barren couples. *Psychology Today*, May, 101–112.

Miles, M.S., & Demi, A.S. (1986). Guilt in bereaved parents. In T.A. Rando (Ed.), *Parental loss of a child*. Champaign: Research Press.

Parkes, C.M. (1965). Bereavement and mental illness. *British Journal of Medicine and Psychology, 38*, 13–26.

Peddicord, D.J. (1982). Perinatal death: some aspects of parental reactions (Doctoral dissertation, Adelphi University, 1982). *Dissertation Abstracts International, 43*, 1263B.

Peppers, L.G., & Knapp, R.J. (1980). *Motherhood and mourning: Perinatal death*. New York: Praeger.
Rando, T.A. (1986). The unique issues and impact of the death of the child. In T.A. Rando (Ed.), *Parental loss of a child*. Champaign: Research Press.
Schiff, H.S. (1977). *The bereaved parent*. New York: Crown.

VI

Conclusion

18

Self-Disclosure and Psychotherapy

George Stricker

Self-disclosure lies at the heart of psychotherapy, the talking cure. It can be defined, somewhat tautologically, as a process by which the self is revealed. That ambiguous definition does not state who is doing the revealing, to whom, or by what means. Each of these ambiguities is critical within the therapeutic relationship. Either the therapist or the patient may be self-revealing, the revelation may be to the other person or to the self, and the means may be verbal or nonverbal, conscious or unconscious.

Fisher, adopting an existential position, describes very clearly that the resistances and transferences that we address in the therapeutic situation are not confined to the therapy. Rather, they are characteristic of the patient's general mode of functioning, and their resolution in treatment is valuable insofar as it can be generalized to the world outside the treatment room. The key resistance is not to the therapist's knowing, but to the patient rediscovering a disavowed portion of himself. The essential secrets are not being kept from the therapist, primarily, but from the self. The therapist is merely a conduit, a way station who encourages and allows the patient to explore ideas, risk disclosures, and come to understand that these secrets are not destructive, can be tolerated by others, and perhaps even can be tolerated by the self. Therefore, the central self-disclosure to be sought is not to the therapist but to the self.

The role of the patient, for Fisher, is simple. He reveals himself to the therapist for the purpose of discovering himself, and by doing so is

George Stricker • Institute of Advanced Psychological Studies, Adelphi University, Garden City, New York 11530.

freed to live a more authentic and fulfilled life. The role of the therapist is less simple. Disclosure is part of a relationship between equals, it can serve to model the comfortable expression of uncomfortable experiences, and it also creates a climate in which self-revelation is acceptable and valued. The therapist must recognize, however, that it is the growth of the patient that is paramount, so that the disclosure is confined to experiences occurring in, or relevant to, the treatment.

As long as the growth of the patient is paramount, there is some question whether a relationship that is inherently asymmetric really is between equals. More likely, two individuals meet who are equal in their humanity and in their adult status, unequal in the particular relationship in which they find themselves, and, by disclosing themselves to each other, they close the gap between themselves in the treatment. Perhaps it might even be said that as equality increases, the need for treatment decreases, and treatment ends well when the two participants are equal in the room, as they are outside it. This statement also suggests that the limits of treatment may be set by the limitations of the therapist, for the patient cannot be taken any further than the therapist has traveled.

Healey takes a historical perspective and views self-disclosure as a part of the Judeo-Christian religious experience. Indeed, as this experience was, and for many people still is, an essential healing experience, the parallel to psychotherapy is compelling. The key to the religious experience lies in the disclosure of the individual to God and of God to the individual. The priest/rabbi serves as the mediator between God and the individual, much as a therapist plays an essential role in the disclosure of the individual to the self. The role of relationship and trust is central to self-disclosure in the religious experience, as it is in the therapeutic experience, and the role of ritual in both experiences cannot be overlooked. The intent of the two experiences may be different, but the process bears striking similarity, as does the central role of the self.

Healey does suggest that one essential difference is that psychotherapy is dyadic (patient and therapist) but religious experience is triadic (individual, spiritual director, God). One may take a sacrilegious view and suggest that psychotherapy is also triadic, and that our principle goal is to bring the patient in closer touch with the God within. This internal God may be variously conceptualized as the superego, the parental introjects, or the authentic self. In any case, the disclosure of the individual to this forbidden internal component, and the acceptance of the dread secrets by that component, carry the seeds of forgiveness, acceptance, and growth. The religious person, through disclosure of sinful or heretical thoughts and feelings, and the acceptance of these, will experience himself as achieving greater communion with his God.

The therapy patient, through disclosure of unacceptable thoughts and feelings, and the acceptance of these, will experience himself as reaching greater internal unity.

Lane and Hull, writing from a psychoanalytic point of view, focus on the issue of therapist self-disclosure in individual therapy. The foundation of psychoanalytic technique was laid by Freud, who espoused, in writing, the total absence of any disclosure, but, in practice, was remarkably active and disclosing. Freud did not consider the possibility that nondisclosure is impossible, in that the absence of a statement constitutes a statement in its own right, so that the silent analyst is presenting a very powerful stimulus to the patient. The counterpoint to Freud was established by Ferenczi, who experimented with a variety of disclosing technical innovations, reaching an extreme with mutual analysis. This approach may be the logical extension of Fisher's concept of a therapeutic relationship between equals, and needs to be moderated by a recognition of the primacy of the patient's needs. Ferenczi also discovered, in his experiments, and as has been noted previously, that the personal limitations of the therapist place a boundary on the growth of the patient. However, the resolution to those limits is not the responsibility of the patient in the therapy (mutual analysis), but of the therapist in his own treatment.

Contemporary developments in psychoanalytic theory allow for the possibility of therapist self-disclosure, leaving unanswered questions concerning the choice, timing, and amount of material to disclose. Nonetheless, there is still the thought that self-disclosure is a dangerous parameter to be employed carefully and judiciously, and that self-disclosure certainly should be limited to those revelations that may demonstrate empathy and acceptance. The range seems to run from Langs, who is a strict adherent to a basic frame, not allowing for any deviation without risk of misalliance, to Khan, whose free use of himself, in the mind of many, carries him beyond the pale of psychoanalysis.

Basescu also focuses on the self-disclosure of the therapist, although he does so from an existential orientation that more closely resembles the approach of Fisher. Basescu cogently argues that the key to the acceptability of the classical psychoanalytic position concerning anonymity/neutrality rests with the relative weight given to the role of fantasy and reality. If the meat of psychoanalysis is the fantasy of the patient, the analyst is best advised to remain neutral and not intrude on that fantasy. However, if reality is given considerable weight, the real relationship becomes more important and the therapist must recognize that any behavior, including anonymity, will have stimulus value and must be taken into account. Neutrality, then, is not identified with anonymity, but with the therapist's attempts to help the patient to understand all aspects of the relationship and to leave all decisions about the patient's life in the hands of the patient. With this conception of neutrality, it is possible to self-disclose and to remain neutral.

Basescu uses the interesting phrase "show and tell" in his title. It points out that some of the self-disclosure is unavoidably shown, such as the therapist's clothing, voice quality, office appointments, etc.; but other aspects of self-disclosure are consciously told. The therapist must be aware of both, and strive for understanding of the motivation behind and impact of both. Just as we ask the patient to strive to understand, it is critical for the therapist to understand the motivation behind self-disclosure. Self-disclosure is not inherently good or bad; it can be well-timed, well understood, geared to the needs of the patient, and highly constructive; it also can be random, defensive, countertransferential, geared to the needs of the therapist, and deleterious to the course of the treatment.

Josephs approaches self-disclosure from the standpoint of self psychology, a particularly relevant theoretical position given the emphasis that has been placed on disclosing to the self. The distinction that is drawn between the verbal self and the experiential self is a crucial one, and one of the primary functions of self-disclosure is to narrow the gap between these two selves, so that the sometimes false, presented self becomes consistent with the authentic, experienced self.

Josephs also emphasizes the essential intersubjectivity of any self-disclosure. In order for self-disclosure to occur, there must be a person who self-discloses and a person who receives the self-disclosure. When the discloser is the patient and the receiver is the therapist, the therapist serves a self-regulatory function, aiding the patient in developing a clearer sense of the meaning and import of the self-disclosure. When the discloser is the therapist and the receiver is the patient, the patient may also serve a self-regulatory function for the therapist but, more importantly, that same information is used to further develop a sense of the experiential self. Two important conclusions follow from this formulation. First, a recognition of intersubjectivity also involves a necessary opting for reality over fantasy, as more value is placed on the quality of the real relationship than on an illumination of the construction of a fantasied relationship. Secondly, the intersubjectivity can be triadic, with the patient, the therapist, and the patient's experienced but not verbalized self all participating. Of course, the therapist's experienced self is also a participant; but that is not the focus of the therapeutic encounter. In this model, the patient will verbalize a self-disclosure, receive information from the response of the therapist, and modify the conception of the experienced self as a result. Similarly, the patient may receive a self-disclosure from the therapist, attempt to integrate it, and, by doing so, reach a modification of the experienced self. If an increase in the patient's self-awareness is a goal of treatment, it can readily be seen that there is a need for an increased disclosure to oneself.

Dryden approaches the topic of self-disclosure through the eyes of a rational-emotive therapist, a departure from the predominant psychoanalytic preference of the majority of the authors of this book. Although the metapsychological premises of the two orientations are vastly different, they do share a high regard for rationality and self-understanding. Thus, self-disclosure is also valued within a rational-emotive and, more generally, a cognitive-behavioral framework, although a primary difference about the role of the unconscious remains.

Perhaps even more than with regard to the role of the unconscious, the two theories differ in their conception of the technique by which the therapist is able to promote change. The rational-emotive therapist is far more active and directive than even the most self-disclosing psychoanalytic therapist would be, but does work toward a more passive position in which the burden of the treatment can be assumed by the patient. In contrast, the psychoanalytic therapist is more likely to begin with maximum passivity and gradually introduce activity and self-disclosures as the judgment is made that the patient would benefit from them. In both approaches, the therapist is an enabler, and the patient's key self-disclosure is to the self, conceived variously by the two orientations.

The approaches agree as to the human equality of the two participants in a therapeutic encounter, but the rational-emotive therapist is far more likely to use that equality, and his own human foibles, as a medium to promote therapeutic growth. The self-disclosure that is a parameter within psychoanalysis is a treatment technique for rational-emotive therapy. Rational-emotive therapists are more likely than psychoanalysts to disclose personal events and their solutions, whereas both are inclined to disclose personal reactions to the patient, and to do so in order to provide information about the impact of the patient. Self-disclosure is used for modeling purposes in both, but in psychoanalysis it is modeled as a process, with the hope that the patient will also begin to explore and feel safe with threatening and unwelcome thoughts and feelings. In rational-emotive therapy, self-disclosure is used to model a successful coping style, to show how the rational-emotive approach can be used effectively to solve personal problems, and to teach the philosophy and technique more directly.

Jackson focuses on unintentional disclosures by the therapist, and does so from a psychoanalytic vantage point. He contrasts those instances of intentional self-disclosure that are planned and generally outside the limits of traditional psychoanalytic practice with examples of unintentional self-disclosure that are unavoidable and present in all therapies, regardless of the orientation of the practitioner. Special events, such as the pregnancy of the therapist, as well as implicit communications, such as are inherent in any personal exchange, fall into the class of unavoidable self-disclosures. The point is made that intentionally providing the patient with information inhibits the ability of the patient to discern for himself, as self-disclosure will occur in any event. The notion of the active patient, rather than a passive and naive patient, suggests that both participants in the treatment are actively and simultaneously construing the other.

If this be the case, self-disclosure is unavoidable, and the only question becomes the mix between reality and fantasy that will contribute to the construal. The more the therapist reveals, the more the patient will have a realistic picture, nonetheless tempered by past experiences and characterological distortions. The less the therapist reveals, the more the patient will construct a picture from these past experiences and characterological distortions, but there will still be input from the unintended disclosures that occur in the therapeutic transactions. The choice between these will be a function of the therapist's theoretical position, personal style, and comfort zone, and it is difficult to suggest that one stance is better than the other. What does seem clear is that the therapist who believes that the patient's productions are entirely transferential is missing the impact of unintentional self-disclosures that occur naturally. At the same time, the therapist who believes that the patient's productions are a veridical reflection of the therapist's stimulus value is ignoring the vast history that leads the individual to cast particular behaviors in uniquely interpreted ways.

Menaker also is concerned with the self-disclosure of the therapist, discusses its implications for transference and countertransference, but does so with an atypical and highly personal style. She expresses more willingness than most of the authors to reveal the details of her life; but the rationale is the very familiar position that it does not do justice to an understanding of the transference to view the necessity of cultivating it, for it will arise in all human relationships. She recognizes the implicit revelations that are part and parcel of all human communication. However, she goes beyond that, revealing herself not only in unavoidable implicit ways, not only by reflecting personal feelings about the patient, but by providing personal information about herself. This is done in the service of creating a relationship in which attunement is present and communicated, and the intersubjectivity of the participants is stressed. As a real human relationship is created, and is enhanced by the self-disclosures that flow in the reciprocal relationship between therapist and patient, a matrix is also created within which previous developmental deficits can be repaired. It is crucial to recognize that the self-disclosures of the therapist are not random, conversational, or self-serving, but are chosen, both carefully and spontaneously, to communicate an empathic understanding of, and bond with, the patient.

There are some issues that cut across therapeutic orientations, and are present whether we view the therapeutic phenomena from a dynamic, behavioral, or existentialist perspective. One of these issues concerns work with nonwhite ethnic minority patients, and this is the topic of concern to Jenkins. The first issue of concern in the treatment of nonwhite ethnic minority patients is the reduction of the disproportionately high attrition rate that is so characteristic in work with these patients. Jenkins asserts that nonwhite ethnic minority patients are highly active in testing the therapist in early sessions, and will not proceed until they are satisfied that they will be treated with understanding, respect, and dignity. Before self-disclosure will be risked, the nonwhite ethnic minority patient must be assured that the climate in the treatment room is more receptive than it is in the dominant society. This, of course, must truly be the case. If so, as we have seen, one approach to providing this assurance, particularly with a patient who is sensitized towards indications of inequality in the relationship, is the use of appropriate self-disclosure by the therapist. The sequence that may ensue consists of self-disclosure by the therapist, which encourages self-disclosure by the patient, which leads to breadth and growth in the authentic, experiential self of the patient.

The principle medium for self-disclosure is language, and this can introduce complications when working with nonwhite ethnic minority patients who, for sociocultural reasons, may have been brought up with, or communicate in, a different language, verbal or nonverbal, than the therapist. The bilingual person has a well-documented problem of gaining access to early developmental issues in a language other than the one in which those issues were experienced. It is also well-known that there is a subtle prejudice towards those who cannot speak our language, the assumption being that these differences are deficits, and are indicative of either a lack of intelligence or the presence of psychopathology. The existence of a parallel problem for bidialectic patients is not as broadly appreciated. Jenkins also contributes the creative suggestion that patients be encouraged to provide self-disclosures in their most comfortable language, even if the therapist does not speak that language, with the experience then being available for discussion between them. This strategy has the dual appeal of facilitating a heightened affective experience for the patient and communicating a respect for the power of the patient's linguistic and sociocultural background.

A second issue that cuts across orientation concerns is the treatment of women, as discussed from a feminist perspective by Brown and Walker. Self-disclosure by the therapist has always been an integral part of the feminist approach to treatment because, consistent with the position of many contemporary psychoanalysts and humanistic therapists, it is seen as empowering for the patient. This disclosure includes personal values and biases as well as life experiences, and is a step in the direction of promoting an egalitarian psychotherapeutic relationship. In order to make an appropriate choice of therapist, patients (always referred to as "clients" in feminist writings) are encouraged to solicit self-disclosure on key value-laden issues.

Placing a premium on self-disclosure also requires careful attention to the risks and ethical considerations raised by such activity, a topic that Brown and Walker address explicitly and clearly. One such issue is boundary management. All self-disclosure must be in the service of the patient's needs, and the ability of the therapist to modulate self-disclosure and seek other, more appropriate, sources of support provides the patient with a mature model of the respect for and value of personal boundaries. A further problem can occur if the therapist overgeneralizes from her own experience and loses touch with the individual predicament of the patient. Not only will this lead to inappropriate solutions, it also will reduce the patient's range of options and control over her fate, thereby undermining two important goals of feminist therapy. A good rule of thumb is the principle that has been enunciated previously, that the self-disclosures of the therapist should not be random, conversational, or self-serving, but should be chosen, both carefully and spontaneously, to communicate an empathic understanding of, and bond with, the patient.

There are special considerations involved when the treatment is not individual therapy with adult patients. One such consideration is in working with children and adolescents, an issue discussed by Papouchis. As a point of departure, Papouchis identifies himself as believing that, with adults, disclosures about reactions to the patient should be sparing and disclosures about personal events should be rare, even though the self-disclosure of the patient is one criterion of successful therapeutic outcome. Nonetheless, with children, the therapist must be mindful of the developmental stage and task, and moderate the use of self-disclosure accordingly. For example, in contrast with the prescription for working with adults, verbal exploration of psychodynamic issues with the latency-age child may be overwhelming and counterproductive, but self-disclosure by the therapist is an empathic response to the child's growing wish to learn about the surrounding world. Similarly, with adolescents, excessive self-examination may not be tolerable for a growing ego, and therapist self-disclosure helps to provide an alternative role model in a more egalitarian setting. With both children and adolescents, the limitations of a developing ego are respected and, while respecting the presence and importance of the parents, the need for an empathic, reality-bound adult is understood.

There is a logical extension of this sensitive, developmentally based approach to the use of self-disclosure. It is clear that children and adolescents usually are caught up in developmental tasks that make the additional burden of self-disclosure sometimes too overwhelming to be therapeutically valuable. It is also clear that, either despite or because of the presence of parents, they often require a clear, empathic adult to be available as a role model and an object of attachment. It is not as clear why the chronological passage of time automatically erases these considerations. For many adults, self-disclosure may also represent a burden that must be tempered by the careful therapist, and the need for an empathic role model or attachment figure has not disappeared with the passing years. It seems likely that the titration of self-disclosure should be geared to developmental needs, regardless of the chronological age of the patient.

At the other end of the developmental spectrum, special considerations are also indicated in working with older adults, the topic of Greenberg's chapter. This chapter is built on a strong research foundation, with much evidence cited that indicates the value of a confidant in the adjustment and happiness of an elderly person. Intimate relationships seem to serve as a buffer against demoralization and depression, and self-disclosure is an important contributor to intimacy. In psychotherapy, some writers view an empathic, supportive relationship, buttressed by the therapist's use of self-disclosure, as an end in itself, providing the elderly patient with gratification that is absent elsewhere in his life. Although this may be of value to some, there are many elderly patients who can benefit from standard psychotherapy, with self-exploration and growth seen as realistic and legitimate goals. For these patients, the considerations governing the use of self-disclosure are much the same as they would be for other adult patients, with judgments about the needs of the patient and the capacity of the therapist determining the introduction, appropriateness, and timing of any self-disclosure. As with any patient, revelations communicating affective attunement are likely to be helpful, and those displaying unresponsiveness or misattunement are not. On the other hand, the patients may not be as free to self-disclose as a younger person might, stemming in part from the norms to which this age cohort was socialized, as well as from more dynamic concerns that might be subject to the same interpretations and interventions as would occur with younger patients.

Consideration must also be given to modalities other than individual therapy. Vinogradov and Yalom present issues in self-disclosure in group therapy. A distinction is made between horizontal self-disclosure, in which the past or the outside is disclosed, and vertical self-disclosure, dealing with intragroup, interpersonal issues. The group often focuses on vertical self-disclosure, whereas individual therapy often is concerned at least equally with horizontal self-disclosure. Among the functions of self-disclosure in a group are to increase cohesiveness and to develop interpersonal learning, effects that they may also have in a nontherapeutic situation. It is this potential to transfer interpersonal learning from the group to real life that is such a critical factor in the efficacy of group therapy. The important point is made that self-disclosure, in order to be constructive, must be tempered by empathy and responsibility. The patient in group therapy must learn to guide self-disclosures by the impact it will have on co-participants, whereas the patient in individual therapy need not be overly concerned by the impact on the therapist. Both the individual and the group therapist certainly should have all self-disclosures (both about himself and about the patient) guided by empathy and responsibility. Although the group therapist is likely to be more self-disclosing than the individual therapist, he, too, must be guided by an understanding of the meaning and impact of each disclosure and must always place the needs of the group above his own needs in determining what and when to disclose.

Much of the material presented to this point was based on clinical experience and theory. There also is a good deal of research evidence relevant to self-disclosure, some of which is directly relevant to therapy and some of which refers to self-disclosure in the world at large. Simon developed a list of the functions of intentional therapist self-disclosure that was based on interviews with eight experienced therapists. These functions, then, are not the idiosyncratic experiences of a single therapist, no matter how skilled, but a compilation of the beliefs and practices of a small number of experienced therapists. However, it must be noted that the high disclosers in this study were primarily identified with a humanistic, nonpsychoanalytic viewpoint, whereas the low disclosers were more likely to be psychoanalytic in orientation. Many of the authors in this volume are perfectly comfortable with a psychoanalytic orientation that incorporates humanistic features and also allows for self-disclosure. Nonetheless, both groups in the study noted similar functions of self-disclosure, differing only in their frequency, content, and motivation for self-disclosure. It is likely that most of these functions would be noted, as well, by the more traditional therapists represented in this volume.

The first function indicated by the therapists is that of modeling. Self-disclosure by the therapist presents the patient with a model of an effective, assertive, high-functioning, and competent human being. It was also noted, much as Papouchis stated, that this was particularly important with adolescents. A second function was to foster the therapeutic alliance. This suggested very early disclosure of demographic information for all therapists, and the use of self-disclosure to resolve therapeutic impasses on the part of some. It also led some low self-disclosers to note that withholding information was sometimes necessary to protect the therapeutic alliance, and it provided a respect for boundaries that sometimes seemed blurred in the high disclosers. The third function was to validate reality. If a patient senses a feeling or event and the therapist, in the service of anonymity, refuses to validate it, the patient is left with an experience of his own lack of attunement to the world, and this is therapeutically counterproductive. The encouragement of the patient's autonomy is a fourth function of therapist self-disclosure. The respect for the equality of the patient that can be conveyed by a self-disclosure provided a good reason for many therapists, although they also noted that an intrusive self-disclosure could be too much of a burden for some patients. This represents another example of the need to be sensitive to boundary issues while engaging in self-disclosure. Finally, the function of self-disclosure for some people was therapist satisfaction, a by-product that must be acknowledged, but a function that surely is not the primary goal of a patient's psychotherapy. It is important to separate the gratification that one can derive from the process and outcome of treatment from the narcissistic self-indulgence that can occur if the focus of the treatment shifts from the patient to the therapist.

Gordon's research did not concern psychotherapy per se, but the role of self-disclosure in Holocaust survivors. Her results attest to the power of self-disclosure in the world outside the treatment room and, by doing so, suggest the value to the patient of a process that can facilitate and encourage self-disclosure. The extent to which a survivor of the Holocaust was able to disclose her terrible experiences was related to the extent to which her daughter was found to be in touch with her own experiences. This intergenerational transmission of skill in self-disclosure is a fascinating finding and points to the value of clear communication to the receiver as well as the sender.

Further, Gordon's use of a measure of referential activity highlights another important aspect of self-disclosure. Referential activity refers to a person's ability to translate experience into language, to be in touch with one's own inner experiences. It suggests that there are two necessary stages for self-disclosure to occur. First, the individual must have a sufficient level of referential activity to be in touch with that experience, thereby disclosing to the self. Having accomplished this, the ability to disclose to others then becomes possible, although some people may choose not to do so. Apparently, parents who choose not to do so risk hampering the growth of their children, who may not develop the referential skills necessary to allow them to progress to the stage where they may choose to disclose to others. This finding also suggests that the therapist who encourages disclosure to the self is facilitating the ability to disclose to others and, by doing so, enabling the patient to achieve greater levels of intimacy in interpersonal relationships.

Frawley, too, describes a research project that shows the importance of self-disclosure in a nontherapeutic situation. Her subjects were victims of childhood incest and thus were also survivors of an early trauma. As with Gordon's Holocaust survivors, the horror of the early trauma is surrounded by a veil of secrecy, one often encouraged, in the case of incest, by the perpetrator. Further, disclosure of incest is often met by disbelief, thus serving to reinforce the "necessity" of silence. Most victims choose not to disclose their experience and, of those who do, most are not believed. This stultification of any attempts at self-disclosure is accompanied by gross failures at intimacy, most particularly in the sexual area, which already has been the scene of overwhelming trauma. The shield that is constructed in order to keep the knowledge of incest in also serves to keep others out.

Frawley provides both research and clinical support for the proposition that victims who engage in disclosure will be more likely to achieve satisfaction in intimate relationships than those who preserve their awful secret. It appears as though self-disclosure has a critical role in nurturing the capacity for intimacy in these victimized women, and the task of the therapist must be to create a climate in which such disclosure is safe and rewarding. Such a climate will be at marked variance with the original parental environment, and will allow for the beginning of a healing process that may compensate for the early developmental defects. It should be noted, of course, that the effects of the self-disclosure are neither painless nor magical. The revelation of a long-held secret is often accompanied by much anguish, and the need for extensive working through is patently obvious. Nonetheless, the results are extremely encouraging, and it does seem as though self-disclosure is a necessary step in the treatment of incest survivors.

Finally, Peddicord describes a research project concerned with another unthinkable area of trauma, grief, and guilt. The perinatal death of a child is an experience of rare heartache. Even if the parents wish to disclose, and the death is an open secret, they often find, even with each other, that their pain is so intense and so individual that others prefer not to hear about it. Much as with Frawley's incest survivors, it is not at all helpful to try to sugarcoat the experience or to deny the individual's sense of guilt and responsibility. It is only by having the therapist (or any concerned other) empathically validate the experience that the sufferer can be free to work it through and move beyond it. It was also demonstrated by Peddicord, as it was by Frawley, that self-disclosure was accompanied by a better level of adjustment to the trauma.

We all want to believe in a just world, so that victims feel that they must have done something to deserve the tragedy that befell them, and others feel more protected from the tragedy if they can blame the victim and, by doing so, insulate themselves from the threat of a similar tragedy. The therapist who enters into the conspiracy of silence will reinforce silence and block the growth of the patient. The therapist who allows the secret to be aired but denies the import, providing reassurance rather than empathy, disqualifies the experience of the victim and adds to the victimization. The patient only learns that the self-disclosure was meaningless and silence was, after all, the best available strategy. It is only the therapist who can appreciate the honestly disclosed feelings of the patient, which are real even if they are also irrational, who can provide the atmosphere that will allow the patient to move beyond the irrational to a more self-accepting view. Thus, self-disclosure is not an end in itself, but it is a necessary step on the path to relatedness and intimacy.

Finally, let us return to some of the questions that were raised in the initial definition of self-disclosure. That definition did not state who is doing the revealing, to whom, or by what means. It should now be clear that both the patient and the therapist engage in acts of self-disclosure, they do so verbally and nonverbally, consciously and unconsciously, and they reveal themselves to each other and to themselves. It is through the self-disclosure of the patient to the therapist that he can begin to recognize previously hidden and unacceptable aspects of himself, to recognize the acceptability of what had been experienced as forbidden secrets, and to grow in a healthier fashion. The self-disclosure of the therapist serves as a model for the patient and also provides information that encourages further disclosures and recognitions. Most importantly, these disclosures and subsequent growth generalize beyond the therapy session, leading to a pattern of relating that can be more spontaneous, authentic, and revealing, and to a level of adjustment and relationships that are more comfortable, fulfilling, and healthy.

Index

MIX
Papier aus verantwortungsvollen Quellen
Paper from responsible sources
FSC® C105338
FSC
www.fsc.org

If you have any concerns about our products,
you can contact us on
ProductSafety@springernature.com

In case Publisher is established outside the EU,
the EU authorized representative is:
Springer Nature Customer Service Center GmbH
Europaplatz 3, 69115 Heidelberg, Germany

Printed by Libri Plureos GmbH
in Hamburg, Germany